CARDIOVASCULAR IMAGING

Yi-Hwa Liu, PhD
Section of Cardiovascular Medicine
Department of Internal Medicine
Yale University School of Medicine
New Haven, Connecticut, USA

Frans J. Th. Wackers, MD
Section of Cardiovascular Medicine
Department of Internal Medicine
Yale University School of Medicine
New Haven, Connecticut, USA

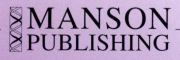

MANSON
PUBLISHING

Copyright © 2010 Manson Publishing Ltd

ISBN: 978-1-84076-109-2

A CIP catalogue record for this book is available from the British Library.

For full details of all Manson Publishing Ltd titles please write to:
Manson Publishing Ltd, 73 Corringham Road, London NW11 7DL, UK.
Tel: +44(0)20 8905 5150
Fax: +44(0)20 8201 9233
Website: www.mansonpublishing.com

Commissioning editor: Jill Northcott
Project manager: Paul Bennett & Kate Nardoni
Copy-editor: Joanna Brocklesby
Design: Cathy Martin, Presspack Computing Ltd
Layout: DiacriTech, Chennai, India
Colour reproduction: Tenon & Polert Colour Scanning Ltd, Hong Kong
Printed by: Grafos S.A., Barcelona, Spain

CONTENTS

4

PREFACE

The purpose of this book is to provide up-to-date technical and practical information about various cardiac imaging techniques for the assessment of cardiac function and perfusion, as well as their potential relative roles in clinical imaging. This book also aims to stimulate use of the new developments of integrated cardiovascular imaging and molecular targeted imaging. It will be the charge of future investigators and clinicians to define the appropriate role(s) for each of the imaging modalities discussed in this book. As distinct from other textbooks, this book provides numerous illustrations of clinical cases for each imaging modality to guide the reader in the diagnosis of cardiovascular diseases and the management of patients based on the imaging modality used. We hope that this book will help the reader to understand the values and limitations of the imaging techniques and to determine which test, in which patient population, and for which purpose would be the most appropriate to use.

Yi-Hwa Liu
Frans J. Th. Wackers

CONTRIBUTORS

James A. Arrighi, MD
Division of Cardiology
Department of Medicine
Brown Medical School
Providence, Rhode Island, USA

Richard T. George, MD
Division of Cardiology
Department of Medicine
The Johns Hopkins University School of
    Medicine
Baltimore, Maryland, USA

Farid Jadbabaie, MD
Section of Cardiovascular Medicine
Department of Internal Medicine
Yale University School of Medicine
New Haven, Connecticut, USA

Albert C. Lardo, PhD
Department of Medicine, Division of Cardiology
    and Department of Biomedical Engineering
The Johns Hopkins University School of
    Medicine
Baltimore, Maryland, USA

Joao A.C. Lima, MD
Departments of Medicine and Radiology
The Johns Hopkins University School of
    Medicine
Baltimore, Maryland, USA

Yi-Hwa Liu, PhD
Section of Cardiovascular Medicine
Department of Internal Medicine
Yale University School of Medicine
New Haven, Connecticut, USA

Robert L. McNamara, MD, MHS
Section of Cardiovascular Medicine
Department of Internal Medicine
Yale University School of Medicine
New Haven, Connecticut, USA

Raymond R. Russell, III, MD, PhD
Section of Cardiovascular Medicine
Department of Internal Medicine
Yale University School of Medicine
New Haven, Connecticut, USA

André Schmidt, MD
Division of Cardiology
Department of Internal Medicine
Medical School of Ribeirão Preto
University of São Paulo
Ribeirão Preto,
São Paulo, Brazil

Albert J. Sinusas, MD
Section of Cardiovascular Medicine
Department of Internal Medicine
Yale University School of Medicine
New Haven, Connecticut, USA

Kathleen Stergiopoulos, MD, PhD
Division of Cardiovascular Medicine
State University of New York at Stony Brook
Stony Brook, New York, USA

Frans J. Th. Wackers, MD
Section of Cardiovascular Medicine
Department of Internal Medicine
Yale University School of Medicine
New Haven, Connecticut, USA

ABBREVIATIONS

A_a	late diastolic velocity
ACC	American College of Cardiology
AHA	American Heart Association
ARVD	arrhythmogenic right ventricular dysplasia
ASD	atrial septal defect
ASNC	American Society of Nuclear Cardiology
ATP	adenosine triphosphate
ATPase	adenosine triphosphatase
AVA	aortic valve area
A-wave	late wave
bFGF	basic fibroblast growth factor
BMI	body mass index
BP	blood pressure
bpm	beats per minute
CAC	coronary artery calcium
CAD	coronary artery disease
ceMRI	contrast-enhanced MRI
CEU	contrast-enhanced ultrasound
CMRI	cardiac magnetic resonance imaging
CoAo	coarctation of the aorta
CT	computed tomography
CW	continuous wave
DCM	dilated cardiomyopathy
DT	deceleration time
DTPA	diethylene triamine pentaacetic acid
D-wave	diastolic wave
E_a	early diastolic velocity
EBT	electron beam tomography
ECG	electrocardiogram
ECM	extracellular matrix
EDV	end-diastolic volume
EF	ejection fraction
ERNA	equilibrium radionuclide angiography
ERO	effective regurgitant orifice
ESV	end-systolic volume
ET	ejection time
E-wave	early wave
FDA	Food and Drug Administration (US)
FDG	[18F]-2-fluoro-2-deoxyglucose
FGF-2	fibroblast growth factor-2
FPRNA	first-pass radionuclide angiography
GBPS	gated blood pool SPECT
GSPECT	gated myocardial perfusion SPECT
HARP	harmonic phase MRI
HCM	hypertrophic cardiomyopathy
HDL	high-density lipoprotein
HIV	human immunodeficiency virus
HU	Hounsfield units
Hz	Hertz
ICD	implantable cardiac defibrillator
ICE	intracardiac echocardiography

IVCT	isovolemic contraction time
IVRT	isovolemic relaxation time
IVUS	intravenous ultrasound
LAD	left anterior descending artery
LCX	left circumflex artery
LDL	low-density lipoprotein
LVEF	left ventricular ejection fraction
LVOT	left ventricular outflow tract
MDCT	multidetector computed tomography
METs	metabolic equivalents
MMP	matrix metalloproteinase
MO	microvascular obstruction
MPI	myocardial performance index
MR	magnetic resonance
MRI	magnetic resonance imaging
MV	mitral valve
PDA	patent ductus arteriosus
PET	positron emission tomography
PFR	peak filling rate
PISA	proximal isovelocity surface area
PMT	photomultiplier tube
PRF	pulse repetition frequency
PS	phosphatidyl serine
PW	pulse wave
QCA	quantitative coronary angiography
Qp/Qs	ratio of pulmonary flow to systemic flow
RCA	right coronary artery
RF	radiofrequency
RV	right ventricle
RVe	regurgitant volume
SPECT	single photon emission computed tomography
SV	stroke volume
S-wave	systolic wave
T	Tesla
TDI	tissue Doppler imaging
TEE	transesophageal echocardiography
TEMRI	transesophageal MRI
TGA	transposition of the great arteries
TGF	transforming growth factor
TID	transient ischemic dilation
TIMP	tissue inhibitor of matrix metalloproteinases
tPA	tissue plasminogen activator
TRV	transient visualization of the right ventricle
TTC	triphenyltetrazolium chloride
TTE	transthoracic echocardiography
TVI	time velocity integral
VEGF	vascular endothelial growth factor
VSD	ventricular septal defect
VTI	velocity time integral

1. An Overview of the Assessment of Cardiovascular Disease by Noninvasive Cardiac Imaging Techniques

Frans J. Th. Wackers   Robert L. McNamara   Yi-Hwa Liu

INTRODUCTION

Noninvasive cardiac imaging has become an integral part of the current practice of clinical cardiology. Chamber size, ventricular function, valvular function, coronary anatomy, and myocardial perfusion are among a wide array of cardiac characteristics that can all be assessed noninvasively. Noninvasive imaging can evaluate many signs and symptoms of cardiovascular disease as well as follow patients with known cardiovascular conditions over time.

During the past three decades several distinctly different noninvasive imaging techniques of the heart, such as radionuclide cardiac imaging, echo-cardiography, magnetic resonance imaging (MRI), and X-ray computed tomography (CT), have been developed. Remarkable progress has been made by each of these technologies in terms of technical advances, clinical procedures, and clinical applications and indications. Each technique was propelled by a devoted group of talented and dedicated investigators who explored the potential value of each technique for making clinical diagnoses and for defining clinical characteristics of heart disease that might be most useful in the management of patients. Thus far, most of these clinical investigations using various noninvasive cardiac imaging techniques were conducted largely in isolation from each other, often pursuing similar clinical goals. There is now an embarrassment of richness of available imaging techniques and of the real potential of redundant imaging data. However, as each noninvasive cardiac imaging technique has matured, it has become clear that they are not necessarily competitive but rather complementary, each offering unique information under unique clinical conditions.

The development of each imaging technique in isolation resulted in different clinical subcultures, each with its separate clinical and scientific meetings and medical literature. Such a narrow focus and concentration on one technology may be beneficial during the development stage of a technique. However, once basic practical principles have been worked out and clinical applications are established, such isolation contains the danger of duplication of pursuits and of scientific staleness when limits of technology are reached.

Each of the aforementioned techniques provides different pathophysiologic and/or anatomic information. Coming out of the individual modality isolation by cross-fertilization is the next logical step to evolve to a higher and more sophisticated level of cardiac imaging. Patients would benefit tremendously if each technique were to be used judiciously and discriminately. Clinicians should be provided with those imaging data that are most helpful to manage specific clinical scenarios.

It can be anticipated that in the future a new type of cardiac imaging specialist will emerge. Rather than one-dimensional subspecialists, such as nuclear cardiologists or echocardiographers, multimodality imaging specialists, who have in-depth knowledge and experience of all available noninvasive cardiac imaging techniques, will be trained. These cardiac imaging specialists will fully understand the value and limitations of each technique and will be able to apply each of them discriminately and optimally to the benefit of cardiac patients. Recently a detailed proposal for such an Advanced Cardiovascular Training Track was proposed (Beller 2006).

Regardless of the technology used, the desired cardiac imaging parameters and the principles for assessment of cardiovascular disease are largely similar.

CARDIAC IMAGING PARAMETERS

Noninvasive diagnostic cardiac imaging is able to obtain information about many important aspects of cardiac integrity, including cardiac anatomy, cardiac pump function, valvular function, and regional myocardial blood flow. Visualization of each cardiac chamber can be obtained from many of the imaging modalities but is particularly useful in echocardiography, MRI, and CT. Determination of chamber sizes and myocardial thicknesses can be extremely valuable clinical information.

Systolic left ventricular ejection fraction (EF) is one of the most important measurements of cardiac pump function. Numerous studies have demonstrated that resting left ventricular EF is an important prognostic variable (Bonow 1993). Other important variables of left ventricular function are diastolic function and left ventricular volume. Left ventricular EF can be determined by each of the imaging modalities discussed in this book. The reader should be able to determine the relative accuracy and limitations of each technique for the purpose of assessing left ventricular function.

The structure and function of cardiac valves are routinely assessed by echocardiography and can also be assessed by MRI. Echocardiography provides excellent temporal resolution to evaluate valvular anatomy at various stages of the cardiac cycle. Cardiac Doppler is used routinely to assess hemodynamics of valvular stenosis and regurgitation. MRI provides excellent spatial resolution, which enables improved imaging of the consequences of valvular disease such as hypertrophy and dilation. MRI also offers valuable information for patients with congenital valvular disease.

STRESS TESTING

Since in the western world the most common form of heart disease is coronary artery disease (CAD), direct or indirect assessment of the regional myocardial blood flow is the most widely performed stress imaging test (Klocke *et al.* 2003). Presently, the most frequently used modality for this purpose is rest–stress radionuclide myocardial perfusion imaging. Myocardial perfusion imaging by contrast echocardiography and MRI is only performed in specialized laboratories. Multislice CT has recently emerged as an additional important noninvasive cardiac imaging technology, useful for evaluating the coronary arteries and cardiac chambers.

One of the main purposes of noninvasive cardiac stress imaging is to clarify whether symptoms are due to underlying heart disease. In the early stages of cardiac disease patients may be relatively asymptomatic at rest but develop symptoms during stress. Thus, an important aspect of cardiac imaging for diagnostic reasons should involve provocative testing, either by physical or by pharmacologic stress, with the aim of reproducing symptoms. However, if physical exercise is inadequate a test may be falsely negative. Since many elderly patients, in particular women, are incapable of performing adequate physical exercise, a relatively large proportion of patients may have to undergo stress testing by pharmacologic means.

Stress testing should be performed using well standardized protocols. In the US physical exercise is predominantly performed using the motorized treadmill, whereas in other countries the stationary bicycle is most frequently used. During treadmill exercise the workload (i.e. speed and incline) is gradually (every 3 minutes) increased until the patient cannot go any further, either because of reproduction of symptoms, fatigue, or other predefined endpoints (*Table 1*). Using bicycle exercise the workload is similarly increased every 3 minutes by 25 Watts. The maximum achievable exercise workload is expressed in duration of exercise (minutes), the number of exercise stages completed, and workload expressed in METs (metabolic equivalents).

Physical exercise

During physical exercise metabolic demand and oxygen requirements of the exercising muscles are increased. In order to deliver the required increased amount of oxygen, cardiac output has to augment by increasing heart rate and myocardial contraction. To meet, in turn, the increased cardiac demand, coronary blood flow has to increase accordingly. If regional coronary myocardial blood flow cannot meet the increased demand due to impaired supply, i.e. significant coronary artery stenosis, regional myocardial hypoperfusion (heterogeneity) occurs, which may cause myocardial ischemia and abnormal

Table 1 Endpoints of stress testing

Absolute indications for terminating stress test:
Severe angina
Signs of poor peripheral perfusion: pallor,
    clammy skin
Central nervous system problems: ataxia,
    vertigo, confusion, gait problems
Hypertension (systolic blood pressure (BP)
    >210 mmHg; diastolic BP >110 mmHg)
Hypotension with symptoms (↓ systolic
    BP >10 mmHg from baseline)
Serious arrhythmia: ventricular tachycardia
    (more than three beats)
ST segment elevation
Equipment malfunction, poor electrocardiogram
    (ECG) tracings
Patient request

Relative indications for terminating stress test:
Reproduction of symptoms, angina
Marked fatigue, shortness of breath, wheezing
Leg cramps, claudication
ST segment depression >2–3 mm
Development of second- or third-degree heart
    block, bradycardia

Table 2 Imaging modalities and stressors

Imaging modality	Preferred stress
SPECT	1. Physical
	2. Vasodilator
	3. Adrenergic
PET	1. Vasodilator
	2. Adrenergic
	3. Physical
Echocardiography	1. Physical
	2. Adrenergic
MRI	1. Vasodilator
	2. Adrenergic
CT	Not applicable

SPECT: single photon emission computed tomography; PET: positron emission tomography; MRI: magnetic resonance imaging; CT: computed tomography.

regional wall motion. For myocardial perfusion imaging this heterogeneity of blood flow is essential to generate abnormal images.

Vasodilator stress

When patients cannot perform adequate physical exercise, pharmacologic stress testing constitutes an alternative diagnostic approach. This may consist of either vasodilator stress with dipyridamole or adenosine, or adrenergic stress with dobutamine. Vasodilator stress causes dilation of the coronary resistance vasculature and is in fact a test of regional coronary blood flow reserve, i.e. the ability of coronary blood flow to meet the increased demand. Under vasodilator stress, myocardial regions supplied by arteries with significant coronary artery stenosis demonstrate less increase in regional myocardial blood flow than the regions supplied by normal coronary arteries, thus resulting in heterogeneity of myocardial blood flow. This heterogeneity of blood flow can be imaged with myocardial perfusion radiotracers. It is important to realize that such heterogeneity indicates regional myocardial hypoperfusion but not necessarily ischemia.

Adrenergic stress

Adrenergic stress with dobutamine stimulates myocardial contraction and increases metabolic demand, resulting also in increased heart rate and enhanced regional wall motion. The increase in workload, heart rate, and regional myocardial blood flow with adrenergic stress is generally less than that with physical exercise. In patients with significant coronary artery stenosis dobutamine stress may cause myocardial ischemia, abnormal regional wall motion, and blood flow heterogeneity.

Choice of imaging modality in stress testing

The three forms of stress described above can be used with any imaging technique. However, some imaging modalities are better suited for a particular stressor (*Table 2*).

CLINICAL INDICATIONS

Noninvasive cardiac imaging for detection of cardiac disease should be performed in appropriate patient populations. This is not only important for the efficient use of tests, but also because reimbursement may be denied if no appropriate clinical indications were documented. Professional societies have published guidelines on how and when to use certain diagnostic tests (Port 1999, DePuey & Garcia 2001, Gibbons *et al.* 2002, Bacharach *et al.* 2003, Klocke *et al.* 2003, Brindis *et al.* 2005). Prior to ordering a diagnostic test physicians should consider the likelihood that a patient has heart disease, as well as the clinical risk of a patient for future coronary heart disease. This can be approximated by Bayesian probability analysis and by calculating the Framingham risk score (Diamond & Forrester 1979, Framingham Score, Pryor *et al.* 1983). Patients with low likelihood of disease and/or at low risk should in general not be evaluated by noninvasive stress testing since the diagnostic yield is low and a relatively high number of false-positive test results may be obtained. The pretest likelihood of having disease can be assessed by step-wise Bayesian probability analysis, considering a patient's symptoms (typical or atypical), gender, and his or her age (Diamond & Forrester 1979). In the American Heart Association (AHA)/American College of Cardiology (ACC)/American Society of Nuclear Cardiology (ASNC) Guidelines, one can find a simple table for the purpose of determining the pretest likelihood of disease. Diagnostic testing is usually considered to be appropriate if the pretest likelihood of disease is intermediate or moderate. To assess the risk for future coronary heart disease the Framingham risk score can be determined on the basis of age, low-density lipoprotein (LDL) and high-density lipoprotein (HDL) cholesterol, blood pressure, presence of diabetes, and smoking (Framingham Score). A patient is considered to be at moderate risk with a 10-year absolute risk of 10–20%. At the present time there appears consensus that in patients with low probability and at low risk for disease, diagnostic testing is inappropriate, whereas in those with high probability and at high risk, direct invasive evaluation is suitable. Although at present algorithms are proposed for how to use various diagnostic technologies in what sequence and in which populations, these proposals are largely based on intuition and extrapolation from data obtained in different patient populations (The 1st National SHAPE Guideline).

PATHOPHYSIOLOGICAL *VS.* ANATOMICAL INFORMATION

Several decades of radionuclide myocardial perfusion imaging have demonstrated that visualization of the relative distribution of myocardial perfusion after stress shows the pathophysiologic consequences of anatomic coronary artery stenosis. Accordingly, myocardial perfusion imaging has more powerful prognostic value than coronary angiography. This should be kept in mind with the present interest in noninvasive visualization of coronary anatomy. The degree of stress myocardial perfusion abnormalities has been shown to correlate strongly with the incidence of future cardiac events (Hachamovitch *et al.* 1996). In contrast patients with normal stress myocardial perfusion imaging, depending on their clinical risk profile, have an excellent short- and long-term prognosis (Elhendy *et al.* 2003).

IMAGE QUANTIFICATION

Cardiac image data acquired via the imaging modalities described herein are digital in nature and thus can be stored in a computer and analyzed quantitatively using special software. Although the left ventricular function and myocardial perfusion can be visually estimated by inspection of the images, this visual analysis is subjective and inevitably results in poor reproducibility. Quantification of nuclear cardiac images, such as single photon emission computed tomography (SPECT), positron emission tomography (PET), and equilibrium radionuclide angiography (ERNA), is quite common in nuclear cardiology and has been proved to be useful for enhancement of reproducibility in assessments of left ventricular function (Lee *et al.* 1985, Germano *et al.* 1995, Faber *et al.* 1999, Khorsand *et al.* 2003, Liu *et al.* 2005) and myocardial perfusion (Faber *et al.* 1995, Liu *et al.* 1999, Germano *et al.* 2000). Quantification algorithms for nuclear cardiac images are normally developed based on the count activities in the myocardium and the geometry of the left ventricle. Although not as well established as in nuclear imaging, echocardiography, cardiac CT, and MRI each has its own standard to quantify chamber size and ventricular function. However, much of the image interpretation remains qualitative. Clearly many future efforts will be placed on improving quantification algorithms. To encourage these efforts, the American Society of Echocardiography has published guidelines for the quantification of chamber sizes and ventricular function (Lang *et al.* 2005).

REPORTING

An important final aspect of assessing the presence or absence of cardiovascular disease by any diagnostic modality is the generation of a report that is understandable by the requesting physician. Reports should be concise and clear and be focused in order to provide an answer to a clinical question. It should be helpful in subsequent clinical management of the patient. Recently standards for the reporting of echocardiography and nuclear cardiac imaging studies have been published (Gardin *et al.* 2001, Hendel *et al.* 2003).

COMPARATIVE STRENGTHS AND WEAKNESSES OF VARIOUS IMAGING MODALITIES

Though it is not possible at present to discuss conclusively the comparative strengths and weakness of each noninvasive imaging modality, some characteristics of each modality can be elucidated. Radionuclide imaging is accessible in most large western medical institutions and has an abundance of data on clinical outcomes to validate interpretation of imaging results. However, time-limited and nonreusable radionuclide agents, specialized training in handling these materials, and relatively large initial capital make radionuclide imaging relatively costly. Echocardiography is the most portable, least expensive, and most available among the imaging modalities, making it ideal for many initial evaluations of heart structure and function. High temporal resolution is of particular value for the assessment of valvular disease and intracardiac shunts. However, spatial resolution is lower than with MRI and CT and the presence and severity of CAD can only be indirectly assessed through the induction of ischemia. MRI has increased spatial resolution with excellent capability to assess chamber size and function. In addition, evaluation of cardiac masses and congenital heart disease is the strength of MRI. However, cost is relatively high and availability remains limited to large centers. CT also has high spatial resolution, but the most incremental value of CT lies in the direct imaging of the coronary arteries. However, akin to MRI, CT is relatively costly and less available than echocardiography and radionuclide imaging. Overall, each modality has individual strengths and weaknesses. Of particular interest is the combination of two imaging modalities to maximize relevant information. For instance, CT and radionuclide imaging can be combined to provide the high spatial resolution of CT for cardiac chamber size and coronary anatomy with the well validated functional assessment of coronary perfusion provided by radionuclide images. Establishing a patient-oriented approach to deciding an imaging strategy which optimizes the strengths of each imaging modality should be the goal of noninvasive cardiac imaging.

It is conceivable that new technologies will emerge for noninvasive cardiovascular imaging. More clinical research is needed to determine which imaging modality provides the desired information most efficiently and effectively, under which clinical circumstances, and in which patient population. For example, each imaging modality visualizes different aspects of a disease, but some provide more comprehensive information than the others. Clinical studies in sufficiently large and well defined patient populations are needed to elucidate which aspect(s) is (are) of clinical relevance. It is of importance that such studies are not limited to comparing the diagnostic yield of imaging modalities at one point in time, but also incorporate intermediate- and long-term follow-up of patients to determine which parameters are of relevance for patient outcome. Cost, availability, accessibility, and reimbursement are also important practical issues that may limit the use of an imaging modality. However, as has been shown in the past for oncology PET and body CT imaging, none of these issues are absolute impediments when clinical research provides solid evidence for clinical effectiveness.

In summary, extensive data exist about the important clinical value of noninvasive assessments of cardiac function and perfusion by multiple imaging techniques. The challenge faced in the near future will be to design algorithms in which each technique will be used in the most effective way.

2. CARDIAC COMPUTED TOMOGRAPHY AND ANGIOGRAPHY

Richard T. George   Albert C. Lardo   Joao A. C. Lima

INTRODUCTION

CT was first introduced in 1972 and the ability to detect human pathology noninvasively using cross-sectional images of the human body transformed nearly all specialties of medicine and surgery. However, it is only recently that technical advances have extended its utility to the diagnosis of cardiac disease. These technical advances have expanded the use of CT to include the assessment of cardiac structure, function, viability, perfusion, and even noninvasive coronary angiography. Cardiac CT is now poised to revolutionize the practice of cardiology.

TECHNICAL CONSIDERATIONS

There are several technical limitations that have, until recently, made cardiac CT impracticable. The heart and each of its chambers is in constant and rapid motion and some of its structures of interest, for example the coronary arteries, are small, ranging between 1 and 5 mm in diameter. Therefore, accurate cardiac imaging requires excellent temporal and spatial resolution. Additionally, the heart can be in different positions, depending on where in the cardiac cycle imaging acquisition takes place. Consequently, images must be gated to the ECG. Cardiac motion is not the only source of motion artifact. In order to control for respiratory motion, patients must hold their breath during a cardiac CT examination, thus acquisition time must be short. Structures of interest within the heart often have the same capability to attenuate X-rays and therefore low-contrast resolution and window width/leveling become important to resolve structures. Accurate coronary imaging requires the optimization of these parameters.

Temporal resolution

The ability to freeze cardiac motion in time is dependent on the effective temporal resolution of the scanning system. Temporal resolution is, simply, how fast a single image of the heart can be obtained. A short time of image acquisition results in a less blurry image of a moving object. A good analogy is the shutter speed of a camera. When a camera has a slow shutter speed, thus a low temporal resolution, photographs of rapid moving objects will appear blurry. On the other hand, a fast shutter speed will result in sharp pictures that clearly show the details of the objects (1).

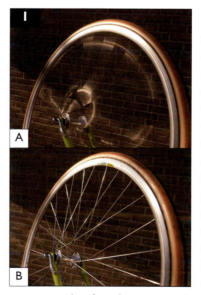

1 Demonstration of temporal resolution using a camera to photograph a rapidly spinning bicycle wheel. (A) The results of a camera with a slow shutter speed, analogous to low temporal resolution. Note that the spokes of the wheel are blurred and cannot be seen individually. (B) The results of a camera with a fast shutter speed and thus high temporal resolution in which each spoke can easily be seen.

CT requires at least 180° of gantry rotation and image acquisition to obtain a three-dimensional slice through the body. However, the resultant temporal resolution of a particular scan depends on more than the gantry rotation time. Heart rate at the time of acquisition (**2**) and a post-processing strategy utilizing the simultaneously recorded ECG, 'retrospective ECG gating' and 'segmental reconstruction', all contribute to the effective temporal resolution.

ECG gating and segmental reconstruction

Due to cardiac motion, successful cardiac imaging requires ECG gating. There are two types of ECG gating, prospective and retrospective. They differ in the way that image data are obtained and also in the type of image data obtained. Thus each of the ECG-gating types has its own advantages and disadvantages.

Prospective ECG gating is the typical gating approach traditionally used in coronary artery calcium scoring, but is now available for CT angiography.

Prospectively, the scanner is programmed to image the patient during a portion of the R-R interval. The window of X-ray exposure can be narrow and result in image data that can be reconstructed at a single phase of the R-R interval or, alternatively, the exposure window can be wide so that multiple phases can be reconstructed from the image data, for example from 60–90% of the R-R interval. Imaging will cover the z-axis distance and the detector array covers for any given scanner. Imaging occurs every other heartbeat with table movement in-between imaged heart beats. The main advantage of prospective ECG gating is a lower radiation dose. However, temporal resolution is limited to approximately half a gantry rotation plus the scanner fan angle and therefore CT coronary angiography is not feasible at higher heart rates. There can also be issues with the misalignment of image slices and contrast enhancement differences seen from the cranial to the most caudal slices. Additionally, arrhythmias occurring during scan acquisition cannot be compensated for in post processing since data throughout the R-R interval are not available.

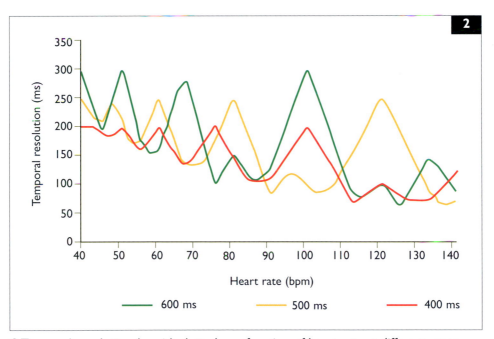

2 Temporal resolution (y-axis) plotted as a function of heart rate at different gantry rotation speeds. Due to the gantry rotation speed and heart rate harmonics temporal resolution varies with heart rate. Lines noted in green (600 ms), yellow (500 ms), and red (400 ms) demonstrate the optimal gantry rotational speed for a given heart rate maximizing temporal resolution. Temporal resolution above applies only to the Aquilion™64 (Toshiba Medical Systems Corporation, Otawara, Japan). MDCT systems vary depending on manufacturer and model.

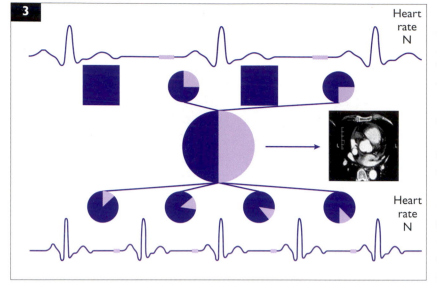

3 Retrospective ECG gating allows for segmental reconstruction that can vary depending on heart rate. With a slow heart rate, as shown on the top trace, adequate temporal resolution is obtained using image data from two R-R intervals. However, with a faster heart rate as shown on the bottom trace, image data from four R-R intervals are required for adequate temporal resolution. Portions of image data are reconstructed from consecutive R-R intervals to complete the 180° dataset required for the reconstructed axial image (arrow).

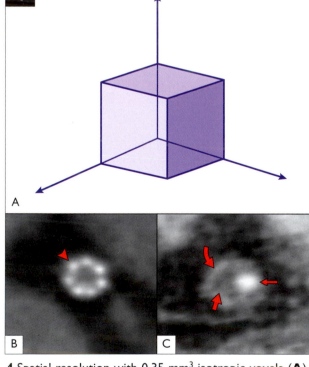

4 Spatial resolution with 0.35 mm³ isotropic voxels (**A**) gives the ability to resolve the struts (arrowhead) of a 2 mm intracoronary stent (**B**) or resolve vessel wall (curved arrow) and lumen (small arrow) and the presence of soft plaque (large arrow) (**C**).

Alternatively, retrospective ECG gating is used in most multidetector computed tomography (MDCT) coronary angiography protocols. During a retrospective ECG-gated protocol, image data are acquired using continuous X-ray exposure to the patient over six to ten heartbeats. Each set of image data is gated to the ECG. Following imaging, one can go back and reconstruct image data from any portion of the R-R interval. Retrospective ECG gating has several advantages. First of all, since image data are available throughout the R-R interval, any cardiac phase is available for MDCT angiography analysis. Since all cardiac phases are available, functional information can be extracted from the image data. Additionally, segmental reconstruction can be performed by taking portions of the image data acquired from several R-R intervals to construct the full 180° of image data needed for a three-dimensional slice (**3**). While retrospective gating has the advantage of acquiring data throughout the cardiac cycle, there is a much higher radiation dose to the patient.

Spatial resolution

Advances that have led to the clinical utility of MDCT in coronary arterial imaging have greatly improved its spatial resolution. Spatial resolution is the distance needed between two separate objects in order to see them as separate objects. The current generation of scanners has the ability to acquire images with slices as thin as 0.5–0.6 mm and containing isotropic voxels as small as 0.35 mm³ (**4**).

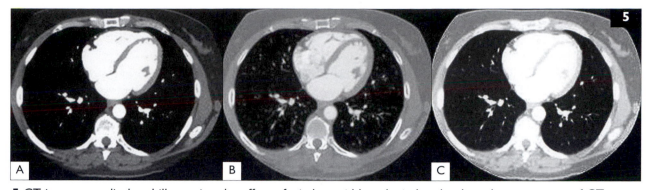

5 CT images are displayed illustrating the effect of window width and window level on the appearance of CT images. (**A**) The window width is set at 350 and the window level is set at 40 and is optimized for soft tissue contrast. Bones, with a high density, are white, while the lungs, with a low density, are black. (**B**) The same image is optimized for examining a wide range of structures. For example, structures with a high attenuation, such as bone, can be examined with a window width of 2500 and a window level of 480. (**C**) The same image with a window width of 1500 and a window level of -600. This allows for high contrast for structures with a low CT attenuation such as the lungs.

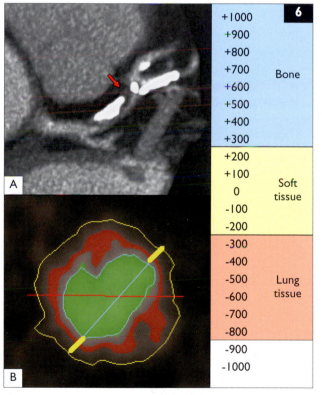

6 Axial image of the proximal left anterior descending artery (**A**) showing a severely calcified vessel and an adjacent soft plaque (arrow). Low contrast resolution and window level allow for the differentiation between the vessel lumen (green) and soft plaque (red) within the vessel wall (**B**). The panel to the right shows the range of CT attenuation coefficients in Hounsfield units illustrating the narrow range for soft tissue.

Contrast resolution

Computed tomographic images reflect the X-ray attenuation of the various tissues. Each pixel in a CT image is assigned a CT attenuation coefficient that is measured in Hounsfield units (HU). Hounsfield units range from −1,000 HU for air to 0 HU for water to several thousand for dense tissues such as bone. Since the human eye cannot resolve with detail a grayscale with such a wide range, CT images are adjusted by changing the window 'width' and window 'level'. The window width is the range of CT attenuation coefficients that will be displayed. The window level is the center around which the range is centered. For example, if the window width is set at 400 and the window level at 300, there will be a grayscale that includes all structures with a CT attenuation coefficient between 100 and 500. All structures with a CT attenuation coefficient less than 100 will be displayed as black and all structures with that greater than 500 will be displayed as white (**5**).

All cardiac structures, excluding calcified vessels, are comprised of soft tissue with similar capabilities to attenuate X-rays. Therefore, an intravascular iodinated contrast agent is required to enhance differences between adjacent structures. Low contrast resolution and a high signal-to-noise ratio are crucial for accurate atherosclerotic plaque imaging (**6**).

ELECTRON BEAM TOMOGRAPHY

Electron beam tomography (EBT) is a unique CT system that was originally manufactured with cardiac imaging in the early 1980s. There have been three generations of EBT scanners and each newer generation has come with improved temporal resolution, which currently stands at 33 ms.

EBT differs from 'helical' or 'spiral' CT mostly because there is no stationary gantry with a rotating X-ray tube and set of detectors. Instead, the only thing that moves is an electron beam and therefore EBT is not constrained to the physical limits of a rotating gantry. EBT uses a high-voltage electron gun that aims a beam of electrons towards a set of tungsten targets beneath the patient. The electron beam is steered by a system of electromagnetic deflection coils toward the tungsten targets that act as an anode and a beam of radiation is produced that passes through the patient to a set of stationary detectors above the patient (7). The electron beam is prospectively gated to the ECG to turn on at a specified phase of the R-R interval. Using two arrays of detectors, two contiguous slices of 1.5 mm, 3 mm, or 7 mm thickness can be obtained per R-R interval. Additionally, the electron beam can sweep multiple targets, up to four, and with two detector arrays the system is capable of obtaining eight slices of the above noted thickness.

EBT is well suited for assessing cardiac function, perfusion, viability, and coronary angiography, but it is best known for coronary calcium screening. Unfortunately, the financial cost of EBT scanners and their limited use for mainly cardiac indications have restricted their availability and have resulted in MDCT becoming the modality of choice for coronary artery calcium scanning. While the majority of this chapter will focus on MDCT, we will discuss some aspects of EBT as well.

MULTIDETECTOR COMPUTED TOMOGRAPHY

MDCT has become the most popular type of CT scanning because of its versatility for imaging any part of the human body. MDCT systems, often referred to as helical or spiral CT, consist of a rotating gantry that contains an X-ray tube opposite to a set of detectors. The patient lies on a scanner table that is capable of moving the patient through the plane of the gantry and thus through the X-ray beam. Images are acquired in spiral fashion (**8**).

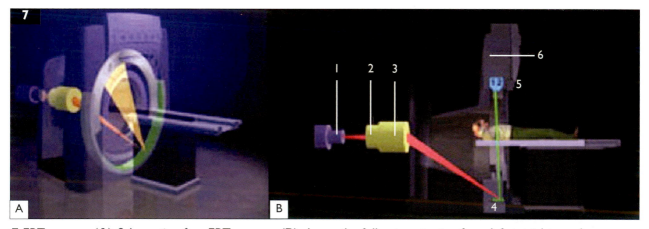

7 EBT scanner (**A**). Schematic of an EBT scanner (**B**) shows the following, starting from left to right: an electron source (1) sends a beam of electrons through a focusing coil (2) and that is then directed by an electromagnetic deflection coil (3) toward one of four target rings beneath the patient (4). The target rings act as an anode and a beam of radiation is produced that passes through the patient to the detectors (5) above the patient (6: data acquisition system.) (Courtesy of GE Healthcare, with permission.)

8 (A) The components of an MDCT gantry. Within the gantry is a row of detectors or collimators opposite to an X-ray tube that rotates around a patient. (**B**) The spiral or helical path of imaging that occurs while the scanner table moves the patient through the gantry.

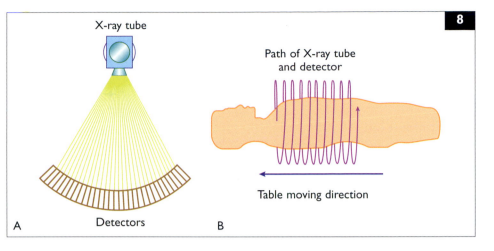

8

X-ray tube

Path of X-ray tube and detector

Table moving direction

A   Detectors   B

Table 3 Typical MDCT protocols for coronary angiography and coronary calcium scoring. Protocols are based on protocols for the Aquilion™64 (Toshiba Medical Systems Corporation, Otawara, Japan) and may vary depending on scanner manufacturer and model

	Calcium scoring	Coronary angiography
Slice collimation	4 mm × 3 mm	64 × 0.5 mm
Rotation time	250 ms	400 ms
Tube voltage	135 kV	120 kV
Tube current	300 mA	250–450 mA
ECG gating	Prospective	Retrospective
Image reconstruction	Half-scan reconstruction	Segmented reconstruction
Intravenous contrast	None	Iodinated contrast ~90–110 mL
Estimated radiation dose	1–3 mSv	12–18 mSv

MDCT scan protocols are optimized for the purpose of the scan and can utilize both retrospective and prospective ECG gating. Retrospective gating is required for coronary arterial imaging and functional imaging, while prospective gating is primarily used for coronary calcium scoring (*Table 3*).

Technical advances over recent years have given MDCT a significant unique advantage over other tomographic imaging modalities in its ability to image with a slice thickness as thin as 0.5 mm. This allows for near isotropic resolution and thus the ability to reconstruct slices in any arbitrary orientation. The present generation of MDCT scanners includes 64 detectors and thus scan acquisition time averages 10–13 s.

While MDCT has unsurpassed spatial resolution, it is more limited in its temporal resolution. MDCT requires a heavy rotating gantry with multiple parts that need to be perfectly aligned for image data acquisition. The physical constraints limit the gantry rotation speed and thus temporal resolution.

Cardiac anatomy

Before discussing the use of cardiac CT for the diagnosis of cardiac pathology, one needs to become accustomed to normal cardiac anatomy as viewed in the axial plane. Radiologists are quite accustomed to examining images throughout the human body in the axial plane which is an orientation that is quite different for the cardiologist or nonradiologist.

CT images are reconstructed and then displayed as if one were looking at the patient from the feet. All body structures that pass through the plane of the gantry are imaged, but not necessarily reconstructed. Often, cardiac images are reconstructed with a limited field of view that excludes many of the structures outside of the heart. Therefore, while the goal may be to evaluate for cardiac disease, it is essential that the images be reconstructed with a full field of view and reviewed by a radiologist for noncardiac pathology. CT images are acquired in the axial plane, but can be reconstructed in any arbitrary plane. Additionally, a three-dimensional volume-rendered image can be displayed (9).

A systematic evaluation of the heart and its surrounding structures is essential for a comprehensive MDCT cardiac examination. Starting with the nonenhanced images from the prospectively gated calcium scan, the coronary arteries, valves and perivalvular structures, aorta, and pericardium are examined for the presence of calcification. Left and right ventricular systolic function are assessed by reconstructing the raw contrast-enhanced imaging data from 0% to 90% of the R-R interval at 10% intervals and an EF is calculated. Cardiac chambers are examined for enlargement. Careful examination of the left ventricular myocardium looking for focal wall motion abnormalities, thinning, or aneurysmal formation, or a hypoenhanced appearance of the myocardium can give clues about the presence of previous myocardial injury. The aortic root and aorta should be examined for the presence of aneurysmal dilation and aortic dissection. Each coronary artery is examined beginning with the right coronary artery (RCA) followed by the left main and left anterior descending artery (LAD), then the left circumflex artery (LCX). While the three-dimensional volume-rendered view is useful for appreciating the course of the coronary arteries and their branches in three dimensions, they should be assessed for stenoses using two-dimensional reconstructions in either the axial plane and/or using multiplanar reconstruction in orthogonal planes. Most often the LAD and LCX are best examined in diastole, but this may vary depending on the heart rate and the amount of

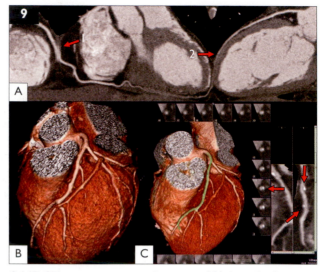

9 MDCT coronary arterial imaging. (**A**) A multiplanar reconstruction starting with the right coronary artery (1) on the left and the left anterior descending artery (2) on the right in a patient with no significant coronary stenoses. (**B**) A three-dimensional volume-rendered image. (**C**) Vessel probing of the left anterior descending artery (green) with short-axis and orthogonal views of the vessel displayed. Several calcified plaques are noted in the left anterior descending artery (arrows).

motion artifact present. The RCA is often more prone to motion artifact and may be best viewed in diastole or end-systole. Multiple phases during the R-R interval should be examined to determine the phase with the least motion artifact. Normal cardiac anatomy viewed in the axial plane is shown in **10**. Left and right dominant circulations are represented in **11**.

MDCT imaging artifacts

Although MDCT has made significant advances towards improving the spatial and temporal resolution, like all imaging modalities it is prone to artifact. Most artifacts are well described and are apparent to the experienced reader. Certain artifacts are the result of anatomical structures or artificial implants that are intrinsic to the patient. Metallic implants such as intracardiac device leads can cause a streak artifact that results in areas of high and low

10 Normal cardiac anatomy as viewed in the axial plane by MDCT. (**A**) Structures just above the origin of the coronary arteries and includes the ascending and descending aorta (1), the bifurcation of the pulmonary arteries (2), and the superior vena cava (3). (**B**) View at the level of the origin of the left main coronary artery. Contrast-filled structures include the left and right atrial appendages (4 and 5), the right ventricular outflow tract (6), and the right and left upper pulmonary veins (7). (**C**) Bifurcation of the left main coronary artery into the left anterior descending (8) and left circumflex (9) arteries. (**D**) Course of the right coronary artery (10) as it passes between the right ventricular outflow tract and right atrium (11). (**E**) The right coronary artery and left circumflex artery in short axis as they course in each

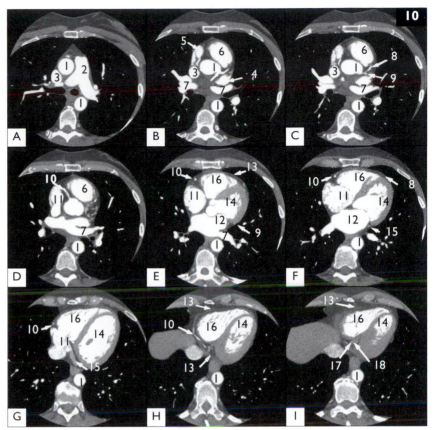

atrioventricular groove. The pericardium (13) is clearly seen. 12 = left atrium; 14 = left ventricle. (**F**) and (**G**) show the coronary sinus (15) as it travels in the atrioventricular groove and empties into the right atrium. (**H**) Course of the right coronary artery posterior to the right ventricle (16). (**I**) The posterior interventricular vein (17) and the posterior descending artery (18) as they begin to course together in the interventricular groove.

11 Three-dimensional volume-rendered images illustrating examples of a left and right dominant coronary arterial tree. (**A**) A left dominant system with the left posterior descending artery (1) originating from the distal left circumflex artery (2) along side the posterior interventricular vein (3). The distal left

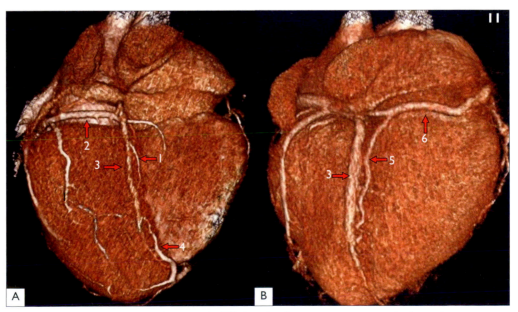

anterior descending artery (4) supplies the distal inferior wall. (**B**) A right dominant system with the right posterior descending artery (5) originating from the right coronary artery (6).

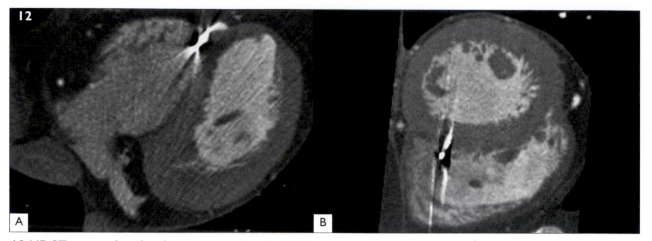

12 MDCT image of artifact from a pacemaker lead. (**A**) View of the lead in the axial plane as it inserts into the right ventricular apex. (**B**) The same patient reconstructed in an oblique view demonstrating the spatial extent of the artifact.

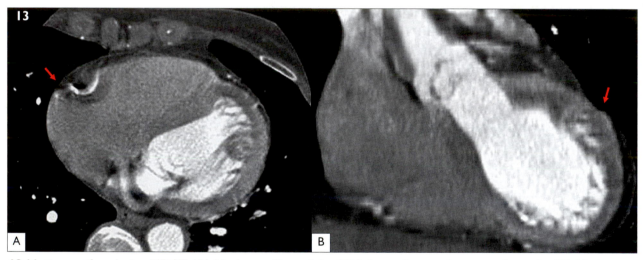

13 Motion artifact during MDCT. (**A**) Motion artifact of the RCA (arrow) secondary to tachycardia. (**B**) Motion artifact secondary to an arrhythmia. In this case, premature ventricular contractions during MDCT imaging cause misalignment of the left ventricular free wall.

X-ray attenuation (**12**). Intracoronary stents, along with coronary calcifications, are associated with blooming artifact that often makes it difficult to see the lumen of the vessel. Motion artifact can often be detected when the surfaces of structures appear distorted and blurred as a result of faster heart rates or arrhythmias (**13**). Reconstruction artifacts can occur in several circumstances. Segmented reconstruction algorithms can result in streaking near structures with high attenuation coefficients like calcium and bone. Reconstruction algorithms that enhance the clarity of edges can falsely increase the brightness in signal density along the edge of a structure.

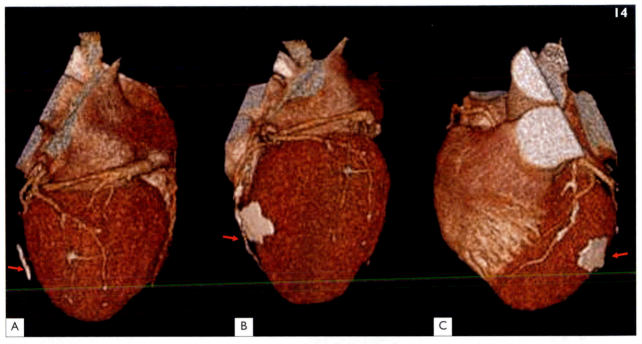

14 Three-dimensional volume-rendered images of the heart from lateral views (**A** and **B**) to an anterior view (**C**) showing focal pericardial calcification (arrows) overlying the anterolateral wall.

CLINICAL CARDIAC COMPUTED TOMOGRAPHY
Pericardial disease

The evaluation of the pericardium is not new to X-ray CT. CT is the gold standard for the diagnosis of calcified pericarditis and is invaluable in the surgical treatment of the disease (**14**). Pericardial effusions are clearly evident on CT. Small effusions are usually located posteriorly and as they enlarge they occupy space anterior to the heart with large effusions eventually surrounding the entire heart. The CT attenuation value of pericardial fluid can assist in differentiating a serous effusion from acute intrapericardial hemorrhage, since a hemorrhagic pericardial effusion typically has higher attenuation values (Olson *et al.* 1989). In the setting of intrapericardial hemorrhage, there may be areas of flocculation.

Pericardial masses can appear in the forms of cysts, diverticuli, or neoplasms. Cysts and diverticuli are differentiated from other masses by their smooth, round, and homogeneous appearance (Wychulis *et al.* 1971). Pericardial tumors can be identified by their anatomical connection to the pericardium. They rarely compress or obstruct the cardiac chambers or great vessels, but when they enlarge they often distort local anatomy.

Myocardial disease

Although CT provides information of left ventricular geometry, wall motion, and wall thickness, the use of MDCT for the diagnosis of primary cardiomyopathies is limited at present. There are case reports noting areas of focally increased contrast uptake in the setting of myocarditis and myocardial fibrosis, but there are no larger studies evaluating MDCT for this purpose (Funabashi *et al.* 2003, Dambrin *et al.* 2004). Using EBT, the features of arrhythmogenic right ventricular dysplasia (ARVD) have been previously described (Dery *et al.* 1986). Similarly, MDCT can

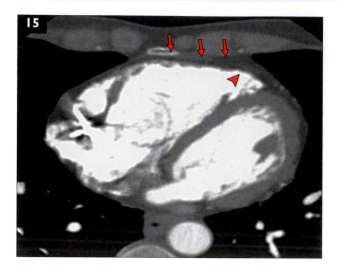

15 MDCT illustrating some of the typical findings in ARVD. The right ventricle is significantly dilated with fatty intramyocardial deposits (arrows) and a scalloped appearance of the right ventricular free wall (arrowhead).

detect typical features associated with ARVD, including right ventricle hypokinesis, bulging of the right ventricular free wall, intramyocardial fat deposits, and a scalloped appearance of the right ventricle wall (**15**). It is reasonable to consider MDCT coronary angiography for the evaluation of a new cardiomyopathy since its high negative predictive value could be used to rule out coronary atherosclerosis as the etiology; this approach has not been rigorously validated, however.

Valvular disease

The high spatial and temporal resolution and the ability of reconstructing ECG-gated MDCT in any arbitrary plane make it an ideal candidate for valvular imaging. Noncontrast MDCT imaging of both the mitral and aortic valves can measure the amount of calcium in the valve leaflets and surrounding structures while contrast-enhanced images can reveal valve motion and anatomy.

Willmann *et al.* carried out a study that included 20 patients with known mitral valve pathology, using four-detector CT. This showed moderate to excellent visibility of all mitral valve structures except for the tendinous chordae in all patients studied (Willmann *et al.* 2002). MDCT evaluation of mitral valve leaflet thickening, calcification, and mitral annular calcification was 100% accurate compared with surgical findings, with excellent correlation to findings found on echocardiography (**16**). Studying mitral regurgitation with 16-detector CT, Alkadhi

et al. demonstrated good correlation between the planimetric measurements of the regurgitant orifice area and results obtained from echocardiography (r = 0.807, p <0.001) and ventriculography (r = 0.922, p <0.001) (Alkadhi *et al.* 2006).

Baumert *et al.* investigated the utility of 16-detector CT in assessing the aortic valve. They found that valve opening was best evaluated in early systole and valve closing in mid-diastole. Using planimetry, aortic valve area as measured by MDCT showed exceptional correlation when compared with transesophageal echocardiography (TEE) (r = 0.96, p <0.0001) (Baumert *et al.* 2005).

Coronary artery disease

Advancements in cardiac CT have made it an ideal candidate for the comprehensive evaluation of CAD and its sequelae. Coronary calcium imaging is well documented in the literature with EBT, and MDCT is now assuming EBT's role in the detection of subclinical atherosclerosis and calcified plaque. Additionally, MDCT imaging of the coronary lumen is a rapidly growing application that is now feasible with the high spatial resolution of today's scanners. Retrospective ECG gating and reconstruction of MDCT images during multiple phases of the R-R interval allow for the assessments of left ventricular systolic function, wall motion, wall thickness, and the sequelae of chronic coronary disease.

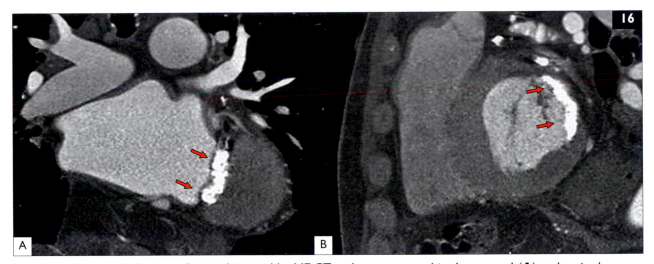

16 Mitral annular calcifications (arrows) imaged by MDCT and reconstructed in the coronal (**A**) and sagittal (**B**) planes.

Coronary artery calcification

Previous studies have documented that atherosclerosis is the only disease known to cause coronary calcification (Blankenhorn & Stern 1959, Frink *et al.* 1970, Wexler *et al.* 1996). While coronary calcification is rare in the first and second decade of life, its prevalence reaches 100% by the eighth decade. Men tend to develop calcifications a decade earlier than women, although this disparity between the sexes disappears by the seventh decade (Janowitz *et al.* 1993).

According to pathological studies, the presence of coronary calcification confirms the presence of atherosclerosis and the amount of calcification is strongly correlated with the total amount of athero-sclerotic plaque (Rumberger *et al.* 1994, 1995, O'Rourke *et al.* 2000). Unfortunately, while there is a positive correlation between the amount of calcium and percent stenosis, the relationship has wide confidence intervals (Tanenbaum *et al.* 1989).

Noninvasive detection of coronary calcification may be performed with EBT or MDCT, but the majority of previous investigations have used the former. Typical EBT calcium scoring protocols use EBT in prospective ECG-gating mode, without iodinated contrast, and acquire images in the axial plane with a 3 mm thickness. Slice acquisition occurs in as little as 50–100 ms. The presence of coronary calcium is confirmed by detecting continuous pixels with a signal density greater than 130 HU. An Agatston score is calculated by determining the area of calcium found in a slice, multiplied by a factor of 1–4 depending on the peak CT attenuation found in each calcified plaque. This is repeated in each 3 mm slice and the sum of all scores represents the Agatston calcium score (Agatston *et al.* 1990).

Coronary artery calcium (CAC) scoring with MDCT will likely become more common in the future with the widespread availability of these imaging systems. While calcium scoring may be performed with either retrospective or prospective ECG gating, the latter is preferred due to a much lower radiation dose. Scan parameters vary between manufacturers and a typical calcium scanning protocol at the authors' institution is shown in *Table 3*. Calcium scoring is performed in a similar fashion to EBT using a threshold of 130 HU to define coronary calcium. As a result of inferior temporal resolution compared with EBT, prospective ECG-gated MDCT calcium imaging can more often be affected by motion artifact. Studies to date show a good correlation between EBT and MDCT, but the correlation at the lower end of CAC scores is not as strong. Reproducibility of scan

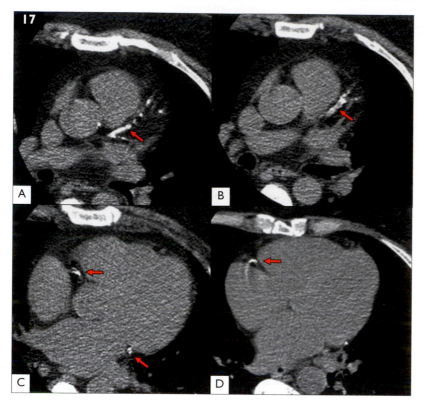

17 CAC imaging using MDCT. (**A**) and (**B**) depict severe calcification (arrows) of the LAD. (**C**) The same patient, showing calcified atherosclerosis in the RCA and LCX (arrows). (**D**) A patient scanned with a heart rate of 95 bpm and the resulting motion artifact of the RCA (arrow).

results does not differ with serial scans using MDCT or EBT (Detrano *et al.* 2005). Figure **17** illustrates CAC imaged by MDCT.

The clinical significance of coronary calcification is well established. The absence of coronary calcification makes the presence of significant atherosclerosis very unlikely (O'Rourke *et al.* 2000, Haberl *et al.* 2001). In contrast, elevated CAC scoring predicts long-term cardiac events independent of traditional risk factors (Agatston *et al.* 1990, Arad *et al.* 2000, Raggi *et al.* 2000, Wong *et al.* 2000). Kondos *et al.* demonstrated, in a population of asymptomatic low- to intermediate-risk adults, that a calcium score >170 had a relative risk of myocardial infarction or cardiac death of 7.24 (95% CI: 2.01–26.15) (Kondos *et al.* 2003). Furthermore, Wayhs *et al.* reported in a study of 98 patients with a CAC score >1000, a 25% annualized rate of myocardial infarction or cardiac death (Wayhs *et al.* 2002). All these studies taken together support the use of calcium scoring as a risk assessment tool, but there is general agreement that a high calcium score alone in an asymptomatic patient is not a cause for referral for invasive angiography. Furthermore, additional studies are needed to define the role of CAC scoring in the scope of traditional risk factor modification efforts.

Coronary angiography
Evaluation of native coronary artery

Technical advancements in temporal and spatial resolution over the past 5 years have made noninvasive coronary angiography feasible with MDCT. Early studies, using four-detector systems, were limited by a 1 mm slice thickness, slow gantry rotation speed, and prolonged breath hold leading to a large number of unevaluable vessels, but showed that CT coronary angiography held promise (Achenbach *et al.* 2000, 2001, Nieman *et al.* 2001, Kopp *et al.* 2002). With the introduction of 12- and 16-detector CT systems, slice thickness became sub-millimeter, breath holding was reduced to approximately 20 s and the diagnostic accuracy improved (Nieman *et al.* 2002a, Ropers *et al.* 2003, Hoffmann *et al.* 2004b, Kuettner *et al.* 2004, Mollet *et al.* 2004). However, there was still an unacceptable number of unevaluable segments: up to 6–17% of segments. Several of these studies documented the advantage of lower heart rates on image quality and beta-blockers became a common component of most MDCT coronary angiography protocols (Giesler *et al.* 2002, Nieman *et al.* 2002b, Schroeder *et al.* 2002, Ropers *et al.* 2003).

The current generation of MDCT imaging systems has the capability to image up to 64 slices simultaneously with a slice thickness of 0.5–0.6 mm and a gantry rotation time of 330–400 ms depending on manufacturer. These features, along with improvements in reconstruction algorithms and software, provide MDCT the spatial and temporal resolution that facilitates the clinical use of MDCT. Typical MDCT coronary angiography protocols use approximately 80–110 mL of intravenous contrast, while breath holds are approximately 10–13 s. As a result of the variability in scanning protocols, patient populations studied, and differences in reporting results on a per-segment, per-vessel, or per-patient analysis, it is difficult to compare 64-slice MDCT studies directly. This section will aim to summarize each of the studies published to date.

Leber *et al.* were the first to report a study of 64-detector CT (Leber *et al.* 2005). They studied 59 patients with stable angina and compared MDCT to quantitative coronary angiography (QCA) and a subset of 18 patients also underwent intravascular ultrasound. They only excluded 13 stented segments and 14 other segments determined to be distal to an occluded vessel. Altogether, they reported results on 798 segments. The overall correlation between the degree of stenosis detected by QCA compared with 64-slice CT was r = 0.54. Sensitivity for the detection of stenosis <50%, stenosis >50%, and stenosis >75% was 79%, 73%, and 80%, respectively, and overall specificity was 97%. In comparison with intravenous ultrasound (IVUS), 46 of 55 (84%) lesions were identified correctly. Sixty-four-slice CT compared well with IVUS with regard to plaque area and percentage of vessel obstruction. Mean plaque areas and the percentage of vessel obstruction measured by IVUS and 64-slice CT were 8.1 mm^2 versus 7.3 mm^2 (p <0.03, r = 0.73) and 50.4% versus 41.1% (p <0.001, r = 0.61).

Raff *et al.* were the next to report their results using 64-detector CT in a group of 70 patients referred for coronary angiography for suspected coronary disease (Raff *et al.* 2005). Fifty percent of the patients studied had a body mass index (BMI) >30, 26% had a calcium score >400, and 25% had a heart rate >70 during scan acquisition. Specificity, sensitivity, and positive and negative predictive values for the presence of >50% stenoses were: by segment (n = 935), 86%, 95%, 66%, and 98%, respectively; by artery (n = 279), 91%, 92%,

80%, and 97%, respectively; by patient (n = 70), 95%, 90%, 93%, and 93%, respectively. Additionally, they found that 83% of segments were suitable for quantitative comparison of CT angiography and invasive angiography. The Spearman correlation coefficient between MDCT and QCA was 0.76 (p <0.0001) and a Bland-Altman analysis demonstrated a mean difference in percent stenosis of 1.3% ± 14.2%.

Leschka *et al.* reported another study of a population with a high prevalence three-vessel disease (Leschka *et al.* 2005). They studied a total of 67 patients with 24 (36%) patients presenting with signs of unstable angina pectoris and 43 (64%) patients presenting before undergoing coronary artery bypass surgery. Without the need to exclude any patients from the analysis, overall sensitivity, specificity, and positive and negative predictive values for classifying stenoses was 94%, 97%, 87%, and 99% respectively on a per-segment basis.

Mollet *et al.* compared 64-slice MDCT to QCA in a group of 52 patients with atypical chest pain, stable or unstable angina pectoris, or non-ST-segment elevation myocardial infarction scheduled for diagnostic invasive coronary angiography (Mollet *et al.* 2004). They reported the following sensitivity, specificity, and positive and negative predictive values for detecting significant stenoses greater than 50% in their segment-by-segment analysis: 99%, 95%, 76%, and 99%, respectively. Interestingly, in the 35% (18/52) of patients with a CAC score >400, MDCT performed well in the detection of significant stenoses. Sensitivity, specificity, and positive and negative predictive values for detecting significant stenoses in patients with a CAC score of 401–1000 (n = 12) were 97%, 93%, 76%, and 99% respectively and with a CAC score >1000 (n = 6) were 100%, 92%, 78%, and 100%, respectively. However, confidence intervals were wide due to the small sample size.

Two additional studies of 64-slice MDCT confirm the above results. In a study of 35 patients with stable angina, Pugliese *et al.* reported, without the need to exclude segments, a sensitivity, specificity, and positive and negative predictive values of 99%, 96%, 78%, and 99%, respectively on a per-segment basis (Pugliese *et al.* 2006). Ropers *et al.* reported a study in a population with a relatively lower prevalence of significant stenoses in 84 patients. They showed sensitivity, specificity, positive and negative predictive values of 93%, 97%, 56%, and 100%, respectively in a per-segment analysis with the need to exclude 4% of segments secondary to calcifications and motion artifact (Anders *et al.* 2006).

Although these early studies of 64-slice MDCT are documenting the improved accuracy and reliability of noninvasive coronary angiography with thinner slice collimation, reported radiation doses have risen and are in the range of 13–21.4 mSv (Mollet *et al.* 2004, Raff *et al.* 2005, Pugliese *et al.* 2006). It is hoped that advances, such as X-ray tube current modulation, will reduce this dose (Trabold *et al.* 2003, Leber *et al.* 2005, Anders *et al.* 2006). Additionally, studies to date were performed in patients with mostly a high pretest likelihood of CAD. Therefore, it is not known how well they will perform in patients with a low or intermediate likelihood of CAD. Additionally, all of the above studies were single-center studies with relatively small groups of patients, thus the field awaits the completion of ongoing multicenter trials. Figures **18–21** illustrate several examples of coronary stenoses detected by MDCT.

Coronary plaque imaging

Early studies documented the heterogeneity of atherosclerotic plaque and the ability of MDCT to differentiate between its components (Kragel *et al.* 1989, Kopp *et al.* 2001, Schroeder *et al.* 2001, 2004, Caussin *et al.* 2003). Additionally, the high correlation between the CAC score and the total atherosclerotic burden has been described (Kragel *et al.* 1989, Kopp *et al.* 2001, Schroeder *et al.* 2001, 2004, Caussin *et al.* 2003). The differentiation between the vessel lumen, vessel wall, hard plaque, and soft plaque requires excellent low contrast resolution and a high signal-to-noise ratio (see **5**). MDCT has a high sensitivity for detecting calcified plaque with sensitivities and specificities of 94–95% and 92–94%, respectively. However, MDCT is less sensitive (53–78%) in the detection of noncalcified plaque (Achenbach *et al.* 2004, Leber *et al.* 2004). Achenbach *et al.* demonstrated a good correlation between MDCT and IVUS in the estimation of

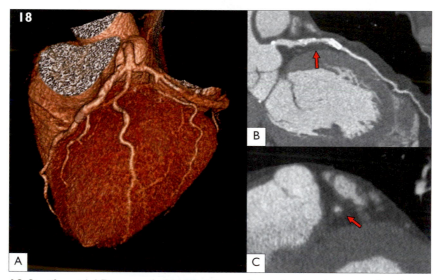

18 Significant LAD stenosis. (**A**) The three-dimensional volume-rendered image illustrates the LAD, ramus intermedius artery, and LCX. (**B**) A greater than 50% stenosis (arrow) in the proximal LAD just prior to an intracoronary stent. (**C**) The LAD stenosis in short axis; note the presence of soft atherosclerotic plaque causing the stenosis (arrow).

19 Chronic RCA occlusion depicted in a three-dimensional volume-rendered reconstruction (**A**) and in a multiplanar reconstruction (**B**) (arrows).

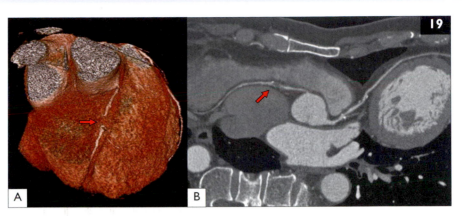

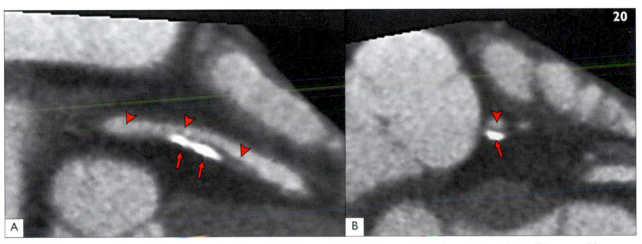

20 Multiplanar reconstruction demonstrating a LAD stenosis in the long axis (**A**) and short axis (**B**) caused by a calcified atherosclerotic plaque (arrows). The vessel lumen (arrowheads) is >50% stenosed.

21 Multiplanar reconstruction of the proximal RCA in a patient with a history of multiple stents. Note the stenosed portion of the RCA between the first and second stents (arrow). Inset shows the RCA in short axis demonstrating a noncalcified stenosis.

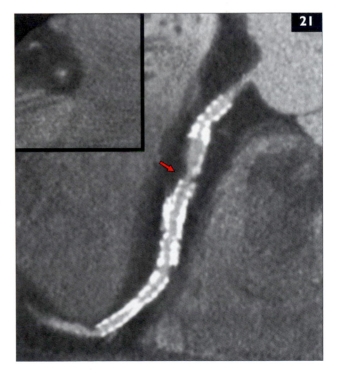

plaque volume (r = 0.8), although MDCT systematically underestimated plaque volume in this study (Achenbach *et al.* 2004). However, this same group reported a moderate correlation (r = 0.55) between MDCT and IVUS in the measurement of plaque cross-sectional area in another study, with a slight overestimation observed by MDCT (Hoffmann *et al.* 2004b). Different imaging systems and methodologies may explain the conflicting results between these two studies. Figures **22** and **23** illustrate calcified and noncalcified plaque.

Coronary artery bypass grafts

While we await studies evaluating the use of 64-slice MDCT for coronary artery bypass graft occlusions and stenoses, four- and 16-slice MDCT has been used for this purpose. Using four-slice CT with a 1 mm slice thickness, Ropers *et al.* reported a study of 65 patients with a total of 182 bypass grafts. They reported sensitivity, specificity, and positive and negative predictive values for detecting bypass occlusions of 97%, 98%, 97%, and 98% respectively (Achenbach *et al.* 2001). However, their accuracy for the evaluation of significant stenoses was poor with only 62% being evaluable. Nieman *et al.* again reported similar high accuracy for evaluating for graft obstruction using four-slice MDCT, but showed less

impressive results when evaluating for graft stenosis and the native coronaries distal to the graft anastomosis (Nieman *et al.* 2003).

More recently, studies using 16-slice MDCT with sub-millimeter slice thickness have been reported. Schlosser *et al.* reported a study of 51 patients evaluating for stenoses and occlusions in 40 arterial and 91 venous grafts and showed a sensitivity of 96%, a specificity of 95%, a positive predictive value of 81%, and a negative predictive value of 99% (Schlosser *et al.* 2004). On the contrary, their assessment of distal anastomosis was hindered since only 74% were evaluable. By excluding the unevaluable distal anastomoses, they reported a sensitivity of 96%, a specificity of 95%, a positive predictive value of 81%, and a negative predictive value of 99%. Another study by Salm *et al.* evaluated 25 patients with a history of coronary artery bypass grafting using 16-slice MDCT (Salm *et al.* 2005). They showed high accuracy in determining the patency of arterial grafts, vein grafts, and nongrafted vessels in 100%, 100%, and 97% of segments, respectively. Additionally, they reported a high sensitivity and specificity for detecting stenoses >50% with a sensitivity/specificity of 100%/94% for vein grafts and 100%/89% for nongrafted vessels. No arterial graft stenoses were presented in this study. Most recently a study by Anders *et al.* evaluated

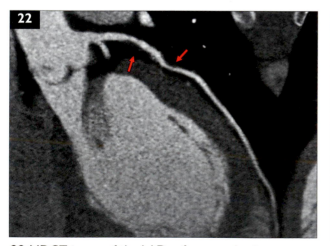

22 MDCT image of the LAD reformatted using multiplanar reconstruction. There are two noncalcified, 'soft' plaques noted in the proximal portion of the LAD (arrows).

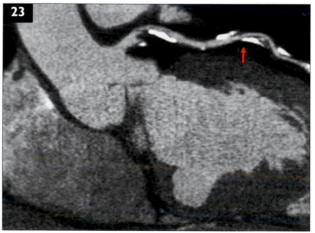

23 MDCT image of the LAD reformatted using multiplanar reconstruction. There are multiple calcified plaques noted along the LAD and one plaque that contains a significant noncalcified component (arrow).

32 patients using 16-slice MDCT (Anders *et al.* 2006). They again confirmed an excellent sensitivity of 100% and specificity of 98% in the detection of occluded vein grafts. They reported results from two observers that concluded that 78% and 84% of grafts were evaluable for stenoses and reported a sensitivity of 80% and 82% and a specificity of 85% and 88% for the detection of high-grade stenoses. Interestingly, due to the number of unevaluable segments and the need for invasive coronary angiography in patients with graft stenoses, the authors concluded that 25% of patients in their study could have avoided invasive angiography as a result of a fully diagnostic and negative graft MDCT angiogram.

These studies illustrate the high accuracy of MDCT for the evaluation of bypass graft occlusion. While stenoses are difficult to assess reliably using MDCT, they can be reliably detected in the setting of a good-quality study. Distal anastomosis and the runoff vessels remain difficult to assess. Further studies with 64-slice MDCT are expected improve upon these earlier studies. Figures **24** and **25** illustrate coronary artery bypass graft imaging by MDCT.

Congenital coronary artery anomalies

Coronary anomalies are uncommon, but not rare, and affect about 1% of the population with 87% presenting as anomalies of origination and distribution and the remainder presenting as fistulae (Yamanaka & Hobbs 1990). While they can often be diagnosed with conventional coronary angiography, their three-dimensional course is best appreciated using MDCT.

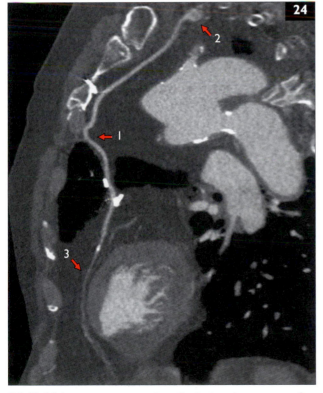

24 Multiplanar reconstruction depicting the course of the left internal mammary artery (1) as it originates from the left subclavian artery (2) and anastomoses with the LAD (3).

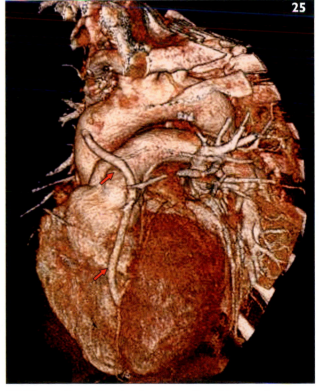

25 Three-dimensional volume-rendered image showing a saphenous vein graft (arrows) originating from the ascending aorta and joining the mid portion of the LAD.

Most anomalies can be considered benign and include:

➤ Separate origins of the LAD and LCX.
➤ Ectopic origin of the circumflex from the right sinus of Valsalva.
➤ Ectopic coronary origin from the posterior sinus of Valsalva.
➤ Anomalous coronary origin from the ascending aorta.
➤ Absent circumflex.
➤ Intercoronary communications.
➤ Small coronary artery fistulae.

However, other anomalies may be associated with potentially serious sequelae such as angina pectoris, myocardial infarction, syncope, cardiac arrhythmias, congestive heart failure, or sudden death. Potentially serious anomalies include (Yamanaka & Hobbs 1990):

➤ Ectopic coronary origin from the pulmonary artery.
➤ Ectopic coronary origin from the opposite aortic sinus.
➤ Single coronary artery.
➤ Large coronary fistulae.

Figures **26–28** illustrate some coronary anomalies.

Cardiac venous anatomy

Advancements in electrophysiology are demanding more accurate imaging of pulmonary venous and coronary venous anatomy. Pulmonary vein isolation procedures for the ablation of atrial fibrillation can substantially benefit from MDCT imaging in pre- and post-procedure. In pre-procedure, the left atrium can be examined for the anatomy of the pulmonary veins and more importantly determine the presence of any supernumerary veins (Jongbloed *et al.* 2005a). Three-dimensional reconstruction of the pulmonary veins can be registered to the electroanatomic maps and assist in complex ablation procedures (Bateman 1995). In post-procedure, MDCT can be used to diagnose the presence of pulmonary vein stenosis (Kuettner 2005). Figure **29** depicts pulmonary vein anatomy.

Cardiac resynchronization therapy with biventricular pacing uses the cardiac veins for placement of left ventricular electrodes percutaneously. Using MDCT Jongbloed *et al.* illustrated the variability of the cardiac venous anatomy in a study of 38 patients (Jongbloed *et al.* 2005a). They showed the following anomalies:

➤ Separate insertion of the coronary sinus and small cardiac vein in 63%.
➤ Continuity of the anterior and posterior venous system at the crux.
➤ The posterior interventricular vein did not connect with the coronary sinus in 8%.

Pre-procedure planning can shorten the length of procedures and determine whether transvenous

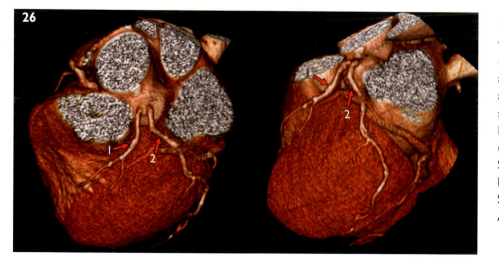

26 Three-dimensional volume-rendered reconstruction illustrating anomalous coronary arteries. Note the separate ostia for the LAD (1) and LCX (2). (Courtesy of Dr. Ruben Sebben, Dr. Jones and Partners Medical Imaging, St. Andrew's Hospital, Adelaide, South Australia.)

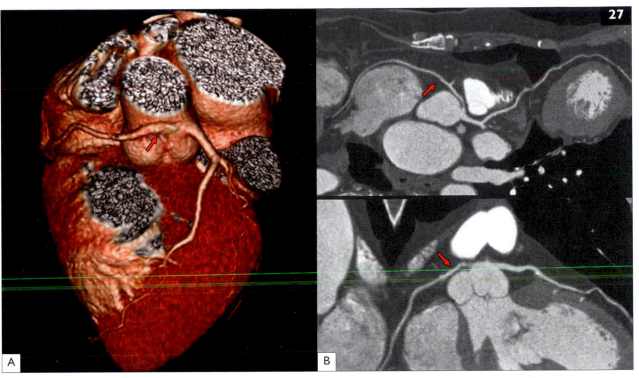

27 Anomalous origin of the RCA. Three-dimensional volume-rendered reconstruction (**A**) and multiplanar reconstructions (**B**) illustrating the anomalous origin of the RCA from the left coronary cusp and coursing between the aorta and the right ventricular outflow tract (arrows).

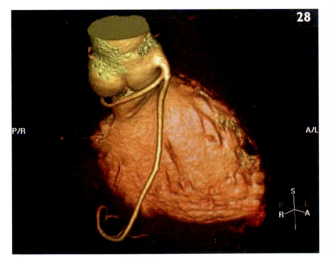

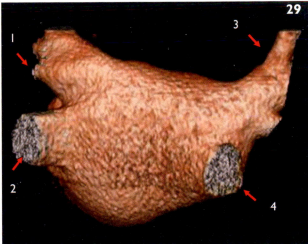

28 Three-dimensional volume-rendered reconstruction illustrating anomalous coronary arteries. Shown is an example of a single coronary artery with the RCA originating from the left main coronary artery. (Courtesy of Dr. Ruben Sebben, Dr. Jones and Partners Medical Imaging, St. Andrew's Hospital, Adelaide, South Australia.)

29 Pulmonary vein anatomy imaged by MDCT. Posterior view of the left atrium depicting the pulmonary veins and their ostia. (1: left upper pulmonary vein; 2: left lower pulmonary vein; 3: right upper pulmonary vein; 4: right lower pulmonary vein.)

pacing lead placement is possible. Figure **30** illustrates normal coronary venous anatomy.

Function

Cardiac MDCT imaging acquires data throughout the cardiac cycle from systole to diastole which allows images to be reconstructed at multiple phases in the R-R interval. Typically, image data are reconstructed from 0% to 90% of the cardiac cycle at 10% intervals. Endocardial and epicardial borders can be outlined using either hand planimetry or various automated border detection algorithms, and myocardial mass, end-systolic and end-diastolic volumes, stroke volume, cardiac output, and EF can be calculated. Studies comparing MDCT and MRI show measurements of stroke volume, end-systolic and end-diastolic volumes, EF, and regional wall motion scores are strongly correlated. Nevertheless, MDCT has a tendency to overestimate volumetric measurements (de la Pena-Almaguer *et al.* 2005, Kuettner 2005, Mahnken 2005). MDCT is well suited to measure right ventricular mass and function (Kim *et al.* 2005). However, compared to MRI, MDCT is inferior in the measurement of dynamic functional parameters such as peak filling rate, peak ejection rate, time to peak ejection rate, and time from end-systole to peak filling rate, due to lower temporal resolution.

Myocardial scar and viability imaging

MDCT and iodinated intravenous contrast are well suited for myocardial viability imaging. Iodinated intravenous contrast agents primarily remain intravascular during the early part of first pass circulation and then later diffuse into the extravascular space (Newhouse 1977, Newhouse & Murphy 1981, Canty *et al.* 1991). These characteristics provide an opportunity to detect hypoenhanced areas early after contrast injection, that signify hypoperfusion, and conversely detect hyperenhanced areas later after contrast injection, that signify damaged myocardium. Signal density measured by MDCT has a direct linear relationship to tissue iodine concentration (Rumberger *et al.* 1991). MDCT can also image the heart with a slice thickness of 0.5 mm with nearly isotopic image resolution. The improved spatial resolution reduces the partial volume artifacts and therefore has the potential for more accurate volumetric sizing of myocardial infarcts as compared with other imaging modalities.

The pharmacokinetics of iodinated intravenous contrast agents provide two opportunities after contrast bolus administration to detect the presence of myocardial infarction, specifically in early and delayed imaging. Infarct imaging during first-pass circulation of intravenous contrast will show the presence of an early defect characterized as an area of hypoenhanced myocardium. Nikolaou *et al.* were the first to demonstrate in a systematic way the significance of early defects using four-detector CT in patients. Compared with biplane ventriculography, MDCT accurately identified the presence of an infarct in 90% of cases (Nikolaou *et al.* 2004). In addition, a recent study using a porcine model of LAD occlusion showed that MDCT could be used to detect acute myocardial infarction (Hoffmann *et al.* 2004a). This study showed that the size of an early perfusion defect correlated well with the extent of myocardial infarction shown by post-mortem triphenyltetrazolium chloride (TTC) staining. More recently, 16-detector CT was compared with delayed enhanced MRI for the detection of chronic infarcts. In a group of 30 patients that underwent MDCT angiography, first-pass MDCT detected 10/11 infarcts noted on delayed-enhanced MRI yielding a sensitivity, specificity, and accuracy of 91%, 79%, and 83%, respectively (Nikolaou *et al.* 2005).

Delayed-enhanced MRI is well validated in the detection of myocardial viability (Gerber *et al.* 2002, Ingkanisorn *et al.* 2004, Thomson *et al.* 2004). Similar to gadolinium, iodinated contrast medium will be preferentially taken up by irreversibly damaged myocytes over time. As such, it is feasible to perform delayed-enhanced MDCT imaging as well. In a canine model of LAD occlusion and reperfusion after 90 minutes, Lardo *et al.* demonstrated that the spatial extent of cell death and microvascular obstruction can be accurately assessed by MDCT (Lardo *et al.* 2006). Using TTC and thioflavin staining to demarcate infarct size and extent of microvascular obstruction, MDCT compared well yielding correlation coefficients of 0.91 and 0.93, respectively (Lardo *et al.* 2004). Mahnken *et al.* compared both early-perfusion deficits and late-enhanced MDCT to delayed-enhanced MRI in a group of 28 patients after reperfusion of an acute myocardial infarction. Late-enhanced MDCT performed 15 minutes after contrast injection was shown to be more accurate than early-enhanced MDCT compared with MRI in detecting both infarct size and location. While late-enhanced MDCT slightly overestimated infarct size,

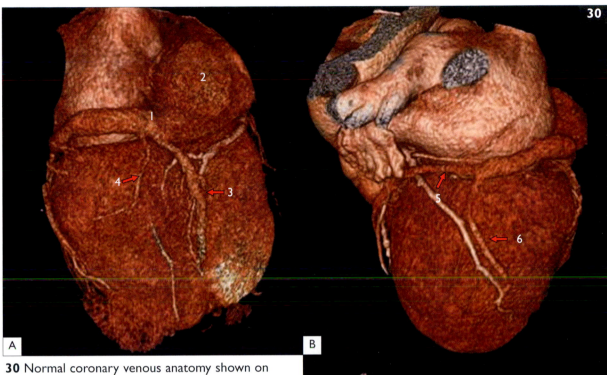

30

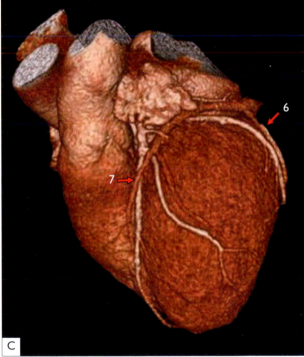

30 Normal coronary venous anatomy shown on three-dimensional volume-rendered images. (**A**) illustrates the coronary sinus (1) as it empties into the right atrium (2). The first tributary of the coronary sinus is the posterior interventricular vein (3) followed by the posterior vein to the left ventricle (4). (**B**) show the great cardiac vein (5) as it gives rise to the lateral marginal vein (6) (**C**) and eventually ends in the anterior interventricular vein (7).

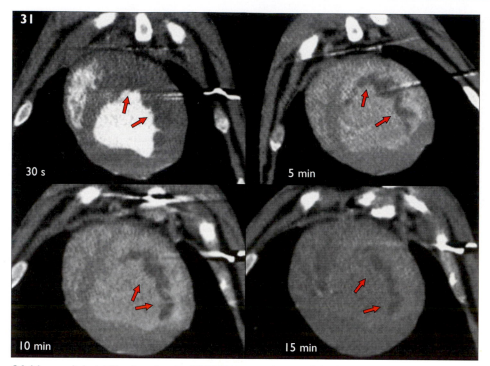

31 Myocardial viability imaging by MDCT in a canine model of acute anterior myocardial infarction. Thirty seconds after contrast injection a hypoenhanced subendocardial perfusion deficit is noted (arrows). Delayed MDCT imaging at 5, 10, and 15 minutes clearly shows a hyperenhanced region in the anterior, anteroseptal, and anterolateral myocardial walls (arrows). The subendocardial area that remains hypoenhanced during delayed imaging represents microvascular obstruction.

early enhancement significantly underestimated infarct size. Figure **31** illustrates both early and late perfusion defects.

Myocardial perfusion imaging

Previously, investigators showed that contrast-enhanced EBT could accurately measure myocardial blood flow. Using serial imaging of a portion of the left ventricle, myocardial blood flow can be accurately quantified by applying various adaptations of indicator-dilution theory (Rumberger *et al.* 1987a,b, Wolfkiel *et al.* 1987, Ludman *et al.* 1993, Bell *et al.* 1999). Likewise, the current generation of MDCT scanning systems can be programmed to image in dynamic mode and track the kinetics of iodinated contrast in real time in the myocardium and left ventricular blood pool. Using dynamic MDCT time–attenuation curves, robust metrics of myocardial blood flow can be derived using upslope and model-based deconvolution methods with excellent correlations with the gold

standard for myocardial blood flow, microspheres (r = 0.93–0.96) (George *et al.* 2007). While serial imaging of the left ventricle over time using dynamic MDCT is technically feasible, its use in patients is limited by incomplete cardiac coverage in the z-axis and a relatively high radiation dose. Future generations of MDCT scanners with larger detector rays will overcome these limitations over the next few years.

Using the current generation of MDCT scanners, recent studies (George *et al.* 2005, 2006b) from the authors' institution have shown in a canine model of LAD stenosis that MDCT angiography, performed during adenosine infusion with the scanner programmed in helical mode, can detect differences in myocardial perfusion (**32, 33**). Furthermore, CT attenuation densities, when measured in the myocardium and normalized to the left ventricle blood pool, have a semi-quantitative relationship with myocardial blood flow. There are limitations to adenosine stress MDCT myocardial perfusion imaging

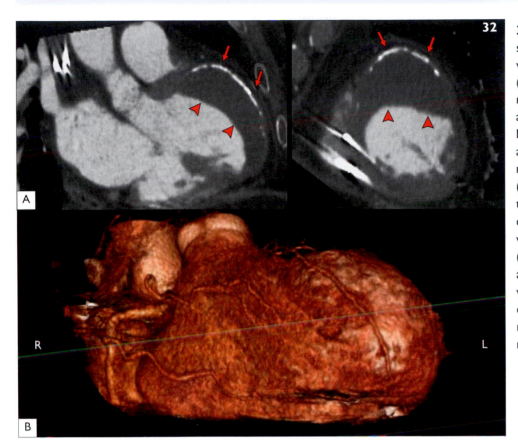

32 Chronic myocardial scar with left ventricular thrombus. (**A**) The left ventricle reconstructed in short- and long-axis views. Note the thin, calcified, aneurismal anterior myocardial scar (arrows). A large thrombus is noted covering the anterior wall from base to apex (arrowheads). (**B**) The aneurismal anterior wall in a three-dimensional volume-rendered reconstruction.

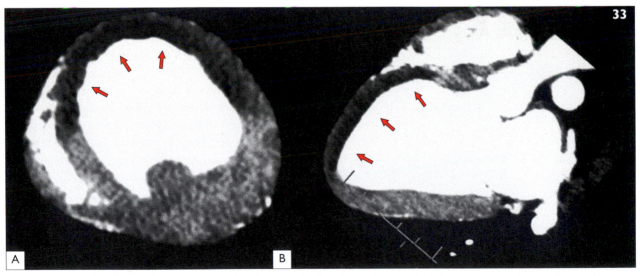

33 Mid-ventricular slice in the axial plane showing a perfusion deficit (arrows) in the anteroseptal, anterior, and anterolateral myocardial territory supplied by the stenosed LAD (**A**). Multiplanar reconstruction showing the extent of the perfusion deficit (arrows) extending from the anteroseptal and anterior walls to the apex (**B**). (Reprinted with permission from George RT, Silva C, Cordeiro MA *et al.* Multidetector computed tomography myocardial perfusion imaging during adenosine stress. *Journal of the American College of Cardiology* 2006 Jul 4;**48**(1):153–160.)

such as adenosine-mediated tachycardia and the current inability to perform rest and stress imaging secondary to the radiation dose. However, further advances in MDCT technology that reduce the radiation dose may overcome these obstacles. Preliminary studies at the authors' institution are demonstrating the accuracy of MDCT myocardial perfusion imaging in patients presenting with chest pain (George *et al.* 2006a) (**34**).

Incidental findings

MDCT imaging of the chest for the evaluation of cardiac disease images not only the heart, but also the surrounding structures. While MDCT coronary angiography does not image the entire chest, the majority of the chest in the z-axis coverage of the examination is included. It is estimated that noncardiac findings are present on 25–61% of MDCT coronary angiography examinations. Furthermore, 5–10% of these findings can be considered of major importance (Haller 2006, Patel 2005, Steinberg 2005). Major findings may include aortic dissection, pulmonary emboli, and malignant tumors in lung, mediastinum, or upper abdominal organs. Intermediate findings include adenopathy, sub-centimeter lung nodules, and solid organ masses. We recommend that nonradiologists consult their radiology colleagues to ensure that each cardiac MDCT examination is evaluated for noncardiac findings. Obviously, immediate attention needs to be made regarding the finding of aortic dissection or pulmonary emboli; however, some findings such as pulmonary nodules, require follow-up CT imaging and/or biopsy (MacMahon 2005).

CONCLUSIONS

Advances in technology have greatly improved the capabilities of X-ray CT, now making MDCT noninvasive angiography and atherosclerotic plaque imaging a reality. These same advances have positioned MDCT to go beyond coronary arterial imaging to a comprehensive evaluation of cardiac disease including function, viability, and perfusion. The current and future generation of MDCT systems have the potential to revolutionize the practice of cardiology and the care of cardiac patients.

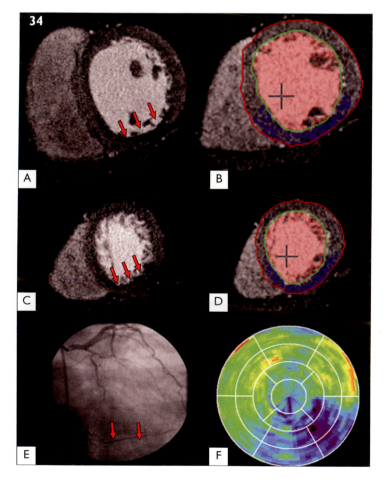

34 First-pass, adenosine-augmented MDCT myocardial perfusion imaging in a patient referred for invasive angiography after SPECT showed a fixed perfusion deficit in the inferior and inferolateral territories. (**A**), (**C**) An inferior and inferolateral subendocardial perfusion deficit in the mid and distal left ventricle, respectively (arrows). Using semi-automated function/perfusion software, myocardium meeting the perfusion deficit signal density threshold of one standard deviation below the remote myocardial signal density is designated in blue in (**B**) and (**D**). Invasive angiography shows a chronically occluded distal RCA with left to right collaterals filling the posterior descending (arrows) and posterolateral branches (**E**). (**F**) 17-segment polar plot of MDCT-derived myocardial signal densities. Note the hypoperfused inferior and inferolateral regions displayed in blue. (Reprinted with permission from George RT, Silva C, Cordeiro MA *et al.* Multidetector computed tomography myocardial perfusion imaging during adenosine stress. *Journal of the American College of Cardiology* 2006 Jul 4;**48**(1):153–160.)

CLINICAL CASES

Case 1: Ulcerated Atherosclerotic Plaque

Clinical history

The patient was a 44-year-old male with a history of heavy cigarette smoking and a complaint of exertional chest pain for several months; he presented to an outside hospital with the sudden onset of substernal chest pain at rest. ECG showed ST segment elevation in the precordial leads. He was treated acutely with tissue plasminogen activator (tPA) and transferred to a tertiary care center. He remained chest pain free following thrombolysis and was referred for a CT angiogram.

Imaging protocol

The patient underwent a noninvasive coronary angiography with the following protocol. Iodinated contrast: iodixanol 120 mL (320 mg iodine/mL); detector collimation: 32 × 0.5 mm; tube voltage: 120 mV; tube current: 400 mA; gantry rotation time: 400 ms; scanning field of view: 320 mm. Using retrospective ECG gating and segmental reconstruction, images were reconstructed every 0.5 mm with a 40% overlap and from 0–90% of the R-R interval at 10% increments and examined for the phase with the least cardiac motion.

Impression

There was a significant obstructive lesion noted in the proximal LAD (arrow). Area within the plaque with a high attenuation density may represent calcification or contrast material entering an ulcerated atherosclerotic plaque (**35**).

Discussion

Although this patient remained chest pain free following thrombolysis, his history of exertional chest pain for several months suggested that he may have obstructive coronary disease. On CT angiography, he was noted to have a tight lesion in the proximal LAD. The mixed appearance of the atherosclerotic plaque suggested either a mixed 'soft' and 'hard' plaque or may suggest plaque ulceration with iodinated contrast entering the fissured plaque.

Management

Based on the patient's clinical history and findings on CT angiogram, the patient was referred for invasive angiography. The invasive angiogram confirmed a 99% stenosis in the proximal LAD. There was no significant obstructive disease in the LCX and RCA. He was treated with angioplasty and a drug-eluting stent. On discharge, in addition to a recommendation to stop smoking cigarettes, he was prescribed the following medical regimen: aspirin and clopidogrel, a beta-blocker, a statin, and an angiotensin converting enzyme inhibitor.

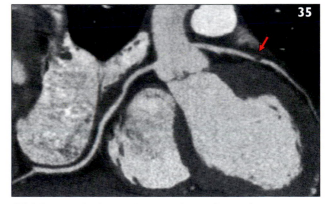

35 Ulcerated atherosclerotic plaque (arrow).

Case 2: Anomalous Origin of the RCA

Clinical history
The patient was a 19-year-old male with a history of tobacco use who had a witnessed cardiac arrest while playing basketball. Bystanders immediately initiated cardiopulmonary resuscitation and defibrillation. He was transported to the hospital and underwent cardiac catheterization to evaluate for obstructive coronary disease or anomalous coronary arteries. Invasive angiography showed an anomalous origin of the RCA (arrow, **36B, C**) from the left coronary cusp (**36A**). However, the course of the RCA could not be adequately determined and the patient was referred for CT angiography to define further the anatomical detail of the coronaries.

Imaging protocol
The patient underwent a noninvasive coronary angiography with the following protocol: iodinated contrast: iodixanol 120 mL (320 mg iodine/mL); detector collimation: 32 × 0.5 mm; tube voltage: 120 mV; tube current: 400 mA; gantry rotation time: 400 ms; scanning field of view: 320 mm. Using retrospective ECG gating and segmental reconstruction, images were reconstructed every 0.5 mm with a 40% overlap and from 0–90% of the R-R interval at 10% increments and examined for the phase with the least cardiac motion.

Impression
The anomalous origin of the RCA (arrow, **36B, C**) from the left coronary cusp was noted to be superior to the origin of the LAD (arrowhead, **36B**). Furthermore, the RCA was noted to be abnormal at its origin with a slit-like ostium and it coursed between the aorta and the pulmonary artery (**36C**).

Discussion
The anomalous origin of the RCA in this patient had two high-risk features that were associated with exercise-induced sudden cardiac death including abnormalities of the initial coronary artery segment and coursing of the artery between the pulmonary artery and aorta (Taylor 1992). Invasive angiography is often inadequate to delineate the course of anomalous coronary arteries and either CT or magnetic resonance angiography are indicated.

Management
Based on the patient's history of aborted sudden cardiac death and a malignant form of anomalous coronary arteries, this patient underwent a single vessel bypass using the right internal mammary artery to bypass the RCA.

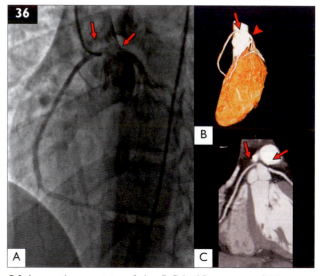

36 Anomalous origin of the RCA. (Courtesy of Marco A.S. Cordeiro, M.D, Ph.D., University of Sao Paulo, Brazil and Johns Hopkins University, Baltimore, MD.)

Case 3: Normal Right Upper Pulmonary Vein and Right Lower Pulmonary Vein

Clinical history

The patient was a 50-year-old male with a 15-year history of paroxysmal atrial fibrillation. Despite trials of several antiarrhythmia medications, the patient was still having frequent episodes of atrial fibrillation associated with shortness of breath. He was referred for an atrial fibrillation ablation procedure. In pre-procedure, he underwent CT angiography to define his pulmonary vein anatomy and construct an electoanatomic map of the left atrium.

Imaging protocol

The patient underwent cardiac CT with the following protocol: iodinated contrast: iodixanol 120 mL (320 mg iodine/mL); detector collimation: 64×0.5 mm; tube voltage: 120 mV; tube current: 400 mA; gantry rotation time: 400 ms; scanning field of view: 320 mm. Using retrospective ECG gating and segmental reconstruction, images were reconstructed every 0.5 mm with a 40% overlap and from 0–90% of the R-R interval at 10% increments and examined for the phase with the least cardiac motion.

Impression

The right upper pulmonary vein (1) and right lower pulmonary vein (2) (**37**) were both noted to be normal in size and origin as shown in the axial view (**37A**) and the three-dimensional volume-rendered view (**37B**). On the left of **37**, there was a single left common pulmonary vein (3) noted.

Discussion

A common left pulmonary trunk is not a rare finding and knowledge of this variant prior to ablation can assist in the positioning of ablation catheters during a pulmonary vein isolation procedure. Avoidance of ablation within the ostium of the pulmonary vein decreases the incidence of pulmonary vein stenosis.

Management

The patient underwent a successful atrial fibrillation ablation with adequate electrical isolation of the pulmonary veins from the rest of the left atrium without complications.

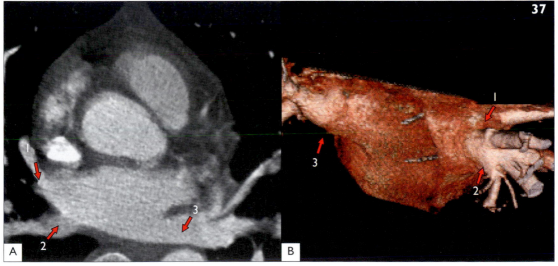

37 Pulmonary veins. Panel A demonstrates the pulmonary vein in the axial view with the right upper (1), right lower (2), and left common (3) pulmonary veins. Panel B demonstrates these same veins in a 3D volume rendered view.

Case 4: Focal Calcification and Thickening of the Pericardium

Clinical history

The patient was a 56-year-old male with a history of CAD, permanent pacemaker, and a mechanical mitral valve replacement; he presented with a complaint of worsening dyspnea on exertion, lower extremity edema, and increasing abdominal girth for approximately 3 years. He had been hospitalized several times with symptoms of congestive heart failure that responded well to diuresis. Transthoracic ECG showed normal left ventricular systolic function and normal mitral valve gradients, but a dilated inferior vena cava suggested an elevated right atrial pressure. Physical examination was notable for an elevated jugular venous pressure and a Kussmaul's sign. In addition to a referral for a right heart catheterization, the patient underwent a noncontrast CT to evaluate for pericardial calcification.

Imaging protocol

The patient underwent a noncontrast MDCT examination with prospective ECG gating using the following protocol: detector collimation: 4 × 3.0 mm; tube voltage: 135 mV; tube current: 150 mA; gantry rotation time: 400 ms; scanning field of view 320 mm. Images were reconstructed every 3.0 mm and examined for the presence of pericardial calcifications.

Impression

There was focal calcification (arrows, **38**) and thickening of the pericardium adjacent to the right atrium and right ventricle. The calcification extended from the insertion of the pericardium at the level of the great vessels to the diaphragm on the right side of the heart.

Discussion

The presence of pericardial thickening and/or calcification noted on CT is extremely valuable in the diagnosis of pericardial constriction. While the absence of calcification does not rule out pericardial constriction, its presence is highly supportive.

Management

Based on this patient's clinical history and the findings of pericardial thickening and calcification, he was referred for right heart catheterization. The study showed Kussmaul's sign and a prominent y-descent on the right atrial tracings, equalization of pressures in all four cardiac chambers, and discordance of the right ventricular and left ventricular systolic pressures during inspiration. These imaging and hemodynamic findings are highly suggestive of constrictive pericarditis. The patient was managed medically with diuretics. However, if he fails to respond with medical management, pericardiectomy may be indicated.

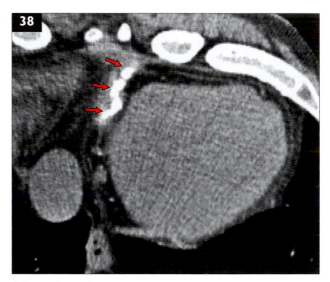

38 Focal calcification and thickening of the pericardium.

Case 5: Patent Stent in the Proximal LAD

Clinical history

The patient was a 61-year-old male, with a history of CAD and a previously placed stent in the proximal LAD, who presented with a complaint of chest pain. Previously, since his angioplasty and following a similar episode of chest pain, he was sent for exercise stress testing with radionuclide imaging that showed an anterior wall reversible perfusion defect. A follow-up catheterization showed no significant obstructive CAD and a patent LAD stent. With the history of a previously abnormal stress test, but normal invasive angiography, he was alternatively referred for MDCT coronary angiography to evaluate for stent patency during this episode.

Imaging protocol

The patient underwent a noninvasive coronary angiography with the following protocol: iodinated contrast: iopamidol 95 mL (370 mg iodine/mL); detector collimation: 64 × 0.5 mm; tube voltage: 120 mV; tube current: 420 mA; gantry rotation time: 400 ms; scanning field of view 320 mm. Using retrospective ECG gating, segmental reconstruction, and a sharp reconstruction kernel, images were reconstructed every 0.5 mm with a 40% overlap and from 0–90% of the R-R interval at 10% increments and examined for the phase with the least cardiac motion.

Impression

There was a patent stent in the proximal LAD with good opacification of the distal vessel (**39**). No in-stent restenosis was noted on this examination. Additionally, left ventricular systolic function was normal and there was only mild nonobstructive coronary disease in the LCX and RCA.

Discussion

CT angiography in the setting of a previously placed stent can be difficult secondary to blooming artifact caused by the stent's metal struts. The image of this stent without artifact and with good confidence is considered to be patent and without in-stent restenosis.

Management

This patient was instructed to continue his current diet and exercise regimen and his medical regimen that included aspirin, beta-blocker, and a statin.

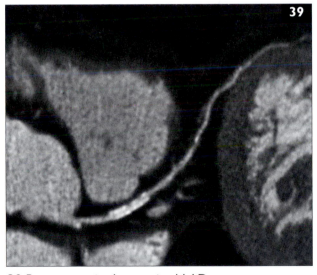

39 Patent stent in the proximal LAD.

3. Nuclear Cardiac Imaging

Raymond R. Russell, III   James A. Arrighi   Yi-Hwa Liu

INTRODUCTION

Nuclear cardiac imaging studies, particularly myocardial perfusion imaging, are a key component of cardiac testing throughout the US and the rest of the world. With advances in imaging technology and the development of new imaging radiopharmaceutical agents, including molecular imaging agents, the clinical importance of nuclear cardiac imaging will be maintained and new indications of the technique will emerge. It is therefore important to understand what the current state of the art of nuclear cardiac imaging is and what its appropriate applications to noninvasive assessment of cardiovascular disease states are.

Nuclear cardiac imaging currently focuses on three clinically important physiological concepts, namely myocardial perfusion, myocardial viability, and ventricular function. In this chapter, we will review the current state of the art in nuclear cardiology, which includes SPECT and PET for evaluation of myocardial perfusion and myocardial viability, planar techniques as well as gated myocardial perfusion SPECT, and gated blood pool SPECT for evaluation of left ventricular function. In addition to descriptions of the methods used to assess each of these factors, the diagnostic and prognostic importance of these factors will be discussed. Following this description of the techniques used in nuclear cardiac imaging, clinical case studies are presented that illustrate the various nuclear cardiac imaging modalities as well as important clinical findings.

MYOCARDIAL PERFUSION IMAGING
An overview of myocardial perfusion imaging

The detection of CAD by myocardial perfusion imaging using radioactive tracers of blood flow has become an essential diagnostic tool. Several modalities are available to assess myocardial perfusion including planar imaging, SPECT, and PET. Of these methods, the most common method is SPECT imaging. Because of the higher sensitivity of SPECT over planar imaging (Fintel *et al.* 1989, Kiat *et al.* 1989, Benoit *et al.* 1996, Cramer *et al.* 1997), planar imaging is generally limited to use in patients that cannot be placed in a SPECT or PET camera (e.g. extremely obese individuals, claustrophobic individuals) and thus this modality will not be discussed further in this chapter.

Routine SPECT and PET myocardial perfusion imaging relies on the identification of flow heterogeneity based on differential uptake of the radioactive flow tracer in the myocardium. Specifically, the flow tracers are taken up by the myocardium relative to regional blood flow, resulting in a lower number of radioactive counts in regions of the heart supplied by a coronary artery with a flow-limiting stenosis compared to a normal coronary artery (**40**). This uptake of the flow tracer is determined, in large part, by the first-pass extraction of the tracer. Because none of the tracers that are approved for clinical use have complete first-pass extraction, especially as the blood flow increases, small differences in blood flow

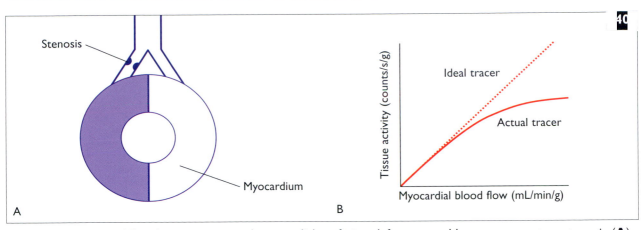

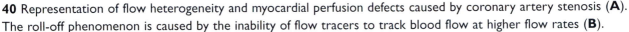

40 Representation of flow heterogeneity and myocardial perfusion defects caused by coronary artery stenosis (**A**). The roll-off phenomenon is caused by the inability of flow tracers to track blood flow at higher flow rates (**B**).

between two areas of myocardium cannot be appreciated using nuclear imaging techniques (**40**). Despite this limitation, known as the 'roll-off' phenomenon, myocardial perfusion imaging with both SPECT and PET agents provides powerful diagnostic and prognostic information, as will be discussed later in the chapter.

Myocardial perfusion imaging can be performed with either single-photon-emitting radiotracers or positron-emitting radiotracers. As their name implies, single-photon-emitting radiotracers release one gamma photon in their decay. It is this gamma photon that passes out of the body and interacts with the scintillation crystal in the gamma camera to produce light that is detected by a photomultiplier tube (PMT), which increases the signal that is ultimately displayed in the image. These images can either be acquired as simple planar images, usually in the anterior, left anterior oblique, and lateral views, or multiple planar images that can be acquired and reconstructed into a three-dimensional SPECT data set (**41**).

In contrast to single-photon emitting radiotracers, positron-emitting radiotracers decay by the release of a positron, a positively charged particle with the same mass as an electron. The positron travels a variable distance based on the energy of the parent isotope before it interacts with an electron in the environment, resulting in an annihilation event, in which two 511-keV photons are produced that travel 180° from each other. It is these two gamma photons that are detected by the PET camera and represent the fundamental difference between PET and SPECT. Specifically, since

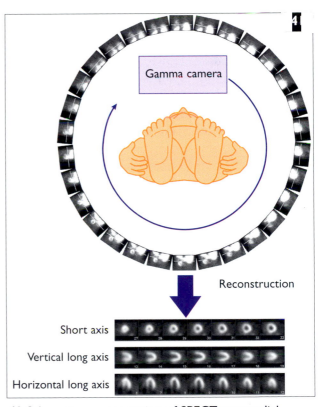

41 Schematic representation of SPECT myocardial perfusion imaging in which multiple planar images are used to construct a three-dimensional data set that can be used to generate tomographic images.

the two gamma photons are released in opposite directions, a true annihilation event should be detected by the PET camera as two signals reach the bank of scintillation crystal/photomultiplier tube detectors at almost the same exact time (**42**). A specialized coincidence detection circuit is used to time the signals coming from the detectors to determine which events are 'true' from those that represent noise. In this way, PET cameras have greater resolution and decreased scatter than clinical SPECT cameras that are used for cardiac studies. However, these benefits come at a cost; specifically, attenuation, which is one of the greatest challenges in nuclear cardiology. It is caused by interactions of the gamma photons with tissue between the point of origin for the gamma photon and the gamma camera, and is twice as severe a problem in PET cameras than in SPECT cameras because there are two gamma photons that must reach the coincidence detectors. As a result, attenuation correction, which is discussed in detail later in the chapter, must be performed to generate acceptable PET images.

Myocardial perfusion radiotracers

There are currently six radiotracers used in the US for perfusion imaging: thallium-201 (^{201}Tl) thallous chloride, technetium-99m (^{99m}Tc) sestamibi, ^{99m}Tc tetrofosmin, rubidium-82 (^{82}Rb) chloride, nitrogen-13 (^{13}N) ammonia, and oxygen-15 (^{15}O) water. Thallium and the technetium-based agents are single-photon-emitting radiotracers and are therefore used with planar gamma cameras and SPECT cameras. The latter three are positron-emitting radiotracers and require PET cameras for imaging and special equipment for tracer production. Importantly, because of their short half-lives, synthesis of ^{13}N ammonia and ^{15}O water require an onsite cyclotron. As a result, there is an increasing interest in the use of ^{82}Rb chloride because it is produced from strontium-82 by a portable generator, improving the accessibility to the tracer. Of note, all of the above radiotracers, except ^{15}O water, are approved by the US Food and Drug Administration (FDA).

Thallium

^{201}Tl was the first radiotracer widely utilized to assess both regional blood flow and myocardial viability. Its primary emission is relatively low in energy, at 79 keV. Its half-life is 73 hr, which is long for a perfusion tracer (*Table 4*).

Myocardial uptake early after intravenous injection of ^{201}Tl is proportional to regional blood flow, and ^{201}Tl has a high first-pass extraction fraction (approximately 85%), minimizing the roll-off of the tracer. Uptake of ^{201}Tl is similar to that of potassium, which is transported across the myocyte sarcolemmal membrane via Na^+/K^+ adenosine triphosphatase (ATPase). After the initial uptake phase, there is a continuous exchange of ^{201}Tl between the myocardium and the extracardiac compartments, driven by the concentration gradient of the tracer between the blood and myocardial compartments. During this phase, termed the 'redistribution' phase, the distribution of

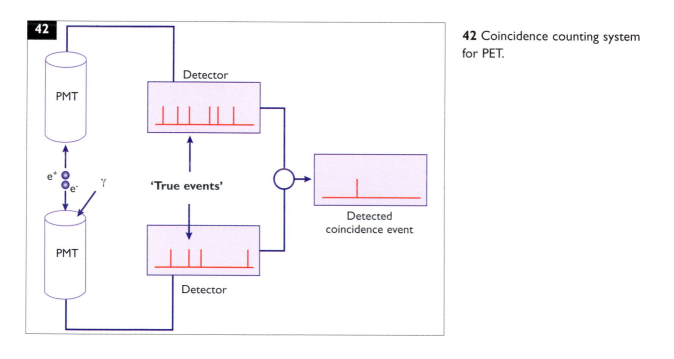

42 Coincidence counting system for PET.

Table 4 Commonly used radiotracers for evaluating myocardial perfusion

Radiotracer	Modality	Energy peak	Half-life
^{201}-thallium chloride	SPECT	79 keV	73 hr
^{99m}Tc-sestamibi	SPECT	140 keV	6 hr
^{99m}Tc-tetrofosmin	SPECT	140 keV	6 hr
^{82}-rubidium	PET	511 keV	76 s
^{13}N-ammonia	PET	511 keV	10 min
^{15}O-water	PET	511 keV	5 min

thallium is proportional to the myocardial potassium concentration and regional blood volume. Defects that are initially seen on the early images may slowly reverse or 'fill in', indicating ischemia and preserved myocardial viability (Pohost *et al.* 1977). In contrast, scarred myocardium does not take up more ^{201}Tl, and initial defects persist over time, resulting in an irreversible (fixed) perfusion defect.

^{99m}Tc-based SPECT radiotracers: sestamibi and tetrofosmin

The technetium-labeled myocardial perfusion agents have a shorter half-life (6 hr) and emit higher-energy (140 keV) photons than ^{201}Tl, thereby improving the image quality while maintaining a relatively low radiation burden to the patient as compared to thallium. The two technetium-based agents in use in the US are ^{99m}Tc-labeled sestamibi and ^{99m}Tc-labeled tetrofosmin. Both agents are initially distributed in the myocardium in proportion to myocardial blood flow. The extraction fraction of both agents is less than that of ^{201}Tl, and sestamibi has a slightly higher extraction fraction as compared to tetrofosmin. However, the clearance of ^{99m}Tc-tetrofosmin from the lungs and liver is faster than ^{99m}Tc-sestamibi, which may improve the quality of early cardiac images. Apart from the imaging characteristics, the most significant difference between technetium-based perfusion tracers and thallium is that technetium tracers display very little redistribution within the first few hours after injection. Thus, the timing of image acquisition relative to isotope injection is more flexible than that with thallium.

PET radiotracers: ^{82}Rb and ^{13}N ammonia

Of the three common PET radiotracers used for the evaluation of myocardial perfusion as mentioned earlier, only ^{82}Rb and ^{13}N ammonia are US FDA approved for diagnostic myocardial perfusion studies.

Like ^{201}Tl, ^{82}Rb is an analog of potassium and is therefore transported into cardiac myocytes by the Na$^+$/K$^+$ ATPase present in the cell surface membrane. However, unlike ^{201}Tl, the half-life of ^{82}Rb is sufficiently short that the radiotracer does not redistribute. The myocardial first pass extraction of ^{82}Rb (65%) is lower than that of ^{201}Tl and is therefore subject to a greater amount of roll-off phenomenon. ^{13}N ammonia has a greater first-pass extraction (80%) and, unlike ^{82}Rb, is metabolically trapped in the cell by incorporation into glutamine by glutamine synthetase. While both PET myocardial perfusion tracers offer the benefit of high spatial resolution with little scatter due to the high energy of the positron-emitting radionuclides and the coincidence detection used for PET, the production of ^{82}Rb by a portable generator has led to more widespread use of this particular PET tracer for myocardial perfusion imaging.

Technical considerations for myocardial perfusion radiotracers

The type of perfusion imaging agents used has important implications with respect to which imaging protocol is appropriate for image acquisition and what the limitations are for the radiotracer. To understand the limitations of the various myocardial perfusion imaging agents, it is important to understand what the characteristics are of a radiotracer that would make it ideal for perfusion imaging. First, an imaging agent needs to track myocardial blood flow accurately over the wide range of values from resting perfusion to maximum vasodilation associated with exercise or pharmacologic vasodilatory agents. As discussed earlier, this ability is determined by the first-pass extraction of the agent. Second, attenuation of the gamma photons from the imaging agent should be minimal. Because the degree of attenuation is related to the energy spectrum of the tracer, higher-energy tracers are less likely to be affected by attenuation. Furthermore, the energy of the tracer must be taken into account when one considers the radiation exposure to the patient. However, as described earlier, PET tracers are a unique exception because the two high-energy 511 keV gamma photons released by the annihilation event must both be detected for an event to be considered a true event and, therefore, the problem of attenuation becomes 'twofold'. Third, the radiotracer should be trapped in the heart following its initial uptake so that 'redistribution' of the tracer does not occur. This allows for greater flexibility in the imaging of the patient after stress testing. Fourth, tracer metabolism should not increase uptake in organs in close proximity to the heart out of proportion to blood flow. An example of this is the uptake of the technetium-based radiotracers, ^{99m}Tc-sestamibi and ^{99m}Tc-tetrofosmin, by the liver, which can decrease the quality of the cardiac image primarily through Compton scatter of gamma photons from the liver. Fifth, the half-life of the tracer should be short enough to allow for rapid serial imaging. Counterbalancing this is the fact that the half-life of the tracer should not be so short that image acquisition is difficult to perform in that a sufficient number of counts cannot be acquired to generate acceptable images.

Image acquisition and processing

The most commonly used SPECT and PET imaging protocols are summarized in **43**. Recommended image acquisition protocols for SPECT studies are outlined in the imaging guidelines published by the ASNC (DePuey and Garcia 2001). For technetium studies, 64 projections over a 180° orbit (from 45° right anterior oblique to 45° left posterior oblique) are acquired. It is also possible to perform 360° acquisitions, which may improve image quality, but also increase acquisition time. The time per projection is 20–30 s. In order to optimize thallium studies, it is generally necessary to image longer per stop (30–40 s); the number of projections may also be decreased from 64 to 32. Adjustments to filtering, i.e. lowering the cutoff frequency for more smoothing of thallium images, are also suggested.

After images are acquired, the raw data consisting of images from all of the projections are converted into tomographic images. This processing involves filtering, image reconstruction, and reorientation of tomographic slices. The image filtering reduces the random photon noise in the image, making it more uniform or 'smooth'. The image reconstruction refers to the process by which a three-dimensional tomographic image is constructed from the multiple projections of two-dimensional images. Two methods of reconstruction are in use: filtered backprojection and iterative reconstruction. In filtered backprojection, two-dimensional raw images are 'projected' back into a three-dimensional image matrix based on geometric models, so as to reconstruct a three-dimensional representation of the objects imaged. Iterative reconstruction algorithms are derived based on the statistical and Poisson noise models to reconstruct the tomographic nuclear image from the acquired projection data. Finally, the tomographic images are reoriented so that the heart is displayed in a standardized format, corresponding to short axis, vertical long axis, and horizontal long axis images (**44**).

The tomographic images are subsequently segmented in the short axis into apical, mid-ventricular, and basal slices. Each of these slices is further segmented into sectors of the left ventricle, with the apical slice divided into four sectors and the mid-ventricular and basal slices each divided into six sectors (**44**). The vertical long-axis slice that contains the apex is also divided into an anterior segment, apical segment, and inferior segment. The 16 short-axis sectors as well as the apical segment from the vertical long axis can be combined to create a 17-segment model of the left ventricle that is commonly used for the circumferential count profiles and polar ('bull's eye') displays of myocardial perfusion (Cerqueira *et al.* 2002). Because each of these segments represents a specific region of the left ventricle, they are also associated with specific vascular territories and it is therefore possible to predict which coronary vessel is responsible for a perfusion defect.

The acquisition of myocardial perfusion images is dependent on multiple factors including characteristics of the patient, the type of stressor used to increase myocardial blood flow, the radiotracer that is used, and the characteristics of the gamma camera that is used to acquire the images. With respect to the first factor, the patient's body habitus can have profound effects on image quality. Specifically, soft tissue attenuation from adipose tissue in obese patients, or breast tissue in women, can result in poor image quality or even create artifacts that can be confused with true perfusion defects. In addition, attenuation of the inferior wall of

43 Commonly used protocols for SPECT and PET myocardial perfusion imaging. Note that for obese patients, SPECT requires 2 days to complete the study while a ^{82}Rb PET study can be completed in 1 hr. EX: exercise.

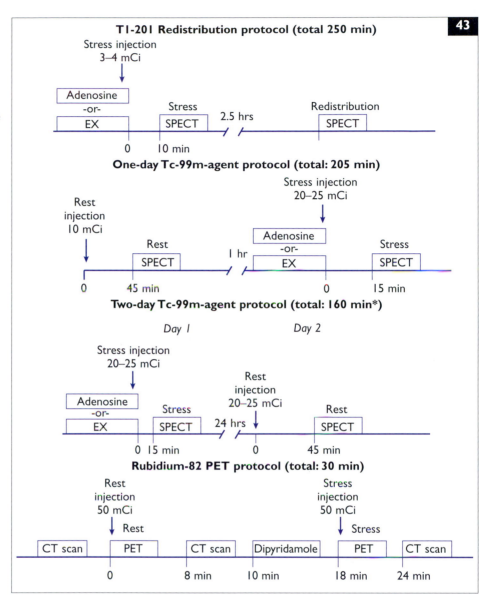

43

Tl-201 Redistribution protocol (total 250 min)

Stress injection
3–4 mCi

Adenosine
-or-
EX | Stress SPECT | 2.5 hrs | Redistribution SPECT

0   10 min

One-day Tc-99m-agent protocol (total: 205 min)

Stress injection
20–25 mCi

Rest
injection
10 mCi

Rest SPECT | 1 hr | Adenosine -or- EX | Stress SPECT

0   45 min   0   15 min

Two-day Tc-99m-agent protocol (total: 160 min*)

Day 1   *Day 2*

Stress injection
20–25 mCi

Rest
injection
20–25 mCi

Adenosine
-or-
EX | Stress SPECT | 24 hrs | Rest SPECT

0 15 min   0   45 min

Rubidium-82 PET protocol (total: 30 min)

Rest
injection
50 mCi

Stress
injection
50 mCi

CT scan | Rest PET | CT scan | Dipyridamole | Stress PET | CT scan

0   8 min   10 min   18 min   24 min

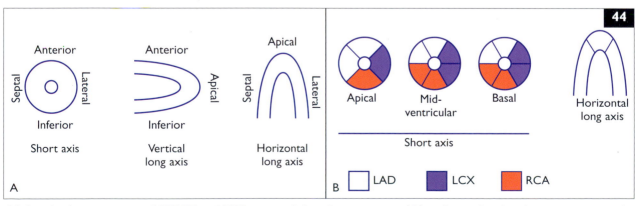

44

Anterior

Septal — Lateral

Inferior

Short axis

Anterior

Inferior

Apical

Vertical
long axis

Apical

Septal — Lateral

Horizontal
long axis

Apical   Mid-ventricular   Basal

Short axis

Horizontal
long axis

A

B   LAD   LCX   RCA

44 Standard orientations of SPECT and PET myocardial perfusion images (**A**) and vascular distributions associated with the 17-segment model (**B**).

the heart by the diaphragm can result in what appears to be inferior scarring. However, these artifacts can generally be minimized by attenuation correction or, in the case of diaphragmatic attenuation, by imaging the patient in the prone position so that the heart is not resting on the diaphragm resulting in greater recovery of radioactivity. The issue of attenuation correction will be discussed later in the chapter.

SPECT myocardial perfusion imaging: principles and techniques

Three of the major radiotracer protocols commonly used for stress/rest SPECT myocardial perfusion imaging are: technetium-only, thallium-only, and dual-isotope. The selection of protocols depends on a number of factors, including physician preference, patient weight, logistics of scheduling, and patient throughput. Single-isotope technetium protocols may be performed on a single day or over 2 days. Single-day protocols initially utilize a lower dose of technetium (7–10 mCi), followed by the first image acquisition. The second set of images is obtained several hours later after a higher dose (25–30 mCi) of the tracer is injected, and the higher counts overwhelm the residual counts from the previous lower dose. Two-day technetium protocols utilize the same dose (20–30 mCi) on 2 separate days. Either stress or resting images can be acquired first, although acquisition of stress images first brings up the possibility of not having to obtain resting images if the stress test and images are normal. This option can both decrease radiation exposure in the patient and increase throughput in the nuclear cardiac imaging laboratory.

Thallium protocols always involve stress first, after an initial injection of approximately 3 mCi of thallium. Early and delayed images then are acquired, sometimes with reinjection of 1 mCi of thallium prior to delayed images. An important aspect of thallium imaging is that the early image, which truly reflects stress perfusion, must be obtained very soon (5–10 minutes) after isotope injection, before significant redistribution of thallium occurs.

Dual-isotope protocols utilize thallium for initial resting perfusion images, followed by stress imaging with technetium-based tracers (Berman *et al.* 1993). The stress technetium images may be obtained while thallium remains in the body because the energy window, which determines which photons the camera records, can be set so that the camera records the higher-energy technetium and ignores the lower-energy thallium photons. These dual-isotope protocols have become popular because they can be performed in somewhat less time than single-isotope SPECT protocols. However, the dual-isotope protocols are associated with the greatest exposure to radiation in patients.

PET perfusion imaging: principles and techniques

The radiotracers commonly used for PET myocardial perfusion imaging are ^{82}Rb and ^{13}N ammonia; ^{15}O water is used in selected centers primarily for quantitative measurements of myocardial blood flow for research purposes (*Table 4*). The relatively short half-lives of the various PET radionuclides have practical implications for myocardial perfusion imaging. At present, stress PET perfusion imaging is limited to pharmacologic stress testing in which the 'stress' conditions can be maintained while the patient is lying down in preparation for rapid acquisition of images. Although some groups are studying the feasibility of exercise stress PET, at present there are no generally accepted protocols. The short half-lives of these tracers, however, allow for the injection of larger doses and for shorter intervals between rest and stress imaging when compared to SPECT imaging with lower radiation exposure from the radiotracer.

In particular, ^{82}Rb acquisitions are very short; rest and stress studies can be performed easily within an hour (**43**), which represents a significant advantage over SPECT. Finally, PET is routinely performed with attenuation correction, which results in more consistent image quality in comparison to SPECT.

Diagnostic accuracy of SPECT and PET

Myocardial perfusion imaging is an important adjunct to stress testing alone, adding incremental diagnostic and prognostic information to stress testing for detecting CAD (Lima *et al.* 2003). A number of studies have assessed the accuracy of SPECT imaging for the detection of CAD and in composite have demonstrated a sensitivity of 88%, a specificity of 70%, and a normalcy rate of 93% (Wackers 2005). Figure **45** summarizes the ranges of sensitivities and specificities that have been reported for the various stress protocols and radiotracers used in SPECT perfusion imaging and demonstrates the wide range of values reported for the different tests.

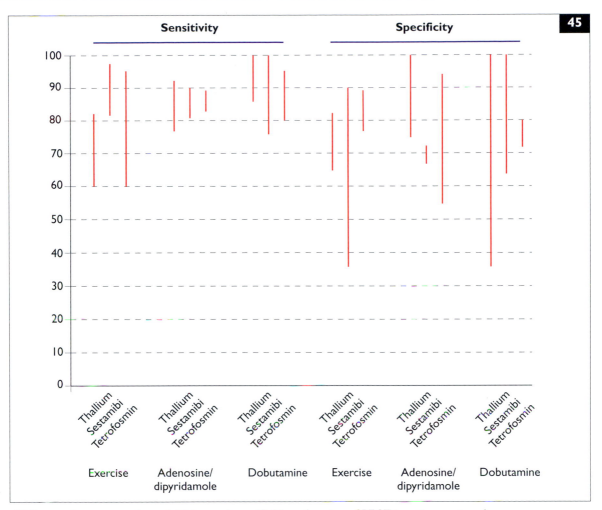

45 Ranges for reported sensitivities and specificities of various SPECT imaging protocols.

In one direct comparison of ^{201}Tl and ^{99m}Tc-sestamibi SPECT, there was a greater sensitivity for ^{99m}Tc-sestamibi compared to that for [201]Tl (93% *vs.* 80%), while the specificity was similar for the two agents (Kiat *et al.* 1989). However, in a study of 2,560 individuals undergoing SPECT perfusion imaging with ^{201}Tl, ^{99m}Tc-sestamibi or ^{99m}Tc-tetrofosmin, the sensitivities and specificities of the three agents were similar (Kapur *et al.* 2002).

The application of PET to the assessment of myocardial perfusion is gaining in popularity and use and may even provide greater accuracy in detecting CAD compared to SPECT (Bateman *et al.* 2006). Direct comparisons of [82]Rb PET and ^{201}Tl SPECT demonstrate that PET has a higher sensitivity (Go *et al.* 1990). A recent study has suggested that PET may be more accurate in the diagnosis of stenoses in specific coronary arteries, and in the detection of multivessel disease (Bateman *et al.* 2006).

Important prognostic information can be obtained from the level of exercise performed on a stress test as well as the hemodynamic response to exercise. However, not all patients can perform an exercise stress test and must undergo a pharmacologic stress test. The pharmacologic agents include those that cause vasodilation through adenosine receptor activation (adenosine and dipyridamole) and those that increase myocardial contractility through β-adrenergic receptor stimulation (dobutamine). As demonstrated in **45**, myocardial perfusion imaging following pharmacologic vasodilation with either dipyridamole or adenosine has similar sensitivities and specificities compared to exercise SPECT. In addition to patients who cannot exercise, myocardial perfusion imaging following vasodilation with adenosine or dipyridamole may prevent septal perfusion defects that can be exaggerated by exercise in patients with left bundle branch block (Burns *et al.* 1991, Vaduganathan *et al.* 1996). Dobutamine myocardial perfusion imaging has also been shown to have a high sensitivity and specificity (Hays *et al.* 1993, Marwick *et al.* 1993, Voth *et al.* 1994, Elhendy *et al.* 2000) as well as a good concordance with exercise SPECT imaging (Herman *et al.* 1994, Marwick *et al.* 1994). The usefulness of adenosine and dipyridamole are somewhat decreased because they are not selective for the A2a adenosine receptors present in the coronary vasculature and cause symptoms including chest pain and shortness of breath. The addition of low-level exercise to adenosine infusion can improve the symptoms associated with adenosine infusion and decrease gastrointestinal radiotracer activity that can complicate myocardial imaging (Mahmood *et al.* 1994, Cramer *et al.* 1996, Samady *et al.* 2002). In addition, new selective A2a receptor agonists have been developed that have fewer reports of symptoms compared to adenosine (Udelson *et al.* 2004, Hendel *et al.* 2005).

Although cardiac SPECT and PET imaging with exercise or pharmacologic stress has yielded a satisfactory accuracy for the diagnosis of CAD, the diagnostic accuracy can be further improved by SPECT and PET image quantification and attenuation correction as described below.

Quantification of SPECT and PET images

The visual assessment of SPECT or PET images is a subjective method of evaluation of myocardial perfusion. This type of visual analysis may result in suboptimal reproducibility of the results. However, the reproducibility can be enhanced with the support of SPECT or PET quantification (Masood *et al.* 2005). An important complement to the visual inspection of images is the quantitative evaluation of perfusion defects. Several quantitative programs are commercially available for perfusion image analysis, and the methods for quantitative image analysis have been found to be highly reproducible (Milcinski *et al.* 1991, Mahmarian *et al.* 1995, Germano *et al.* 2000), improving the detection of CAD (Tamaki *et al.* 1984, DePasquale *et al.* 1988, Mahmarian *et al.* 1990, Acampa *et al.* 1998).

The clinical utility of nuclear cardiology studies is partly due to the inherently quantifiable nature of nuclear imaging. In particular, quantification provides accurate and reproducible assessment of myocardial perfusion defect size and severity. Several quantification methods and computer software have been developed for SPECT and PET cardiac images (Garcia *et al.* 1990,

Berman *et al.* 1993, Alazraki *et al.* 1994, Liu *et al.* 1999, Kirac *et al.* 2000, Slomka *et al.* 2005). These quantification methods are designed primarily based on the concept of circumferential count profiles extracted from the emission tomographic images, although the data displays vary among the different software packages. A patient study processed with four widely used SPECT and PET quantification programs is shown in **46**. This comparison serves to illustrate the representative display of quantitative myocardial perfusion from the various programs; the most reasonable practice is to choose one program to use for quantification and to gain understanding of the strengths and weaknesses of that particular program.

Attenuation correction for SPECT and PET

Photon emissions from the radioactive decay (e.g. SPECT) or from the annihilation of the positrons (e.g. PET) in the myocardium are inevitably attenuated by the extracardiac tissue such as breast and diaphragm. Breast attenuation in cardiac emission tomography is quite common in women (Goodgold *et al.* 1987, Hansen *et al.* 1996), and may create false anterior perfusion defects, while diaphragmatic attenuation mostly occurs in men, and may cause false inferior defects. Obesity is another major cause of photon attenuation. The attenuation artifacts in part account for the suboptimal specificity of SPECT in the detection of myocardial perfusion abnormalities. These attenuation artifacts, however, can be alleviated by incorporating nonuniform attenuation correction into SPECT and PET image reconstruction.

The basic method of attenuation correction involves acquisition of transmission and emission images and an attenuation map is generated from the transmission images based on the production of an image from the ability of external radiation, generated either by an X-ray tube or a gamma-ray-emitting radioactive line source, to penetrate objects to varying degrees related to the physical composition of the objects. The generated attenuation map is subsequently applied to PET or SPECT reconstruction for attenuation correction. Because PET cameras rely on coincidence detection, nonuniform attenuation correction is required for PET imaging to compensate for the positron annihilation events that are not 'counted' by PET cameras because one of the two coincident 511 keV gamma photons is prevented from reaching the detectors by attenuating

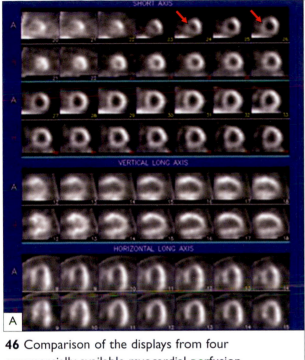

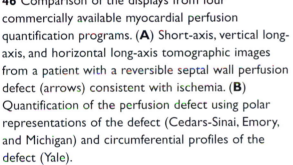

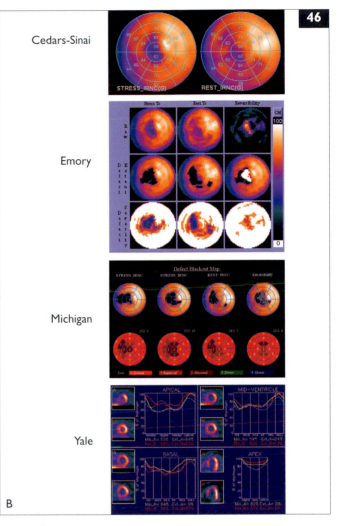

46 Comparison of the displays from four commercially available myocardial perfusion quantification programs. (**A**) Short-axis, vertical long-axis, and horizontal long-axis tomographic images from a patient with a reversible septal wall perfusion defect (arrows) consistent with ischemia. (**B**) Quantification of the perfusion defect using polar representations of the defect (Cedars-Sinai, Emory, and Michigan) and circumferential profiles of the defect (Yale).

tissue. As a result, all PET cameras are manufactured with some form of attenuation correction built into them. In contrast to PET, attenuation correction for SPECT is not used routinely in nuclear cardiac imaging, although it has drawn substantial attention recently in the nuclear cardiac imaging community and is increasingly being used (Narayanan *et al.* 2003, Masood *et al.* 2005).

The concepts of attenuation correction used in SPECT and PET are similar in that the attenuation map is generated from the transmission scans and is subsequently applied to SPECT or PET image reconstruction. However, unlike PET imaging, the transmission images for SPECT can be acquired either sequentially or simultaneously with the emission images using external point, line, or sheet transmission sources. The most widely used transmission sources for SPECT imaging are gadolinium (^{153}Gd) and americium (^{241}Am) because of their long half-lives. Although SPECT attenuation correction using the external transmission sources have been US FDA approved and used in nuclear cardiac imaging for more than a decade, transmission images acquired using the external sources are not of high quality and therefore the attenuation maps generated from these transmission images are not necessarily optimal.

Recently, hybrid SPECT/CT and PET/CT imaging systems have become available and popular for nuclear cardiac imaging. X-ray CT images obtained from these hybrid imaging systems not only provide the anatomical information about the organs imaged but also allow for a sophisticated nonuniform attenuation correction. Using X-ray CT transmission images for attenuation correction in SPECT or PET reconstruction may be preferred because superior image quality attenuation maps can be obtained from the CT images. It has been reported that cardiac

SPECT using CT-based attenuation correction may facilitate the clinical image reading and improve the diagnostic accuracy in the detection of myocardial perfusion abnormality (Hendel *et al.* 1999, Araujo *et al.* 2000, Kjaer *et al.* 2002, Links *et al.* 2002, Banzo *et al.* 2003, Narayanan *et al.* 2003, Grossman *et al.* 2004, Heller *et al.* 2004, Fricke *et al.* 2005, Masood *et al.* 2005, Utsunomiya *et al.* 2005).

While most SPECT/CT and PET/CT systems utilize a low-dose, nondiagnostic quality CT image for the attenuation map, the development of multislice CT systems offers the potential of developing hybrid cameras that combine the ability to perform SPECT or PET imaging and obtain CT scans that can be used not only for attenuation correction but also for coronary artery calcium scoring and CT angiography.

Prognostic value of SPECT perfusion imaging

One of the greatest strengths of myocardial perfusion imaging is its robust prognostic power. Multiple studies have evaluated the prognostic value of SPECT myocardial perfusion imaging in a wide variety of patient populations and in a number of clinical centers. A recent meta-analysis of 21 studies evaluating the prognostic value of SPECT included 53,762 individuals and supports the concept that myocardial perfusion SPECT imaging adds incremental prognostic value concerning cardiac mortality and myocardial infarction to the prognostic information provided by clinical variables, exercise testing variables, and angiographic findings (Mowatt *et al.* 2005). Several studies have demonstrated that normal myocardial perfusion imaging is associated with an excellent prognosis and an annual cardiac event rate of <1% (Machecourt *et al.* 1994, Marie *et al.* 1995, Geleijnse *et al.* 1996, Iskander & Iskandrian 1998, Hachamovitch *et al.* 2003, Shaw *et al.* 2003, Schinkel *et al.* 2005). In the presence of multiple cardiac risk factors, such as diabetes, hypertension, advanced age, and male gender, while the absolute risk may be higher than in healthy individuals, patients with normal SPECT perfusion studies have a more favorable prognosis than those with abnormal studies (Hachamovitch *et al.* 2003). At the other end of the spectrum, important prognostic information concerning both cardiac death and myocardial infarction is gained from the extent and severity of perfusion defects in patients either with no prior history of CAD or with a history of prior myocardial infarction (Machecourt *et al.* 1994, Alkeylani *et al.* 1998, Hachamovitch *et al.* 1998, 2005, Elhendy *et al.* 2004, Leslie *et al.* 2005).

The application to special populations has supported the diagnostic and prognostic power of myocardial perfusion imaging. Specifically, the use of imaging in diabetic patients is of growing importance because of the incidence of diabetes and the fact that cardiovascular disease is the leading cause of death in diabetic patients. Furthermore, diabetic patients with abnormal myocardial perfusion studies have poorer outcomes compared to nondiabetic patients with similar perfusion defects (Hachamovitch *et al.* 2005). Asymptomatic diabetic patients are of particular interest, since the prevalence of abnormal myocardial perfusion images is much higher than in nondiabetic individuals (Zarich *et al.* 1996, De Lorenzo *et al.* 2002, Wackers *et al.* 2004, Zellweger *et al.* 2004). Overall, the prevalence of silent ischemia in diabetic individuals is 20–60%.

Other specific groups may benefit from myocardial perfusion imaging based on their high rate of cardiac mortality, including patients with chronic kidney disease (Feola *et al.* 2002, Patel *et al.* 2003, Dussol *et al.* 2004, Hase *et al.* 2004), women (Friedman *et al.* 1982, Hachamovitch *et al.* 1996, Amanullah *et al.* 1997, Santana-Boado *et al.* 1998, Mieres *et al.* 2003), African-Americans (Akinboboye *et al.* 2001), Hispanics (Shaw *et al.* 2005), and Asians (Galasko *et al.* 2005). In addition, patients presenting with congestive heart failure can be evaluated with myocardial perfusion imaging to help determine if the heart failure is due to ischemic or nonischemic causes (Danias *et al.* 2004, Yao *et al.* 2004).

Additional prognostic information is provided by myocardial SPECT perfusion imaging based on the presence of high-risk features. Specifically, an elevated lung:heart ratio, which is correlated with an increased pulmonary artery capillary wedge pressure (Patel *et al.* 2004) is a sensitive marker of severe CAD (Bacher-Stier *et al.* 2000, Romanens *et al.* 2001, Daou *et al.* 2002). In addition, left ventricular transient ischemic dilation (TID), which is caused by a diffuse decrease in subendocardial tracer uptake, is due to the left ventricular cavity appearing larger on the stress perfusion images than on the resting images. TID is associated with a high burden of CAD and poor prognosis (Abidov *et al.* 2003, 2004).

Prognostic value of PET perfusion imaging

PET myocardial perfusion imaging offers several advantages in comparison to SPECT myocardial perfusion imaging. First, in obese patients, image quality tends to be better with PET because of the greater recovery of radioactive counts thanks to the high-energy 511-keV gamma photons produced by the PET tracers as well as the use of attenuation correction with PET cameras. Second, the protocols used for imaging patients tend to be shorter for PET myocardial perfusion imaging because of the short half-lives of ^{13}N (10 minutes), ^{15}O (5 minutes), and ^{82}Rb (1.3 minutes). Related to the issue of radiotracer half-life, the radiation exposure of the patient with PET studies is generally lower than that with SPECT myocardial perfusion studies.

As with SPECT myocardial perfusion imaging, PET perfusion imaging can provide prognostic information in addition to diagnostic information. While normal dipyridamole ^{82}Rb PET studies are associated with a high event-free survival, there is a step-wise increase in the cardiac event rate in patients with defects of increasing severity (Marwick *et al.* 1997). This is true even in patients with normal PET imaging but ischemic ECG changes during dipyridamole infusion (Chow *et al.* 2005), in contrast to patients with normal SPECT images but ischemic ECG changes during adenosine or dipyridamole stress testing, in whom there is an increased risk of myocardial infarction and need for revascularization (Abbott *et al.* 2003, Klodas *et al.* 2003). One study has demonstrated the ability of dipyridamole ^{82}Rb PET to identify asymptomatic patients at risk for restenosis following angioplasty (Van Tosh *et al.* 1995).

ASSESSMENT OF MYOCARDIAL VIABILITY

The method that remains the 'gold standard' for the assessment of myocardial viability is the evaluation of flow and metabolism by cardiac PET. In this method, both regional metabolic activities assessed by the uptake of [18F]-2-fluoro-2-deoxyglucose (FDG), and resting myocardial perfusion assessed with either ^{13}N or ^{82}Rb, are determined and the relationship between metabolism and flow is assessed. FDG uptake and retention are dependent on an intact sarcolemma and the presence of adenosine triphosphate (ATP) to phosphorylate FDG by hexokinase, which traps the FDG within the cardiac myocyte. In normal myocardium, there will be homogeneous uptake of both FDG and the flow tracer. In regions of the heart with perfusion defects that show little or no reversibility, if FDG uptake is decreased to a similar extent as perfusion, the defect is matched and represents scar, with little chance of improvement in function following revascariztion. In contrast, if there is a mismatch between FDG uptake and the perfusion defect, then the region is considered to have viable, but jeopardized myocardium that will benefit from revascularization (Tillisch *et al.* 1986, Tamaki *et al.* 1989, 1995, Carrel *et al.* 1992, Lucignani *et al.* 1992, Marwick *et al.* 1992, Gropler *et al.* 1993, Knuuti *et al.* 1994, Baer *et al.* 1996, Gerber *et al.* 1996, Maes *et al.* 1997). Furthermore, FDG-PET can also be used to predict which patients will have an improvement in heart failure symptoms and exercise capacity with revascularization (Eitzman *et al.* 1992, Di Carli *et al.* 1994, 1995). The sensitivity, specificity, and positive and negative predictive values of FDG-PET in predicting an improvement in left ventricular function are 88%, 73%, 76%, and 86%, respectively, based on a meta-analysis of these prior studies (Bax *et al.* 1997c).

While PET assessment of flow and metabolism to evaluate viability may be the gold standard, there are several hurdles to the widespread use of this technique to identify viable myocardium. The first is the need for a cyclotron for FDG production and the second is the need for a PET camera for imaging of the PET tracers. Because of the relatively longer half-life of ^{18}F compared to other PET tracers, a regional distribution system has been established to provide FDG to imaging centers that are geographically remote from cyclotron generators. To deal with the second issue of the need for a PET camera, which is more expensive than a SPECT camera, SPECT cameras can be equipped with special ultra-high-energy collimators for SPECT imaging of PET tracers. In this way, FDG images can be obtained by single photon imaging and perfusion images can be acquired with standard SPECT myocardial perfusion imaging agents (Burt *et al.* 1995, Martin *et al.* 1995, Sandler & Patton 1996, Chen *et al.* 1997, Bax *et al.* 1998, Sandler *et al.* 1998, Srinivasan *et al.* 1998). These FDG-SPECT studies have been shown to have good concordance with FDG-PET studies and identify patients that will benefit from revascularization (Bax *et al.* 1997a, b).

In addition to FDG-based methods for assessing myocardial viability, SPECT methods based on uptake of ^{201}Tl or ^{99m}Tc-sestamibi can be used to identify viable myocardium. Because ^{201}Tl uptake is mediated by the sarcolemmal Na^+/K^+ ATPase, it requires the presence of cytosolic ATP and an intact sarcolemma, in a manner analogous to that for FDG uptake and retention. A variety of imaging protocols, including rest/redistribution, rest/redistribution/reinjection, and stress/redistribution/reinjection, have been employed for ^{201}Tl viability imaging, and all of these methods have high levels of concordance with flow/metabolism assessment with PET (Bonow *et al.* 1991, Dilsizian *et al.* 1993, Altehoefer *et al.* 1994, Bax *et al.* 1998).

With respect to the use of ^{99m}Tc-sestamibi in viability assessment, studies have demonstrated a direct relationship between ^{99m}Tc-sestamibi uptake and the degree of myocardial fibrosis. Based on this relationship, a ^{99m}Tc-sestamibi perfusion defect that contains <50% of the maximal myocardial counts is associated with a lack of functional improvement with revascularization (Maes *et al.* 1997). The sensitivity of ^{99m}Tc-sestamibi for detecting viable myocardium can be increased with the administration of nitroglycerine to increase collateral blood flow (Greco *et al.* 1996, 1998, Batista *et al.* 1999, Senior *et al.* 2002, Kostkiewicz *et al.* 2003, Tzonevska *et al.* 2005).

ASSESSMENT OF LEFT VENTRICULAR FUNCTION

The assessment of left ventricular function is an essential part of cardiac evaluation risk stratification of a patient. Left ventricular function is an important predictor of survival in patients with either ischemic or nonischemic congestive heart failure (Hammermeister *et al.* 1979). In addition, transient left ventricular dysfunction induced by ischemia during exercise stress testing has important prognostic implications. Left ventricular function is one of the major determinants of survival in patients with CAD and is important in determining the need for cardiac defibrillator implantation (Hammermeister *et al.* 1979, Multicenter Postinfarction Research Group 1983, Zaret *et al.* 1995, Kober *et al.* 1996, O'Connor *et al.* 1997). Accurate monitoring of left ventricular EF is also important in patients before and after receiving anthracycline chemotherapy. While left ventricular function can be assessed with any of the noninvasive modalities discussed in this book, radionuclide techniques provide reproducible, quantitative, and relatively quick methods for assessment of left ventricular systolic and diastolic function.

Left ventricular systolic and diastolic function can be assessed by a variety of nuclear techniques, including gated planar blood pool imaging either immediately after injection of radiotracer (first-pass radionuclide angiography, FPRNA) or after equilibration of the tracer with the blood pool (equilibrium radionuclide angiography, ERNA), gated myocardial perfusion SPECT (GSPECT) or gated blood pool SPECT (GBPS).

The general principle of acquisition for all nuclear techniques except first-pass studies is the concept of ECG gating, which links images to various time points, or 'frames,' in the cardiac cycle. Data from multiple cardiac cycles are summed until sufficient counts are obtained to ensure adequate image quality. Gated blood pool or reconstructed SPECT or PET slices can then be displayed as a movie or 'cine' loop, to allow for visual and quantitative assessment of left ventricular function. The accuracy of this calculation depends on a number of factors, including the adequacy of the ECG-gated signal, the lack of heart rate variability, and adequate count statistics. The nuclear approaches to assessments of the left ventricular function are described below.

FPRNA approach

It is possible to assess both right and left ventricular function using planar gated blood pool studies based on FPRNA in which the initial transit of radiotracer through the right ventricle, pulmonary circulation, and left ventricle is imaged (**47**). However, FPRNA is technically challenging because acceptable data can only be acquired if there is a rapid and compact bolus injection of the tagged red blood cells and the gamma camera is oriented properly (Daou *et al.* 2004). The overlap of the right and left ventricles on equilibrium studies, which limits its applicability for assessment of right ventricular function, is not a problem with FPRNA.

Proper acquisition techniques are critical for FPRNA. In particular, the radiotracer must be administered in a concentrated, continuous manner and a gamma camera with high count rate capability must be used. Almost any ^{99m}Tc-labeled radiopharmaceutical can be used for FPRNA, as long as it can be injected rapidly, produce

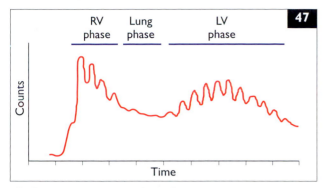

47 Time–activity curve for a first-pass radionuclide angiocardiographic assessment of right and left ventricular function demonstrating the right ventricular (RV), lung, and left ventricular (LV) phases of the bolus of radiotracer.

adequate counts, and have acceptable radiation exposure. ^{99m}Tc-pertechnetate, red blood cells, or myocardial perfusion tracers (e.g. sestamibi, tetrofosmin) are used frequently, since the technique is often combined with ERNA or SPECT myocardial perfusion studies for the purpose of assessing right ventricular function. Exercise radionuclide angiography can be obtained by this technique using a portable gamma camera, with correction for motion using a fixed radioactive point source on the patient's chest. Other radiotracers, such as ^{99m}Tc-diethylene triamine pentaacetic acid (DTPA) or sulfur colloid can be used if FPRNA is obtained alone.

FPRNA images typically are acquired in the 30° right anterior oblique projection, to optimize separation of the atria and great vessels from the ventricles (Bodenheimer *et al.* 1978). The optimal framing interval depends on the heart rate. A region of interest initially is placed on the entire heart, to determine right and left ventricular phases. Subsequently, regions of interest are placed on the right and left ventricles, for calculation of the EF. In general, for optimal calculation of EF, data are used from two to three cycles from the right ventricular phase and four to six cycles from the left ventricular phase.

Left ventricular EF obtained by FPRNA will have a statistical error of between 2% (for normal ventricular function) and 10–20% (for depressed ventricular function). Functional information obtained with first-pass techniques shows good correlation to EF measured by other imaging techniques (Folland *et al.* 1977, Ashburn *et al.* 1978, Hecht *et al.* 1978, Wackers *et al.* 1979, Johnson *et al.* 1995). Because the first-pass technique usually involves acquisition of only

a single view, its utility for analysis of regional wall motion is limited.

Although FPRNA has largely been replaced by ERNA, gated SPECT, and echocardiography, the technique remains potentially useful as an adjunct to equilibrium gated blood pool imaging or to SPECT perfusion studies (using rest injection of ^{99m}Tc-labeled perfusion tracers) for assessment of right and/or left ventricular function.

ERNA approach

Systolic left ventricular function as measured by the left ventricular EF, and diastolic function as measured by the peak filling rate (PFR), can be determined by equilibrium radionuclide angiography (Zaret *et al.* 1971). In the ERNA technique, red blood cells are labeled with ^{99m}Tc in order to visualize the left ventricular blood pool. ECG-gated planar images are acquired in three standard views for routine diagnosis: left anterior oblique, anterior, and lateral. The primary view used for ERNA quantitative analysis is the left anterior oblique view. The left anterior oblique view has a clear separation of the two ventricles which allows for calculations of the left ventricular EF. In the left anterior oblique view the left ventricle displays as a spherical shape and as such the counts-derived left ventricular volume can be calculated based on the spherical model of the left ventricle. To determine left ventricular blood pool counts, the regions of interest are drawn on the end-systole and end-diastole frames. The means of generating the regions of interest of the left ventricle in the cardiac cycle can be manual, semi-automatic, and automatic. Discussion of these three regions of interest approaches is beyond the scope of this chapter. In brief, the left ventricle time–activity curve is generated from the end-diastole to end-systole based on the total counts in the regions of interest. Ultimately, the left ventricle EF is derived from the peak and nadir values of the time–activity curve and the PFR is calculated by the first derivative of the time–activity curve.

Gated planar ERNA remains the mainstay for the serial, quantitative assessment of left ventricular function in patients receiving anthracycline-based chemotherapy. This stems in part from the reproducibility of the method compared to echocardiographic and other scintigraphic methods of evaluation of left ventricular EF. In addition, other scintigraphic methods to determine left ventricular EF (e.g. GSPECT and GBPS) require greater acquisition time than a single planar ERNA obtained in the left anterior oblique view. Furthermore, a greater number of time points with higher count statistics can be sampled per R-R interval with planar ERNA than with GSPECT or GBPS, providing more accurate assessment of left ventricular EF.

GSPECT approach

Gated SPECT myocardial perfusion imaging does not rely on radio-tagging of the blood pool. Rather, assessment of left ventricular function is based on identifying the borders of the left ventricular myocardium or changes in count density in the left ventricular wall based on the changes in count recovery associated with myocardial thickening (Najm *et al.* 1989, DePuey *et al.* 1993, Yang & Chen 1994, Boonyaprapa *et al.* 1995, Germano *et al.* 1995, Everaert *et al.* 1996, Smith *et al.* 1997, Brigger *et al.* 1999, Itti *et al.* 2001, Liu *et al.* 2005). Consequently, gated SPECT myocardial perfusion images can be used to determine left ventricular EF. In this method, edge detection algorithms are used to determine the left ventricular cavity at end-systole and end-diastole from ECG-gated SPECT perfusion images. Several studies have demonstrated that GSPECT provides an acceptable estimate of left ventricular EF. Gated SPECT and gated PET myocardial perfusion imaging allow for the assessment of left ventricular function in addition to the perfusion data from the 'static' or ungated images. It is also important to assess regional left ventricular function and wall motion, and these are evaluated qualitatively by review of cine images.

GSPECT has offered the ability to combine the assessment of myocardial perfusion and the assessment of global and regional wall motion and has become the preferred myocardial perfusion imaging modality, providing significant incremental prognostic information to the myocardial perfusion images (Johnson *et al.* 1997, Smanio *et al.* 1997, Sakamoto *et al.* 2004). Evaluation of regional wall motion from GSPECT myocardial perfusion images can also decrease the number of false-positive studies arising from either diaphragmatic or breast attenuation based on the presence of normal wall motion.

The left ventricular EF calculated from gated myocardial perfusion SPECT has been shown to correlate with the left ventricular EF determined by planar equilibrium gated blood pool imaging and first-pass gated blood pool imaging (Chua *et al.* 1994, Williams & Taillon 1996, Calnon *et al.* 1997, He *et al.* 1999, Vaduganathan *et al.* 1999, Vallejo *et al.* 2000b). However, SPECT measurements of left ventricular EF can be unreliable if there is a dense perfusion defect or if there is scatter from extracardiac activity (DePuey *et al.* 1999, Manrique *et al.* 1999, Vallejo *et al.* 2000a, b; Navare *et al.* 2003, Liu *et al.* 2005).

GBPS approach

Recent developments in SPECT imaging have allowed for tomographic acquisition of GBPS images. The evaluation of left ventricular EF by GBPS has been shown to be comparable to that by ERNA. However, in contrast to ERNA, GBPS is associated with superior assessment of both right and left ventricular anatomy and function (Akinboboye *et al.* 2005) and thus allows for the assessment of right and left ventricular function. The left ventricular EF determined by GBPS correlates well with other assessments of left ventricular function (Van Kriekinge *et al.* 1999, Vanhove *et al.* 2003, Higuchi *et al.* 2004, Nichols *et al.* 2004, Akinboboye *et al.* 2005, Kim *et al.* 2005). Unlike gated myocardial perfusion SPECT, GBPS provides a reliable assessment of left ventricular EF in patients with dense myocardial infarcts (Akinboboye *et al.* 2005). GBPS has been used in a variety of specific patient populations, including evaluation of left ventricular dyssynchrony in patients with heart failure, evaluation of systemic ventricular function in patients with complex congenital heart disease, and assessment of right ventricular function and morphology in patients with ARVD (Casset-Senon *et al.* 1998, Adachi *et al.* 2003, Fauchier *et al.* 2003).

The application of GBPS to the assessment of right ventricular disorder extends past the simple evaluation of left ventricular EF and right ventricular EF used in determining response to therapy. In patients with right ventricular dysfunction, GBPS can be used to assess right ventricular enlargement, asynchronous right ventricular contraction, and increased contraction dispersion in addition to right ventricular EF. GBPS has been used to evaluate the functional response to accessory pathway radiofrequency ablation (Chevalier *et al.* 1999).

CLINICAL CASES

The following cases illustrate various aspects of nuclear cardiac imaging, including the detection of ischemia and scar by both SPECT and PET methods, common artifacts, and the assessment of left ventricular function. The myocardial perfusion images displayed in this chapter follow the standard convention established by the ASNC, with stress images displayed on the top row of images and resting images displayed below the stress images. Images are displayed in a standardized short-axis orientation, a vertical long-axis orientation, and a horizontal long-axis orientation (**44**). Furthermore, the 17-segment model of the left ventricle that corresponds to vascular territories is used to identify regional myocardial perfusion defects.

Case 1: SPECT with Normal Stress/Rest Perfusion

Clinical history

The patient was a 45-year-old male referred for stress testing after he had experienced several episodes of syncope. His cardiac risk factors included a history of smoking. His physical examination was unremarkable.

Imaging protocol

The patient exercised for a total of 11 minutes on a Bruce protocol achieving a workload of 12.9 METs. The patient's resting heart rate was 72 beats per minute (bpm) and increased to 179 bpm at peak exercise (97% of his age predicted maximal heart rate). His resting blood pressure was 108/72 mmHg and increased to 144/80 mmHg at peak exercise. He did not develop chest pain during exercise. His ECG showed no changes diagnostic for ischemia. He was injected with 16.4 mCi of ^{99m}Tc-sestamibi at peak exercise and 27.3 mCi of ^{99m}Tc-sestamibi at rest as part of a 1-day imaging protocol and underwent SPECT imaging. His resting left ventricular EF by gated SPECT was normal.

Impression

There were no perfusion defects present in either the stress or rest images (**48**).

Discussion

The patient exercised at an excellent workload during the stress test without evidence of ischemia either on the ECG or on the myocardial perfusion images. It is very unlikely that the syncopal episodes that the patient experienced were due to myocardial ischemia causing arrhythmias. Furthermore, based on the normal stress test and large retrospective studies, the patient's annual risk of experiencing a myocardial infarction or cardiac death is <1%. While a normal stress test confers an excellent prognosis for a variety of patient populations, the annual cardiac event rate will still vary between groups based on the presence of cardiac risk factors such as diabetes (Hachamovitch *et al.* 2003).

Management

The patient was referred for ambulatory electro-cardiographic monitoring to document any arrhythmias that might have caused the syncopal episodes.

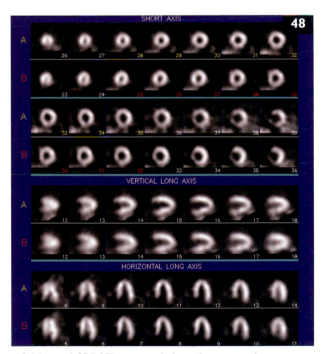

48 Normal SPECT myocardial perfusion study.

Case 2: Normal SPECT with Stress Perfusion

Clinical history

The patient was a 57-year-old male referred for stress testing because of a 5-month history of nonexertional left-sided chest pain. His cardiac risk factors include a history of hypertension and hyperlipidemia and a family history of CAD. The patient was obese with a BMI of 32 kg/m^2, but his physical examination was otherwise unremarkable.

Imaging protocol

The patient exercised for a total of 9 minutes and 15 s on a modified Bruce protocol achieving a workload of 10.1 METs. The patient's peak heart rate was 147 (90% of his age predicted maximal heart rate). He had a normal blood pressure response to exercise and developed no chest pain during exercise. His electrocardiogram showed no changes diagnostic for ischemia. He was injected with 25.0 mCi of ^{99m}Tc-sestamibi at peak exercise and underwent SPECT imaging. His resting left ventricular EF by gated SPECT was normal.

Impression

There were no perfusion defects present in the stress images (**49**).

Discussion

The patient was appropriately referred for stress testing given his risk factor profile and symptoms. Given the lack of ischemic ECG changes during exercise at a high workload during the stress test as well as the normal perfusion images and normal left ventricular EF, resting images were not obtained (Worsley *et al.* 1992).

Management

Based on the results of the stress test, the patient's referring physician placed him on antihypertensive medications and a statin for primary prevention of CAD and counseled him on the importance of weight reduction and exercise.

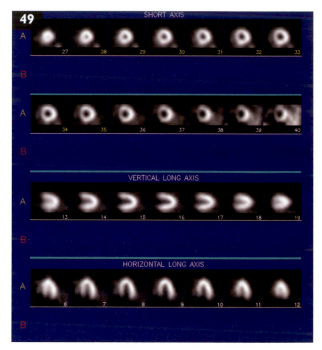

49 Normal SPECT myocardial perfusion study requiring no resting imaging.

Case 3: SPECT Showing Ischemia

Clinical history

The patient was a 55-year-old male referred for stress testing because of increasing exertional central chest pressure. His cardiac risk factors included a history of hypertension and hyperlipidemia. The patient's physical examination was normal. Of note, the last episode of chest pain occurred while walking from the parking lot to the stress testing laboratory and was relieved by resting.

Imaging protocol

The patient exercised for a total of 6 minutes on a Bruce protocol achieving a workload of 7.0 METs. The patient's resting heart rate was 75 bpm and increased to 149 bpm (90% of his age predicted maximal heart rate). His resting blood pressure was 150/102 mmHg and increased to 180/120 mmHg in response to exercise. The patient developed his typical chest pain during the stress test and his ECG showed 2–3 mm flat ST-segment depressions in precordial leads V4 and V5 5 minutes into exercise. He was injected with 16.4 mCi of ^{99m}Tc-sestamibi at rest and 26.9 mCi of ^{99m}Tc-sestamibi at peak exercise and underwent SPECT imaging. His resting left ventricular EF by gated SPECT was normal.

Impression

There was a large, dense anterolateral perfusion defect on the stress images (arrows, **50**) that is absent on the resting images. This was consistent with an anterolateral area of ischemia.

Discussion

The patient had evidence of anterolateral ischemia on the myocardial perfusion imaging consistent with significant stenoses affecting the LAD and LCX. It is of note to mention that while ST-segment depressions on ECGs obtained during stress testing are diagnostic for myocardial ischemia, they do not generally localize the area of ischemia. Specifically, the inferolateral

ECG leads (II, III, aVF, V4, V5, and V6) are the most sensitive leads for diagnosing ischemia, but can indicate anterior ischemia as well as lateral or inferior ischemia. This explains why no ischemic changes were noted in the anterior precordial leads, V1, V2, and V3, despite scintigraphic evidence of anterior ischemia. In contrast, ST elevations during stress testing are more accurate in predicting the vessel with a critical lesion (Fuchs *et al.* 1982).

Management

The patient was referred for cardiac catheterization, which revealed high-grade stenoses of the LAD and LCX. The patient underwent successful angioplasty and stenting of the lesions with resolution of symptoms.

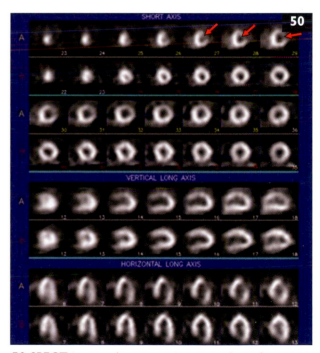

50 SPECT images demonstrating anterolateral ischemia.

Case 4: High-risk SPECT Study

Clinical history

A 70-year-old male with a history of hypertension, diabetes, and hypercholesterolemia was referred for stress testing because of increasing chest pain with exertion. The pain was described as a pressure sensation in the center of the chest that initially occurred when the patient walked up several flights of stairs or when carrying several bags of groceries. However, over the past 2 weeks, the pain was occurring when he walked about 30 meters. The pain would always resolve if he stopped exerting himself and never occurred at rest.

Imaging protocol

The patient performed treadmill exercise for 5 minutes and 15 s on a Bruce protocol, achieving an estimated workload of 7.0 METs. His resting heart rate was 70 bpm and increased to 111 bpm at peak exercise (74% of his age predicted maximal heart rate). The resting blood pressure was 136/86 mmHg and decreased to 114/76 mmHg at peak exercise. The patient developed his typical chest pain at 2 minutes and 45 s of exercise as well as 2 mm flat ST-segment depressions in leads III, aVF, V5, and V6. The test was terminated because of the hypotensive blood pressure response during exercise. The patient was closely monitored following exercise and his ECG changes resolved 4 minutes into the recovery period.

Imaging was performed with the injection of 24.7 mCi of ^{99m}Tc-sestamibi at peak exercise and 24.8 mCi of ^{99m}Tc-sestamibi at rest as part of a 2-day imaging protocol. Gated SPECT images were acquired which demonstrated a left ventricular EF of 26% in the images acquired after exercise and a left ventricular EF of 50% in the images acquired after resting injection.

Impression

The SPECT images show moderate-sized anteroseptal and inferior perfusion defects in the stress images (arrows, **51**) that resolved in the resting images. Of note, the left ventricular cavity appears to be larger in the stress images compared to the resting images. In addition, the right ventricle is readily visualized on the stress images but is barely visible on the resting images. These findings are consistent with ischemia in two distributions, the LAD and the RCA, with evidence of a high burden of ischemia based on the TID of the left

ventricle and transient visualization of the right ventricle (TRV). Furthermore, these ischemic defects occurred at a low workload with associated signs (hypotension), symptoms (angina), and electrocardiographic evidence of myocardial ischemia.

Discussion

The findings of this study, including evidence of ischemia at a low workload, multivessel ischemia, TID, TRV, and transient left ventricular dysfunction, confer a high risk (~8–10% annual risk of myocardial infarction or cardiac death) of a cardiac event. The TID is attributed to decreased radiotracer uptake in the subendocardial region due to diffuse ischemia, making the left ventricular cavity appear larger (Weiss *et al.* 1987). The TRV is thought to be due to right ventricular strain caused by left ventricular dysfunction resulting in an increase in the pulmonary capillary wedge pressure and increased right-sided pressures (Williams & Schneider 1999).

Management

Based on the results of the stress test, the patient was referred for cardiac catheterization and was found to have triple vessel disease. The patient subsequently underwent coronary artery bypass grafting.

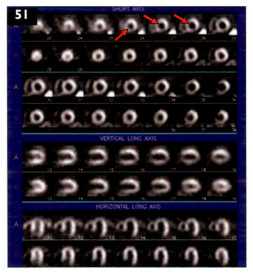

51 SPECT images showing anteroseptal and inferior ischemia and high-risk markers of TID of the left ventricle and transient right ventricular visualization.

Case 5: SPECT Showing Scar

Clinical history
A 60-year-old female with a history of hypertension and hypercholesterolemia was hospitalized after experiencing an episode of syncope. The patient was referred for stress testing for further evaluation of the syncopal episode.

Imaging protocol
The patient underwent an adenosine ^{99m}Tc-tetrofosmin SPECT myocardial perfusion study because of leg pain and the inability to exercise. Her resting heart rate was 63 bpm and increased to 80 bpm at peak adenosine infusion. Her blood pressure increased from 132/80 mmHg to 142/80 mmHg at peak adenosine infusion. There were no ECG changes during adenosine infusion. The patient underwent resting imaging with 25.9 mCi of ^{99m}Tc-tetrofosmin and stress imaging with 26.1 mCi of ^{99m}Tc-tetrofosmin. Gated SPECT imaging demonstrated preserved left ventricular EF with anterior akinesis.

Impression
There was a moderate-sized anterior perfusion defect extending from the apex to the mid-ventricular level on both the stress and rest images, there was minimal improvement in the defect (arrows, **52**). These findings were consistent with a moderate-sized anterior scar.

Discussion
Scarring following myocardial infarction can predispose patients to the development of ventricular tachycardia that uses the viable tissue around the scar as part of the arrhythmogenic circuit. In the case of this patient, the identification of an area of scarring suggests that further evaluation for the presence of such a reentrant circuit should be carried out.

Management
The patient underwent electrophysiologic testing, revealing the presence of inducible ventricular tachycardia, which was thought to be responsible for the syncopal episode. The patient subsequently underwent placement of an implantable cardiac defibrillator (ICD).

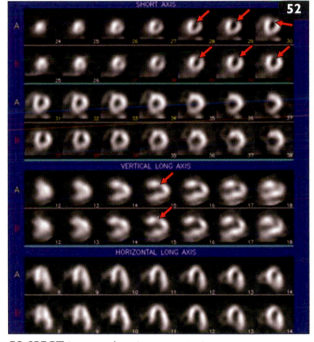

52 SPECT images showing an anterior scar.

Case 6: SPECT Showing Scar Mixed with Ischemia

Clinical history

A 45-year-old male with no significant past medical history was brought to the emergency department following a motor vehicle accident when the patient lost consciousness. In the emergency department, an ECG revealed ST elevations in V1 through V4 consistent with an acute anterior wall myocardial infarction. The patient was taken as an emergency to the cardiac catheterization laboratory and found to have a totally occluded LAD. However, because of the presence of extensive chest wall trauma, angioplasty and stenting of the occluded artery were not performed because of the risk of bleeding from the use of antiplatelet agents and anticoagulants that would be required. The patient was treated medically and was referred several weeks later for stress testing.

Imaging protocol

The patient underwent an adenosine ^{99m}Tc-tetrofosmin SPECT myocardial perfusion study because of the inability to exercise adequately following the trauma. The resting heart rate was 74 bpm and increased to 80 bpm at peak adenosine infusion. His blood pressure decreased from 120/78 mmHg to 112/70 mmHg at peak adenosine infusion. There were no ECG changes during adenosine infusion. The patient underwent resting imaging with 15.8 mCi of ^{99m}Tc-tetrofosmin and stress imaging with 25.2 mCi of ^{99m}Tc-tetrofosmin. Gated SPECT imaging demonstrated a mildly depressed left ventricular EF with anteroseptal hypokinesis.

Impression

There was a large anteroseptal perfusion defect extending from the apex to the base of the heart (arrows, **53**). Comparing the stress images to the resting images, there was some improvement in the defect, although it did not normalize. These findings were consistent with an extensive area of scar mixed with ischemia.

Discussion

A 'mixed' or 'partially reversible' perfusion defect indicates the presence of both regions of nonviable scar tissue and viable myocardium that was ischemic. In this particular patient, there was still a significant amount of viable myocardium present in the anteroseptal wall.

Management

The patient underwent repeat coronary angiography, which revealed recanalization of the LAD, although there was a 90% stenosis in the proximal segment of the artery. The patient underwent angioplasty and stenting of the vessel without complications.

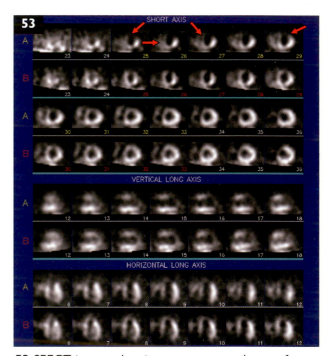

53 SPECT images showing an anteroseptal area of scar mixed with ischemia.

Case 7: SPECT Complicated by Attenuation

Clinical history

A 48-year-old male with a history of hypertension and tobacco use was referred for stress testing because of complaints of intermittent chest pressure. The pain occurred both at rest and with exertion and resolved spontaneously. The patient's physical examination was unremarkable.

Imaging protocol

The patient exercised for 9 minutes 38 s on a Bruce protocol with an estimated workload of 10.1 METs. The test was terminated because of patient fatigue. The resting heart rate was 67 bpm and increased to 169 bpm at peak exercise (98% age predicted maximal heart rate). The resting blood pressure was 130/85 mmHg and increased to 165/85 mmHg at peak exercise. There were no ECG changes during exercise. Myocardial perfusion imaging was performed with the injection of 15.1 mCi of ^{99m}Tc-sestamibi at rest and 25.6 mCi of ^{99m}Tc-sestamibi at peak exercise as part of a 1-day imaging protocol. Gated SPECT imaging was performed. Based on the gated SPECT studies, the left ventricular EF was 58% and there were no regional wall motion abnormalities.

Impression

The SPECT images show a small defect in the inferior wall that is present in both the stress and rest studies (arrows, **54**). The planar images show that when the patient was repositioned from the supine position (the position normally used for myocardial perfusion imaging) to the left lateral decubitus position, there was greater recovery of counts in the inferior wall, indicating the presence of diaphragmatic attenuation

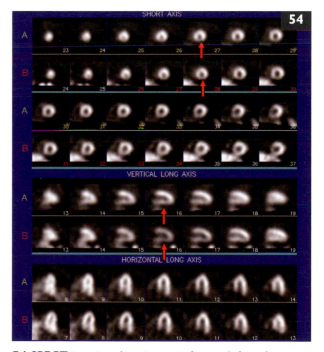

54 SPECT imaging showing an inferior defect that was due to diaphragmatic attenuation (arrows).

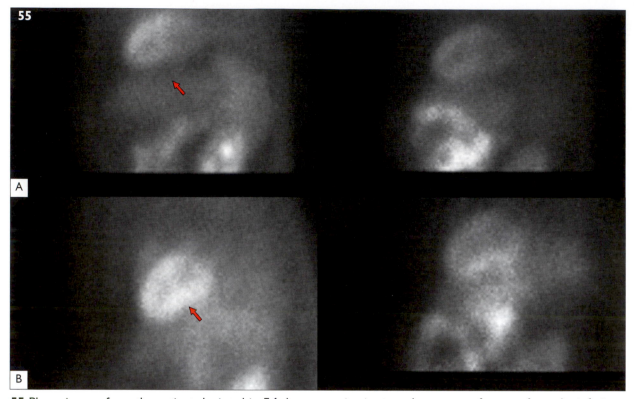

55 Planar images from the patient depicted in **54** demonstrating improved recovery of counts from the inferior wall when the patient was placed in the decubitus position, indicating the presence of diaphragmatic attenuation. (**A**) Left lateral view in supine position (left image, stress; right image, rest). (**B**) Left lateral view in decubitus position.

(arrows, **55**). Based on the planar images, combined with the lack of a wall motion abnormality in the inferior wall, the inferior wall defect was due to diaphragmatic attenuation and therefore this was a normal perfusion study.

Discussion

Two of the most important factors affecting image quality of SPECT myocardial perfusion scans are tissue attenuation and photon scatter. Tissue attenuation is caused by the absorption of gamma photons from the radiotracer by surrounding tissue so that fewer photons reach the gamma camera. The three most common forms of tissue attenuation are diaphragmatic attenuation, breast attenuation, and generalized attenuation due to obesity. Diaphragmatic attenuation, which is due to the close proximity of the left hemidiaphragm to the inferior wall of the heart, can be identified by imaging of the patient in the left lateral decubitus position, when the heart will fall away from the diaphragm. Other ways to identify diaphragmatic attenuation include the presence of normal motion of the inferior wall when there is a fixed defect (DePuey & Rozanski 1995). If a fixed defect is due to the presence of scar tissue, there should be a wall motion abnormality (hypokinesis, akinesis, or dyskinesis) associated with it. In addition, diaphragmatic attenuation can be identified by prone imaging of the patient or by the use of attenuation correction. In the case of the current patient, this study was performed with a SPECT camera equipped with a low-resolution CT scanner that allowed for attenuation correction based on the absorption of X-rays from the CT scanner. The artifacts caused by photon scatter are discussed in the next case presentation.

Management

The patient continued his current antihypertensive therapy and was counseled on smoking cessation. No further cardiac evaluation is required at this point.

Case 8: SPECT Complicated by Motion

Clinical history

A 45-year-old male with a history of diabetes, hypertension, hyperlipidemia, and a previous renal transplant was referred for preoperative evaluation prior to pancreatic transplant. The patient denied chest pain or shortness of breath.

Imaging protocol

The patient exercised on a treadmill for a total of 10 minutes, 52 s, reaching stage 4 of a Bruce protocol with an estimated workload of 12.9 METs. Resting heart rate was 85 bpm and increased to 181 bpm at peak exercise (103% of the age predicted maximal heart rate). His resting blood pressure was 124/70 mmHg and increased to 224/100 mmHg at peak exercise. The patient did not experience chest pain during stress. There were no ECG changes diagnostic for ischemia during stress. Myocardial perfusion imaging was performed with the injection of 15.5 mCi of ^{99m}Tc-sestamibi at rest and 25.7 mCi of ^{99m}Tc-sestamibi at peak stress. Rotating cine images used to evaluate the quality of the study with respect to motion and extracardiac radiotracer uptake demonstrated a significant degree of cardiac motion. Gated SPECT imaging was performed. Based on the gated SPECT studies, the left ventricular EF was 56% and there were no regional wall motion abnormalities.

Impression

The SPECT images obtained following exercise show artifacts caused by patient motion during image acquisition (**56**). These include a fragmented appearance to the left ventricle and the presence of blurring of the anterior wall creating the 'hurricane' sign (arrows, **56**). The artifact produces an image that looks like the National Oceanic and Atmospheric Administration's symbol for a hurricane. There are no such motion artifacts noted on the resting images.

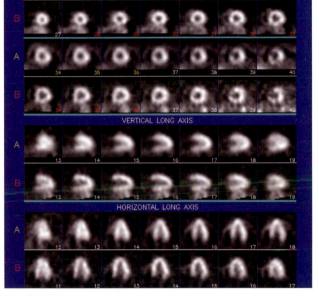

56 SPECT images complicated by motion artifacts ('hurricane' sign, arrows).

Discussion

Patient motion can affect image quality due to artifacts. This study produced two of the more common motion artifacts (Cooper *et al.* 1992). Because of the significant motion effect on study interpretation, one of the quality control measures for myocardial perfusion studies is to assess the degree of motion, as was done in this study.

Management

The patient underwent repeat stress perfusion imaging in which there was minimal motion. There were no perfusion defects noted in the new stress test and no further cardiac evaluation was required.

Case 9: SPECT Complicated by Subdiaphragmatic Radioactivity

Clinical history

A 69-year-old male with a history of a previous inferior wall myocardial infarction was referred for stress testing because of new onset chest pain with associated shortness of breath during exertion. The patient denied any resting symptoms and his physical examination was unremarkable.

Imaging protocol

The patient performed treadmill exercise for 7 minutes and 32 s, achieving stage 3 of a Bruce protocol with an estimated workload of 10.4 METs. The resting heart rate was 90 bpm and increased to 166 bpm at peak exercise (110% of the age predicted maximal heart rate). The resting blood pressure was 110/60 mmHg and increased to 130/80 mmHg at peak exercise. There were no ECG changes during the stress test and the test was terminated because of fatigue. The patient underwent stress imaging after the injection of 16.1 mCi of ^{99m}Tc-sestamibi at peak exercise and resting imaging after the injection of 26.0 mCi of ^{99m}Tc-sestamibi. The gated SPECT study demonstrated a normal left ventricular EF, but evidence of inferolateral hypokinesis on the post-stress images.

Impression

The stress images show a large inferolateral perfusion defect (**57**) in the same locations as the hypokinesis noted on the gated SPECT images (not shown). However, the resting images are complicated by severe uptake of radiotracer in the liver and intestines (arrows, **57**), which obscures the inferolateral wall. This makes it impossible to determine if the inferolateral defect is fixed (i.e. scar) or has a component of reversibility (i.e. ischemia). Therefore, this is a nondiagnostic study.

Discussion

Along with attenuation, photon scatter from radiotracer in extracardiac tissues is the most common cause of artifacts in nuclear cardiac perfusion images (Pitman *et al.* 2005). This is especially true for the technetium-based myocardial perfusion imaging agents, ^{99m}Tc-sestamibi and ^{99m}Tc-tetrofosmin, which are cleared by the hepatobiliary system. It is also more common in pharmacologic stress tests in which the vasodilating

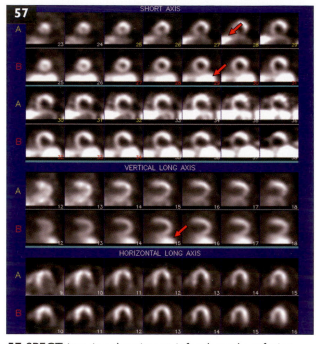

57 SPECT imaging showing an inferolateral perfusion defect on the stress images that is obscured by intense subdiaphragmatic radiotracer uptake (arrows).

agent tends to increase blood flow to all organs, including the liver. Note that the interference from subdiaphragmatic radioactivity in the stress images in this patient is less than that seen in the resting images because there is increased blood flow to the heart with relative shunting of blood away from the splanchnic circulation with exercise. Had this been a pharmacologic stress test, the stress images would likely have been as poor as the resting images. Furthermore, if one was to base interpretation of the study solely on the quantification, one would incorrectly conclude that the defect is reversible because of the photons scattering into the region of the inferolateral wall from the gastrointestinal tract. To overcome this artifact, several options are available. First, the images can be reacquired 30 minutese later with the hope that the radioactivity in the gastrointestinal tract has moved away from the heart. However, this does not always solve the problem. Second, a radiotracer that is cleared by the kidneys and therefore does not accumulate in the liver to the same extent, such as the single-photon-emitting tracer, ^{201}Tl, or the positron-emitting tracer, ^{82}Rb, can be used.

Management

The patient underwent repeat stress testing with ^{82}Rb and PET. The study, which was not complicated by subdiaphragmatic radiotracer uptake, demonstrated that the inferolateral perfusion defect was present on both the stress and resting images and therefore represented a scar with no evidence of ischemia. The patient was maintained on his cardiac medications, which included a beta-blocker, aspirin, and a statin.

Case 10: SPECT with Extracardiac Findings

Clinical history

A 67-year-old male with a history of smoking and hypertension was referred for a cardiac evaluation prior to surgery for lung cancer. The patient denied any history of chest pain but did have exertional shortness of breath.

Imaging protocol

The patient underwent an adenosine ^{99m}Tc-tetrofosmin SPECT myocardial perfusion study. The resting heart rate was 73 bpm and increased to 85 bpm at peak adenosine infusion. His blood pressure increased from 114/82 mmHg to 126/86 mmHg at peak adenosine infusion. There were no ECG changes during adenosine infusion. The patient underwent resting imaging with 15.9 mCi of ^{99m}Tc-tetrofosmin and stress imaging with 26.2 mCi of ^{99m}Tc-tetrofosmin. The gated SPECT images demonstrated normal resting left ventricular function.

Impression

There were no perfusion defects noted on the myocardial perfusion study. However, there was a focal area of radiotracer uptake adjacent to the lateral wall of the left ventricle at the base of the heart (arrows, **58**). This extracardiac activity was also seen on the rotating raw images (circles, **59**). This area of focal radiotracer uptake corresponds to the location of the patient's lung mass.

Discussion

While the focus of nuclear cardiac stress tests is obviously the detection of myocardial ischemia, it is important to remain observant for extracardiac findings. Focal uptake of ^{99m}Tc-sestamibi can be observed in breast cancers as well as lung cancers and is related, in part, to the high degree of vascularity that tumors can have (Williams *et al.* 2003). Interestingly, the product of the multidrug resistance gene, P-glycoprotein, can export ^{99m}Tc-sestamibi out of cells, and loss of ^{99m}Tc-sestamibi uptake from a tumor can be used to identify tumors expressing P-glycoprotein.

Management

Because no perfusion defects were noted on the stress test, the patient underwent left lobectomy without further cardiac evaluation.

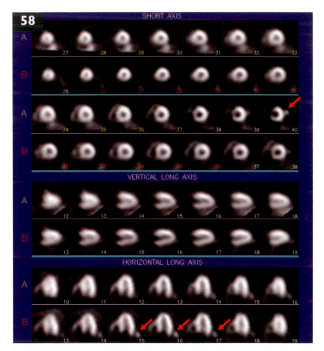

58 SPECT images demonstrating focal extracardiac uptake of radiotracer by a lung tumor (arrows).

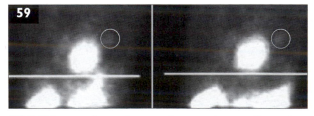

59 Still images from the rotating raw images from the patient depicted in **58** showing the focal radiotracer uptake (circles).

Case 11: PET Showing Ischemia

Clinical history

An 81-year-old female with a history of hypertension and dyslipidemia was referred for a dipyridamole ^{82}Rb PET study because she complained of increasing dyspnea on exertion. Specifically, 2 months prior to the study, she was able to walk up two flights of stairs without experiencing shortness of breath. However, since that time, she had noted progressive worsening of dyspnea on exertion to the point that she was unable to walk up a flight of stairs without stopping to catch her breath.

Imaging protocol

The patient underwent a dipyridamole ^{82}Rb PET perfusion study with the infusion of 47.9 mg of dipyridamole over 4 minutes. The resting heart rate was 68 bpm and increased to 84 bpm at peak dipyridamole infusion. The blood pressure was 141/70 mmHg at baseline and decreased to 116/64 mmHg at peak dipyridamole infusion. The patient developed 2–3 mm of ST depression in leads II, III, aVF, and V4–V6 as well as 2 mm of ST elevation in aVL, V1, and V2 during dipyridamole infusion. These ECG changes resolved with treatment with 100 mg of aminophylline and sublingual nitroglycerine. The patient underwent rest imaging following the injection of 37.1 mCi of ^{82}Rb and stress imaging following the injection of 37.5 mCi of ^{82}Rb.

Impression

The stress PET images show a large perfusion defect in the anteroseptal region extending from the apex to the base of the heart (arrows, **60**) that improves in the resting images. This reversible defect was associated with transient ischemic dilation of the left ventricle. Based on the gated PET images the resting left ventricular function was normal but with transient hypokinesis of the anteroseptal region in the stress images. The PET images, combined with the ECG changes during dipyridamole infusion, were consistent with a large area of ischemia in the distribution of the LAD. Furthermore, there were high-risk features to the study including transient ST elevation in the anteroseptal leads consistent with transmural ischemia and the presence of TID of the left ventricle.

Discussion

One of the most common complaints of patients with CAD referred for myocardial perfusion imaging is shortness of breath. Furthermore, the presence of dyspnea identifies a group of patients referred for stress testing who are at increased risk of cardiac death and all-cause mortality (Abidov *et al.* 2005). In the case of this patient, the worsening of her symptoms suggested progression of her CAD. This is a high-risk PET perfusion study.

Management

Because of the high-risk nature of the study, the patient was admitted for observation and further evaluation. The patient underwent cardiac catheterization, which revealed a subtotal occlusion of the proximal LAD but no other significant stenoses. The patient underwent angioplasty and stenting of the LAD lesion without complication and was discharged the next day.

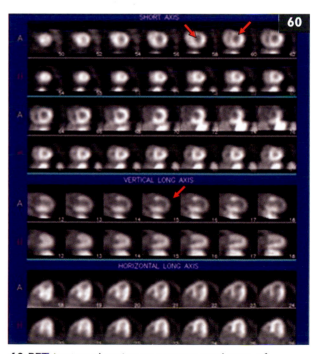

60 PET images showing an anteroseptal area of ischemia (arrows).

Case 12: PET with Normal Perfusion

Clinical history

A 57-year-old male with a history of hypertension, dyslipidemia, and type 2 diabetes mellitus was referred for a dipyridamole ^{82}Rb PET study for the assessment of exertional chest pain. The chest pain was described as sharp and substernal and was relieved by resting. The patient was obese (height: 173 cm; weight: 120 kg; BMI: 40.1 kg/m^2), but otherwise his physical examination was unremarkable.

Imaging protocol

The patient initially underwent an adenosine ^{99m}Tc-tetrofosmin SPECT myocardial perfusion study. The resting heart rate was 86 bpm and increased to 119 bpm at peak adenosine infusion. His blood pressure increased from 112/82 mmHg to 130/88 mmHg at peak adenosine infusion. There were no ECG changes during adenosine infusion. The patient underwent resting imaging with 26.7 mCi of ^{99m}Tc-tetrofosmin and stress imaging with 26.0 mCi of ^{99m}Tc-tetrofosmin. The SPECT images are of poor quality because of the patient's body habitus (**61**).

Because of the poor quality of the SPECT images, the patient underwent a dipyridamole ^{82}Rb PET perfusion study with the infusion of 68.1 mg of dipyridamole over 4 minutes. The resting heart rate was 89 bpm and increased to 91 bpm at peak dipyridamole infusion. The blood pressure was 144/93 mmHg at baseline and decreased to 138/86 mmHg at peak dipyridamole infusion. There were no ECG changes during dipyridamole infusion. The patient underwent rest imaging following the injection of 47.8 mCi of rubidium and stress imaging following the injection of 48.0 mCi of rubidium.

Impression

There were no perfusion defects noted on the PET myocardial perfusion study (**62**).

Discussion

While the SPECT images are of poor quality because of severe attenuation of the 140-keV gamma photons from ^{99m}Tc-tetrofosmin, the PET images are of much better quality resulting in an improvement in the sensitivity and specificity of the detection of myocardial

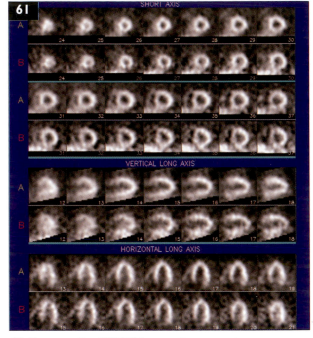

61 Poor-quality SPECT images from an obese individual.

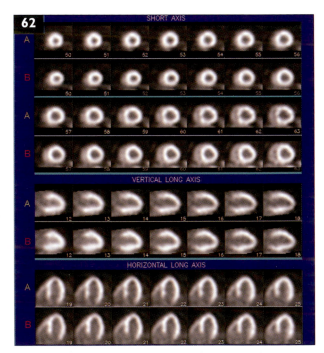

62 PET images for the patient with poor-quality SPECT images depicted in **61**. There are no perfusion defects present.

perfusion defects (Bateman *et al.* 2006). This improvement in quality comes from the fact that positron emitting radionuclides, such as ^{82}Rb, produce two high-energy 511-keV gamma photons through an annihilation event caused by the collision of the positron with an electron in the local environment. These higher-energy gamma photons are better able to penetrate tissue and reach the camera detectors than are the gamma photons from lower-energy radionuclides. In addition, all PET cameras are equipped with hardware that allows for attenuation correction. Therefore, in obese patients, cardiac PET may enable the acquisition of improved myocardial perfusion images.

Management

The patient was instructed to continue his primary preventative therapy, which included hypoglycemic agents to control his blood sugar, an angiotensin converting enzyme inhibitor and diuretic for control of his blood pressure, and a statin to treat his dyslipidemia.

Case 13: PET Showing a Scar

Clinical history

A 64-year-old male with a history of myocardial infarction and percutaneous transluminal coronary angioplasty 17 years prior to the current study was referred for a dipyridamole ^{82}Rb PET study for preoperative cardiac evaluation for the removal of a bladder tumor. The patient denied any symptoms of chest pain or shortness of breath.

Imaging protocol

The patient underwent a dipyridamole ^{82}Rb PET perfusion study with the infusion of 69.9 mg of dipyridamole over 4 minutes. The resting heart rate was 94 bpm and was unchanged at peak dipyridamole infusion. The blood pressure was 122/74 mmHg at baseline and decreased to 82/38 mmHg at peak dipyridamole infusion. The patient had no symptoms or ECG changes during dipyridamole infusion. The patient underwent rest imaging following the injection of 48.9 mCi of ^{82}Rb and stress imaging following the injection of 48.8 mCi of ^{82}Rb.

Impression

The stress PET images show a large perfusion defect in the anteroseptal region extending from the apex to the base of the heart that are unchanged in the resting images (arrows, **63**). Based on the gated PET images (not shown) the resting left ventricular function was moderately depressed with global hypokinesis, which was more severe in the anteroseptal region. The PET images were consistent with a large area of anteroseptal scar without evidence of significant ischemia. Furthermore, the CT images acquired for attenuation correction demonstrate the presence of an apical aneurysm with evidence of calcification (arrow, **64**).

Discussion

There is a wide spectrum of severity of scarring that can be seen following myocardial infarction. In this patient, it has taken the most extreme form of transmural scarring. In addition to the functional compromises caused, it also predisposes the patient to the development of life-threatening ventricular tachyarrhythmias and the development of mural thrombus.

Management

Because there was no evidence of ischemia, no further cardiac evaluation was necessary prior to this patient's surgery. However, given his depressed resting left ventricular function, close peri-operative monitoring of his volume status was recommended.

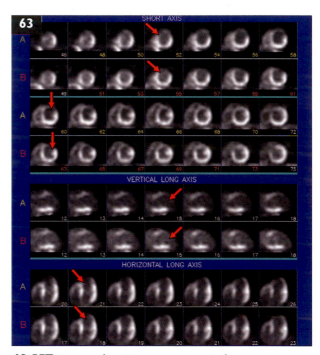

63 PET images showing an anteroapical scar.

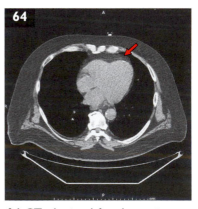

64 CT obtained for the patient shown in **63**, which was used for attenuation correction of the PET study. Note the area of calcification (arrow), which represents a calcified aneurysm.

Case 14: PET Showing Viable Myocardium

Clinical history

A 70-year-old male with a history of anterior wall myocardial infarction and severe anterior wall hypokinesis (left ventricular EF: 35%) was referred for evaluation of myocardial viability. Coronary angiography revealed a complex, heavily calcified stenosis in the LAD.

Imaging protocol

The patient underwent a resting ^{82}Rb PET perfusion study with an injection of 51.2 mCi of rubidium. Following perfusion imaging, the patient received intravenous injections of insulin to maximize myocardial glucose uptake and subsequently was injected with 7.3 mCi of the glucose analog, FDG, and underwent imaging of myocardial glucose uptake.

Impression

The resting PET images show a large perfusion defect in the anteroseptal region extending from the apex to the base of the heart (arrows, **65**). The FDG images demonstrate enhanced glucose uptake (arrowheads, **65**) in the same anteroseptal region in which there is a perfusion defect. The PET images demonstrate a mismatch between flow (^{82}Rb imaging) and metabolism (FDG imaging), which indicates the presence of viable myocardium in the anteroseptal region.

Discussion

Viability assessment based on the comparison of flow and metabolism by PET imaging, and more recently also by SPECT imaging of PET tracers (Sandler & Patton 1996), identifies viable myocardium based on the fact that viable myocardium that is chronically hypoperfused will demonstrate glucose uptake that is enhanced relative to the perfusion defect (mismatch). This is in contrast to a region of myocardial scar in which

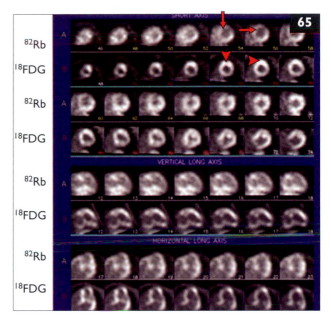

65 PET viability study showing uptake of FDG (arrowheads) in the anteroseptal region which has reduced perfusion (arrows) consistent with viable but hibernating myocardium.

there is a similar decrease in both flow and metabolism (match). Detecting the presence of viable myocardium is useful in identifying patients who will have a significant improvement in left ventricular regional wall motion and overall left ventricular function following revascularization (Tillisch *et al.* 1986).

Management

Based on the presence of viable myocardium, the patient underwent percutaneous coronary intervention with debulking of the calcified lesion in the LAD with subsequent successful angioplasty and stenting of the lesion.

Case 15: ERNA with Normal Left Ventricular Function

Clinical history

A 56-year-old female with a history of leukemia undergoing chemotherapy was referred for assessment of left ventricular function prior to receiving a dose of doxorubicin. Her cumulative doxorubicin dose to date was 250 mg/m².

Imaging protocol

A sample of the patient's red blood cells was labeled with 32.8 mCi of ^{99m}Tc-pertechnetate using the *in vitro* method. Gated planar images were acquired in three standard views (left anterior oblique, anterior, and lateral).

Impression

The gated ERNA images demonstrate normal left ventricular systolic function with an EF of 59% (66; lower limit of normal ERNA left ventricular EF: 50%) and normal left ventricular diastolic function with a PFR of 2.75 end-diastolic volumes (EDV)/s (lower limit of normal: 2.50 EDV/s). The heart chamber sizes were all normal and the left ventricular EDV was normal at 71 mL (upper limit of normal EDV: 140 mL).

Discussion

Left ventricular function, usually assessed as the EF, is a very important prognostic factor in patients with CAD (Zaret *et al.* 1995). In addition, the determination of EF is crucial for assessing cardiotoxicity in patients receiving anthracycline chemotherapeutic agents, such as doxorubicin. Gated blood pool imaging, such as ERNA, provides a reproducible method for determining left ventricular function.

Management

Because there was no evidence of cardiotoxicity, the patient received her next round of chemotherapy with plans to monitor her left ventricular function.

End-diastole

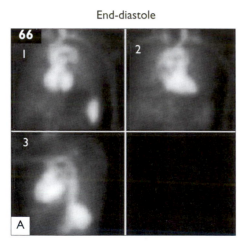

End-systole

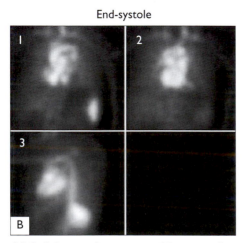

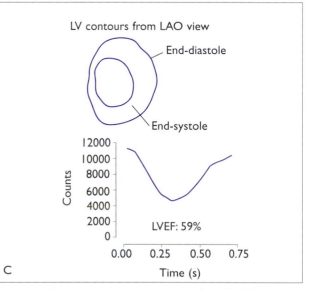

66 Still frames from an equilibrium radionuclide angiographic study obtained at end-diastole (**A**) and end-systole (**B**) from an individual with normal left ventricular function. The changes in the left ventricular cavity are shown in outline in the upper panel of (**C**) and the count-activity curve based on the radioactivity in the left ventricle is shown in the lower panel of (**C**) (1: left anterior oblique; 2: anterior; 3: lateral.)

Case 16: ERNA with Depressed Left Ventricular Function

Clinical history

A 24-year-old female with a history of breast cancer who had a previous history of receiving doxorubicin chemotherapy (cumulative doxorubicin dose to date was 500 mg/m^2) was referred for assessment of left ventricular function.

Imaging protocol

A sample of the patient's red blood cells was labeled with 30.1 mCi of ^{99m}Tc-pertechnetate using the *in vitro* method. Gated planar images were acquired in the left anterior oblique, anterior, and lateral positions.

Impression

The gated ERNA images demonstrate severely depressed left ventricular systolic function with an EF of 28% and impaired left ventricular diastolic function with a PFR of 2.13 EDV/s (**67**). The heart chambers were enlarged and the left ventricular EDV was increased, at 168 mL.

Discussion

This case demonstrates the utility of assessing left ventricular function by ERNA. The decreased left ventricular EF and PFR are consistent with impaired systolic and diastolic function secondary to doxorubicin cardiotoxicity (Singal & Iliskovic 1998).

Management

Based on the depressed left ventricular function, no further chemotherapy was planned for the patient. In addition, she was started on angiotensin converting enzyme inhibitor and diuretic therapy to treat her heart failure.

End-diastole

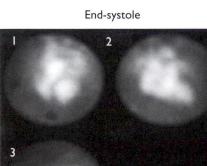

End-systole

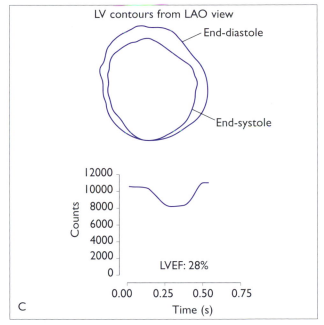

67 Still frames from an equilibrium radionuclide angiographic study obtained at end-diastole (**A**) and end-systole (**B**) from an individual with doxorubicin cardiotoxicity. The changes in the left ventricular cavity are shown in outline in the upper panel of (**C**) and the left ventricular count-activity curve based on the radioactivity in the left ventricle is shown in the lower panel of (**C**). Note the minimal changes in the ventricular cavity between end-systole and end-diastole. (1: left anterior oblique; 2: anterior; 3: lateral.)

Case 17: Gated SPECT with Normal Perfusion and Normal Left Ventricular Function

Clinical history

A 57-year-old female with a history of diabetes was referred for stress testing with a history of increasing shortness of breath. Of note, her fasting blood glucose concentration was 11.66 mmol/L and her hemoglobin A1C content was 9.7%.

Imaging protocol

The patient exercised on a treadmill for a total of 7 minutes, 25 s, reaching Stage 3 of a Bruce protocol with an estimated workload of 10.1 METs. Resting heart rate was 70 bpm and increased to 155 bpm at peak exercise (95% of the age predicted maximal heart rate). Her resting blood pressure was 128/84 mmHg and increased to 190/90 mmHg at peak exercise. The patient did not experience chest pain during stress. There were no ECG changes diagnostic for ischemia during stress. Myocardial perfusion imaging was performed with the injection of 16.3 mCi of ^{99m}Tc-sestamibi at rest and 25.4 mCi of ^{99m}Tc-sestamibi at peak stress. SPECT imaging showed no perfusion defects. The gated SPECT images revealed a normal resting left ventricular function and no wall motion abnormalities.

Impression

The gated SPECT study shows normal myocardial perfusion with normal global and regional left ventricular function (**68**).

Discussion

As compared with gated blood pool imaging with ERNA, gated SPECT can be used to assess left ventricular function based on radiotracer accumulation in the heart muscle rather than in the blood pool. The EF is determined by identifying the left ventricular cavity. Several studies have demonstrated a good correlation between the EF determined by ERNA and the EF determined by gated SPECT. However, there are situations in which gated SPECT is not as accurate, including in the presence of dense perfusion defects and in small hearts (Vallejo *et al.* 2000b).

Management

The patient required no further cardiac evaluation, based on the results of the stress test. She was counseled on tight glycemic control for her diabetes.

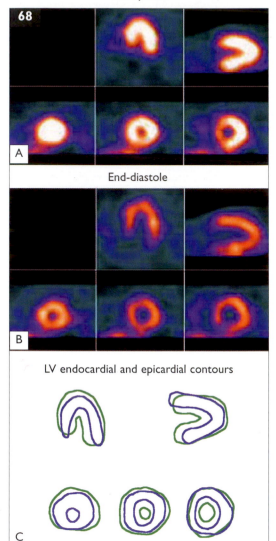

End-systole

A

End-diastole

B

LV endocardial and epicardial contours

C

68 Gated SPECT assessment of left ventricular function in a patient with normal myocardial perfusion and normal left ventricular function. Still frames from end-systole and end-diastole are shown in (**A**) and (**B**) and (**C**) shows the outline of the left ventricle at end-systole (green) and end-diastole (blue).

Case 18: Gated SPECT with Scar, Depressed Left Ventricular Function

Clinical history

An 87-year-old male with a history of a prior anterior wall myocardial infarction and ischemic cardio-myopathy was referred for stress testing because of increasing shortness of breath and lower extremity edema. Of note, the patient had stopped taking his furosemide.

Imaging protocol

The patient underwent an adenosine ^{99m}Tc-tetrofosmin SPECT myocardial perfusion study. The resting heart rate was 85 bpm and increased to 96 bpm at peak adenosine infusion. His blood pressure decreased from 138/80 mmHg to 86/42 mmHg at peak adenosine infusion. The baseline ECG showed a left bundle branch block pattern, which did not change during adenosine infusion. The patient underwent resting imaging with 16.5 mCi of ^{99m}Tc-sestamibi and stress imaging with 27.0 mCi of ^{99m}Tc-sestamibi. The gated SPECT images showed a large anteroseptal perfusion defect on both the stress and rest images. Left ventricular function was severely depressed and there was evidence of anteroseptal akinesis. Compared to a gated myocardial perfusion stress test obtained 2 years before the current study, there has been no significant change in either the size of the perfusion defect or left ventricular function.

Impression

The gated SPECT study shows evidence of a large anteroseptal scar, consistent with the patient's history of a previous anterior wall myocardial infarction (arrows, **69**). As a result of this myocardial infarction, there has been adverse remodeling affecting the entire ventricle.

Discussion

In this patient, a myocardial perfusion study was obtained to determine if the patient's new symptoms were due to new areas of ischemia or a further decrease in left ventricular function. As discussed above, a more accurate determination of left ventricular function may be obtained by ERNA, which would be important if the patient is being considered for placement of an ICD.

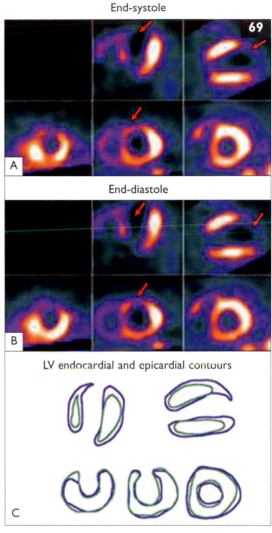

End-systole

End-diastole

LV endocardial and epicardial contours

69 Gated SPECT assessment of left ventricular function in a patient with a large anteroseptal scar (**A**, **B**, arrows) and severely depressed left ventricular function. Note the minimal thickening and movement of the left ventricle based on the outlines of the left ventricle at end-systole (green) and end-diastole (blue) (**C**).

Management

Based on the results of the perfusion study, it suggests that the patient's symptoms were not due to new ischemia, but rather due to his medical noncompliance. After diuresis, the patient felt better. He also underwent an ERNA, which demonstrated a left ventricular EF of 25% and the patient was referred for ICD placement.

4. ECHOCARDIOGRAPHIC IMAGING

Robert L. McNamara   Farid Jadbabaie   Kathleen Stergiopoulos

INTRODUCTION

The application of ultrasound to view cardiac structures is commonly attributed to Inge Edler, a Swedish cardiologist, in 1953. Although by today's standards, these instruments were very limited, within a decade many common cardiac conditions, such as mitral stenosis, aortic stenosis, tumors, and pericardial effusion could be diagnosed. The original technique evaluated only the amplitude of the sound wave and was termed A-mode. By assigning values to different brightnesses in the display the imaging technique became B-mode. When using the information across time to evaluate the motion of cardiac structures the technique was called M-mode, which remains an important diagnostic tool. The development of the linear scanner facilitated the translation of these images into two-dimensional display. Subsequent introduction of the sector scan enabled the two-dimensional images to be viewed in real time. In the early cardiac ultrasound history, Japanese investigators applied Doppler principles in the evaluation of pressure gradients across the aortic valve. Since then spectral Doppler has become a practical diagnostic tool. Assigning colors to specific velocities and simultaneously displaying these colors on the two-dimensional images lead to the development of color flow Doppler. These major echocardiographic techniques, M-mode, two-dimensional, spectral Doppler, and color Doppler, constitute the basis of the present standard transthoracic echocardiographic examination.

These standard techniques can also be applied in more specific ways. As gases are echodense (bright), imaging the heart after the introduction of small bubbles into the bloodstream is called contrast echocardiography. Stress echocardiography images patients in two dimensions before and after a stress test to assess wall motion. Combining multiple two-dimensional planes by precise mapping results in a three-dimensional display. By placing the ultrasound crystals on a smaller probe and inserting the probe down the esophagus, the heart can be imaged from the posterior perspective and from positions much closer to the heart. This technique is termed transesophageal echocardiography (TEE).

Approximately one in ten people over the age of 65 receive some form of echocardiography each year (Lucas *et al.* 1999), making rest echocardiography one of the most widely used imaging tools in cardiology. In addition to these officially documented and billed studies, focused studies using hand-held machines are increasingly popular in emergency departments, intensive care units, and even in outpatient clinics. Although other noninvasive modalities such as nuclear imaging, CT, MRI, and PET are also available to image the heart, echocardiography is rapid, portable, and relatively inexpensive. Advances in image quality, development of new uses (such as the relatively new application of tissue Doppler imaging), and the increase in prevalence of patients with cardiovascular disease ensures the continued growth in the use of echocardiography.

Indications for transthoracic echocardiography (TTE) are broad and include most cardiovascular diagnoses and many noncardiovascular ones. The American College of Cardiology and the American Society of Echocardiography published guidelines in 2003 (Cheitlin *et al.* 2003). The wide evaluation spectrum of left ventricular function which includes global EF, segmental wall motion, cardiac valve stenosis, regurgitation, or vegetations and pericardial effusion, may be the main reason that the majority of patients are referred for echocardiography. Other indications of echocardiography may include the examination of right ventricular size and function and the estimation of pulmonary artery pressures, particularly for patients with pulmonary abnormalities. Estimation of chamber sizes and wall thicknesses and evaluation of congenital heart disease are also common in echocardiography.

Stress echocardiography is usually performed to identify segmental wall motion abnormalities at rest or with stress (either after exercise or by pharmacological means) to evaluate patients with known or suspected CAD. The ability to visualize valvular function with exercise provides a relatively unique but less common use of echocardiography. TEE provides high-resolution images and is particularly important for evaluation of cardiac sources of emboli for patients with stroke, examination of the cardiac valves for patients with suspected endocarditis, visualization of prosthetic valves, and identification of abnormalities of the aorta.

These examinations are performed both for patients without known cardiac abnormalities for diagnostic purposes and for patients with known cardiac disease. A murmur on physical examination often prompts evaluation for valvular heart disease. Patients with shortness of breath, chest pain, fatigue, arrhythmias, or palpitations will often undergo echocardiography to assess left ventricular function. Persistent fevers and/or bacteremia, particularly for patients with indwelling catheters, are often evaluated for suspected endocarditis. Patients with known valvular heart disease are frequently followed with serial examinations (e.g. yearly) to identify progression of disease before symptoms develop. Patients with myocardial infarction are routinely assessed for prognosis. Potential progression of a previously identified pericardial effusion can also be evaluated serially.

As mentioned previously, the portability of echocardiography enables its use in a multitude of settings. In addition to the traditional studies performed within the echocardiography laboratory, complete studies are frequently performed for patients in intensive care units. TEE is often performed during cardiac as well as occasionally noncardiac surgery. Although frequently undocumented, focused examinations are increasingly being performed for patients in the emergency department, for patients in the hospital on work rounds, and for patients in outpatient clinics when a full imaging laboratory is not easily accessible. As the imaging systems become smaller, lighter, and less expensive, their uses will likely increase.

PHYSICS AND IMAGE GENERATION
Physics
Echocardiography is the technique of obtaining dynamic real-time images of cardiac structures using reflections of transmitted ultrasound waves. A basic knowledge of ultrasound physics and instrumentation is necessary for optimal use and understanding of the applications and limitations of this technique. Sound waves are areas of compression and rarefaction in the molecules that are created by vibrations of the sound source and propagated through the physical medium. These compression and rarefactions are best described by a sine wave.

Sound waves are characterized by amplitude or loudness, frequency or the number of cycles per second or Hertz (Hz), and wavelength or the distance between two consecutive peaks. Speed of travel of sound through the medium or propagation velocity, is determined by density of the medium. Propagation velocity through blood and soft tissue is faster than air and is approximately 1540 m/s. The relationship between frequency (f), wavelength (λ) and propagation velocity (V) can be formulated as:

$$V \, (m/s) = f \, (Hz) \times \lambda \, (m). \qquad (1)$$

Sound waves with frequencies between 20 Hz and 20 KHz are audible and can be heard by humans. Ultrasound waves are sound waves with frequencies above 20 KHz. Ultrasound waves commonly used in medical imaging have a frequency range of 1–40 million Hertz or mega Hertz (MHz).

At tissue interfaces, ultrasound waves can be transmitted straight through, reflected (transmitted back), or refracted (transmitted at a different angle). The reflected sound waves can be received by the transducer and generate real-time images. These interactions are determined by acoustic impedance, or capacity of transmitting sound for each tissue. Acoustic impedance (Z) is the product of tissue density (ρ) and velocity of propagation through the tissue (V):

$$Z = \rho \cdot V. \qquad (2)$$

The amount of ultrasound energy reflected depends on the difference in acoustic impedance at either side of the interface as well as the angle of incidence of sound beams. The larger the difference of acoustic impedance and the more perpendicular to the interface, the higher the percentage of reflected ultrasound beam.

With passage of ultrasound waves through the tissue, there is a steady loss of ultrasound energy. This energy loss, or attenuation, is largely due to heat conversion from tissue friction and ultrasound dispersion from scatter. The higher the ultrasound frequency and the farther the distance traveled, the greater the attenuation.

Image generation

Ultrasound signals are generated by the piezoelectric crystal in the transducer. Once exposed to an electric current, the polarized molecules in the crystal change alignment with the direction of electricity. Exposure to alternate electric current leads to vibration of the crystal and creation of the ultrasound waves. Piezoelectric crystals in current-phased array transducers contain multiple smaller crystal elements, each individually creating an ultrasound wave. These waves create a front that is the ultrasound beam. Electronic control of timing of activation on each crystal allows for electronic steering and focusing of the ultrasound beam.

Ultrasound wave is generated in a pulsatile form. The shape of the waves and the number of cycles in each pulse are set for characteristics of each individual machine and determine penetration and image resolution. The frequency at which this ultrasound pulse is generated is called pulse repetition frequency (PRF). Once a pulse is generated, there is adequate 'listening time' allowing for return of the reflected pulse. Vibrations from reflected ultrasound waves in the crystal create alternate electric currents that can be further processed into real-time images.

Given relatively constant speed of sound in the tissues, the time required for return of the reflected signal determines the depth of structure from the transducer and the amplitude represents the strength of returning signals. Therefore, the location and intensity

of reflected signals can be displayed as horizontal spikes (A-mode) or dots with varying degree of brightness (B-mode) along the vertical axis of display. The sizes of the spikes or degree of brightness correlate to strength of returning signals. B-mode signals can also be displayed over time (M-mode), creating an image with very high temporal resolution (~2,000 frames/s).

Two-dimensional images are created by sweeping the updated B-mode images along the tomographic plane. Since finite time is required to generate each B-mode line (scan line), the rate of creating a single two-dimensional image (or frame) depends on the number of scan lines and the depth of the structure. Thus, there is a trade off between the number of scan lines and the frame rate. Temporal resolution in the two-dimensional images depends on both the number of scan lines (scan line density) and the frame rate. Typically 100–200 scan lines/frame and 30–60 frames/s are required to display motion of cardiac structures adequately. Other determinants of two-dimensional image quality are axial and lateral resolution. Axial resolution is the ability to distinguish two neighboring points along the direction of ultrasound beam. Ultrasound wave frequency (transducer frequency) is the most important determinant of axial resolution. Lateral resolution, or the ability to distinguish two neighboring points across the direction of ultrasound beam, is equal to the beam size at any given point along the path of ultrasound beam. Lateral resolution is highest at focal zone. As the ultrasound beam diverges with depth, lateral resolution will subsequently decline.

Doppler imaging is an integral part of an echocardiographic examination and is based on the principle that frequency of sound produced by a moving object is higher when the object is moving toward the observer than when the object is moving away from the observer. This phenomenon is due to compression of sound waves in the direction toward the motion and expansion in the direction opposite to the motion. Using the same principle, the reflected ultrasound waves traveling from red blood cells would have higher frequency if blood flow is toward the transducer and have lower frequency if the flow is in the opposite direction. The difference in transmitted (F_T) and received (F_R) frequencies, or Doppler shift, is related to the velocity (V) of red blood cells, the speed of travel of sound in the blood (C), and the angle (θ) between the directions of blood flow and ultrasound wave beam (angle of incidence) as expressed below:

$$F_R - F_T = V \frac{2 F_T \cos(\theta)}{C}. \qquad (3)$$

The angle of incidence is critically important in the measurement of the velocity. When flow is parallel to ultrasound beam (0° or 180°) $\cos(\theta)$ is equal to one. However, as θ increases, the measured velocity would be under estimated. At 90°, $\cos(\theta)$ is zero and there would be no Doppler shift recorded. The frequency difference between transmitted and reflected ultrasound signals is analyzed using Fourier analysis. All detected velocities are displayed as pixels in a time–velocity plot known as spectral Doppler.

In pulse wave (PW) Doppler, pulses of ultrasound are transmitted and received by the same crystal after allowing for required travel time from the transducer to the depth of interest and return. By setting the time interval between the pulses (PRF), reflected signals from a desired depth (sample volume) can be obtained. Therefore, PW Doppler can provide information on blood flow velocity from a specific location. Maximum Doppler shift measured by PW Doppler is limited by the sampling rate (or PRF). The maximal detectable Doppler shift frequency also known as Nyquist limit is equal to one half of the PRF.

In continuous wave (CW) Doppler, two separate crystals are used for transmission and reception of ultrasound signals, eliminating the need for ultrasound pulsation. All the velocity information along the path of ultrasound beam is obtained without limitation on the maximal blood flow velocities detected. However, velocity at specific locations along the path of the beam cannot be obtained.

Color Doppler is a special technique for real-time display of velocity and direction of blood flow superimposed on a two-dimensional image. Velocity information is obtained through multiple PW Doppler sampled volumes and displayed in a color scale. By convention, shades of red are assigned for flow towards the transducer and blue for flow away in the opposite direction. The constructed color map is then superimposed on the two-dimensional image. Similar to PW Doppler, color Doppler images are limited by Nyquist limit, with high velocities creating a mosaic of colors. Temporal resolution of color Doppler images is lower than regular two-dimensional images due to the time required for obtaining both color information and two-dimensional image. Usually, the image resolution is optimized by using a smaller color window or a narrower image sector.

Standard transthoracic echocardiographic views

Standard TTE images are obtained by placing the transducer over the acoustic windows on the chest wall. For image orientation, the American Society of Echocardiography recommends that the location of transducer (apex of the image sector) is displayed at top of image, left ventricular lateral wall toward the right of the screen, and right ventricle toward the left of the screen.

In the parasternal window, the transducer is placed in the third or fourth intercostal space adjacent to the left sternal border. The parasternal long-axis view is an image plane across mitral and aortic valves, left atrium, portions of left ventricle along anteroseptal and inferolateral (posterior) walls, and right ventricular outflow tract (**70**). This view is particularly useful for visualization of structures in the base of the heart. By tilting the transducer medially and caudally, the parasternal view of the right ventricular inflow can be obtained. In this view, the image plane is across the right atrium, tricuspid valve, and proximal portions of the right ventricle.

By rotating the transducer clockwise, one can obtain imaging planes across the parasternal short axis of the left ventricle at multiple levels perpendicular to the long axis of the heart. In the short-axis view of the

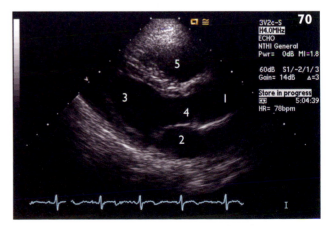

70 Parasternal long-axis view. (1: aorta; 2: left atrium; 3: left ventricle; 4: left ventricular outflow tract; 5: right ventricle.)

base of the heart, a cross-section of aortic valve, and, anterior to it, a section of tricuspid valve and right ventricular outflow tract including pulmonic valve can be seen (**71**). By tilting the transducer apically along the long axis of the left ventricle, short-axis views across the mitral valve and a mid-ventricular short-axis view across the papillary muscles and apex can be obtained (**72**).

In the apical window, the transducer is placed at the apex of the heart. The image plane in this window extends from the apex to the base along the long axis of the left ventricle. The apical window is particularly useful for the assessment of regional wall motion as well as Doppler evaluation of flow across the aortic, mitral, and tricuspid valves. In the apical four-chamber view, the imaging plane is adjusted to obtain a horizontal cut through both left and right ventricles. In this view, the lateral walls and apex of both ventricles as well as the interventricular septum are visualized (**73**). By tilting the transducer superiorly, an apical five-chamber view can be obtained. In this view the image plane includes the aortic valve and small portion of the aorta (**74**).

The apical two-chamber view is obtained by a 90° counterclockwise rotation of the transducer from an apical four-chamber view. In this view a vertical cut through the left ventricle (anterior and inferior walls), mitral valve, and left atrium is obtained (**75**). The apical three-chamber view is obtained by a further counterclockwise rotation of the transducer to include

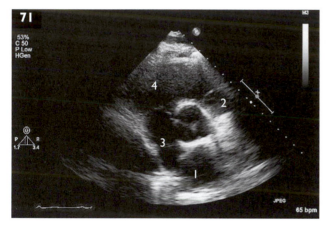

71 High parasternal short-axis view. (1: left atrium; 2: pulmonary artery; 3: right atrium; 4: right ventricle.)

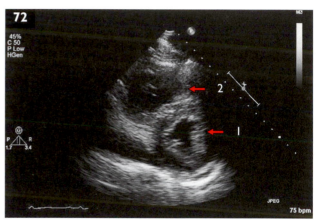

72 Parasternal short-axis view. (1: left ventricle; 2: right ventricle.)

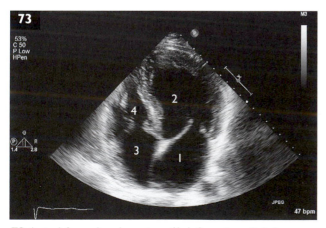

73 Apical four-chamber view. (1: left atrium, 2: left ventricle; 3: right atrium; 4: right ventricle.)

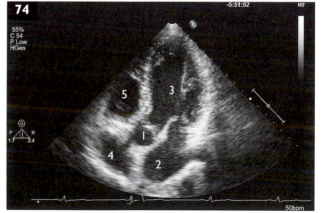

74 Apical five-chamber view. (1: aorta; 2: left atrium; 3: left ventricle; 4: right atrium; 5: right ventricle.)

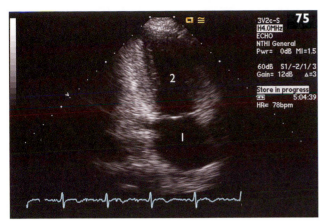

75 Apical two-chamber view. (1: left atrium; 2: left ventricle.)

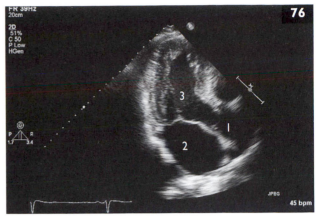

76 Apical three-chamber view. (1: aorta; 2: left atrium; 3: left ventricle.)

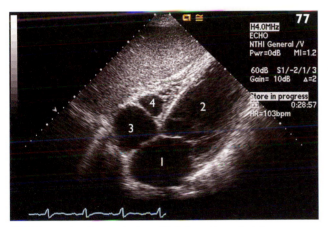

77 Normal subcostal view. (1: left atrium; 2: left ventricle; 3: right atrium; 4: right ventricle.)

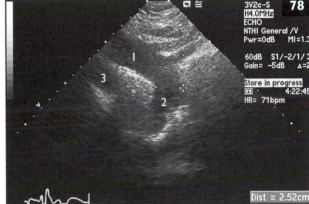

78 View from the suprasternal notch. (1: aorta; 2: descending aorta; 3: pulmonary artery.)

a long-axis cut through the aortic valve and ascending aorta as well as portions of the right ventricular outflow tract. The anterior septum and posterior walls of the left ventricle can be seen as well (**76**).

For the subcostal view window, the transducer is placed below the xyphoid process and the ultrasound beam is directed towards the left shoulder with the marker pointing to the left of the patient. The subcostal four-chamber view is similar to the apical four-chamber with the image plane across both the left and right ventricles (**77**). By a counterclockwise rotation of the transducer, a subcostal short-axis view is obtained and can be adjusted to include the inferior vena cava and hepatic veins.

The suprasternal window is obtained by placing the transducer in the suprasternal notch and pointing inferiorly (**78**). The image plane is adjusted to obtain a long-axis cut through the aortic arch and ascending and descending aorta. In this view, take-off of head vessels from the aortic arch are seen. This view is best used for the assessment of the aortic arch and flow in the proximal descending aorta.

M-MODE AND TWO-DIMENSIONAL ECHOCARDIOGRAPHY IN EVALUATION OF CARDIAC DISEASES
Chamber sizes
Many cardiac diseases are caused by increase in size of the heart chambers. Quantitating these changes is important in echocardiography. The American Society of Echocardiography has published guidelines for the

quantification of the chamber sizes (Lang *et al.* 2005). Initially M-mode was used due to the high spatial resolution and high timing precision. In the parasternal long-axis view, linear measurements for right ventricular end-diastolic dimension, left ventricular end-diastolic dimension, left ventricular end-systolic dimension, and left atrial end-diastolic dimension are often obtained using the 'leading edge' technique. This technique specifies that each point of the measurement be placed on the near edge (closest to the transducer) of the bright echo corresponding to the appropriate interface. For left ventricular cavity measurements these interfaces are located between the interventricular septum and the ventricular cavity and between the left ventricular cavity and the posterior wall. However, M-mode only provides information along the lines originating from the transducer (**79**). Unless the desired chamber size is exactly parallel to one of these lines, the measurement will be inaccurate. Often the measurements obtained from M-mode overestimate the chamber sizes as compared to those obtained from two-dimensional echocardiography.

Two-dimensional echocardiography offers the flexibility of measuring along any line within the image plane. Improved image resolution and easier determination of precise timing during viewing have increased the use of two-dimensional echocardiography for the determination of the same chamber measurements that can be obtained from M-mode. Although the parasternal long-axis view displays the left ventricle

relatively perpendicular to the ultrasound waves in the majority of patients, many patients' hearts are displayed at a significant angle (so called 'vertical hearts'). Measurements made from two-dimensional echocardiography provide superior accuracy for the chamber size. Frequently, the measurements from M-mode and two-dimensional echocardiography can be discordant by 10–20%. In addition to this superior accuracy, two-dimensional linear measurements can be obtained in multiple views. The parasternal view often does not provide a fair representation of the right ventricle due to its complex shape. Right ventricular short-axis measurements as well as a long-axis measurement can be obtained from the four-chamber view (Lang *et al.* 2005). Normal right ventricular size is approximately two-thirds that of the left ventricle. The left atrium often enlarges more in a longitudinal direction than in the short-axis direction that is measured in parasternal views. The apical four-chamber view and, less often, the apical two- and three-chamber views are used to measure the longitudinal axis of the left atrium. The right atrium is not well characterized by parasternal views. Measurements are made in the apical views similar to those for the left atrium.

Two-dimensional imaging not only improves accuracy in linear measurements but adds the capability of area measurements. Using geometric assumptions, the combination of measurements from one or two views can be used to estimate the chamber volumes, in particular left ventricular diastolic and systolic volumes. The simplest technique applies only linear measurements. For instance, left ventricular volume can be assumed to be a sphere, a cylinder on top of a cone, a truncated ellipse, or a bullet. The disadvantage of these techniques is the assumption of symmetric contraction. Not only do different walls contract to different degrees in the normal heart, but cardiac function after a myocardial infarction typically shows regional variation. Thus, left ventricular volumes obtained using linear measurements in patients with ischemic heart disease may be significantly flawed. Nevertheless, two-dimensional echocardiography enables one to trace directly an outline of the endocardial walls. Currently, the most common method for determining left ventricular volume is based on the geometric assumption that the left ventricle is a stack of thin disks (**80, 81**). By outlining the endocardial walls in two-chamber and

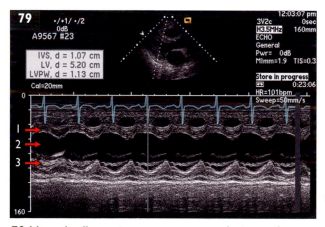

79 M-mode, illustrating measurements during end-diastole. (1: interventricular septum; 2: left ventricle; 3: left ventricular posterior wall.)

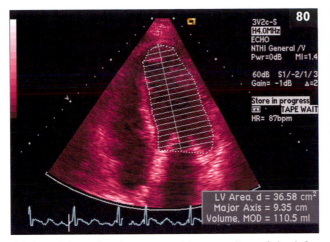

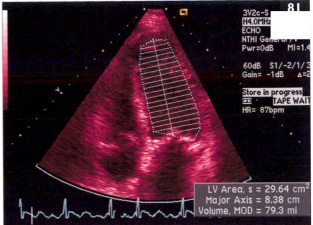

80 Apical four-chamber view with an outline of the left ventricle during diastole. Left ventricular volume is estimated by the Simpson's method of disks.

81 Apical four-chamber view with an outline of the left ventricle during systole. Thus, with the volume of 110.5 mL during diastole and 79.3 mL during systole, the EF is (110.5 - 79.5)/110.5 = 28%.

four-chamber views along with a linear measurement of the long axis, the individual volumes of multiple 'disks' within the left ventricular cavity can be estimated and subsequently combined to obtain total left ventricular volume. While this method usually provides a more accurate volume than that using only linear measurements, obtaining views that include the true apex remains difficult, particularly in the two-chamber view. Shortening of the apex may significantly underestimate left ventricular volume. Once the estimates of the left ventricular volumes are obtained for both diastole and systole, assessment of stroke volumes and EF can be calculated. Stroke volume is the difference between the left ventricular diastolic volume and the left ventricular systolic volume. EF is the stroke volume divided by the left ventricular diastolic volume (see Left ventricular systolic function).

In addition to left ventricular volumes, other chamber volumes can also be obtained using the method described above. While the single linear measurement of left atrial size obtained from the parasternal long-axis view has been standard, an estimate of left atrial volume is increasingly being performed. As with left ventricular volume, left atrial volume can be estimated using only linear measurements or a combination of area tracing and linear measurements obtained from the apical views (**82**). Although less frequently performed, a similar estimate for right atrial volume can be obtained. Linear measurements or the 'multiple disks' method

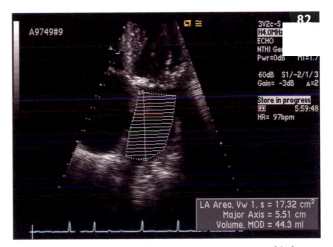

82 Four chamber-view showing measurement of left atrial area. By combining the area measured in the two-chamber view, a left atrial volume can be estimated.

in the apical view have been employed to estimate right ventricular volume, but the accuracy is limited by the irregular shape of the right ventricle.

Left ventricular systolic function

Left ventricular systolic function is a powerful predictor of prognosis in the majority of cardiovascular disorders including ischemic heart disease, heart failure, and valvular disease. Echocardiography enables both qualitative and quantitative assessments of left ventricular systolic function with the use of M-mode, two-dimensional, and Doppler techniques. Left ventricular volume and EF as well as global and

Table 5 Left ventricular functions associated with ejection fraction

Left ventricular function	Ejection fraction
Hyperdynamic	>70%
Normal	50–70%
Mildly decreased	40–45%
Moderately decreased	30–35%
Severely decreased	<30%

regional function can be accurately assessed at the bedside (*Table 5*).

Several quantitative methods for the calculations of left ventricular volumes and EF have been described (Schiller *et al.* 1989). All of these methods are based on the geometric assumption of a symmetric shape (hemi-ellipsoid or cylinder and hemisphere) for the left ventricular cavity during various phases of the cardiac cycle. The cubed method is the most simplified approach and assumes the left ventricular cavity as a symmetric hemi-ellipsoid where the long-axis length is twice the short-axis diameter. The hemi-ellipsoid volume is therefore approximated as $V = D^3$, where D is the left ventricular internal diameter obtained from the parasternal long-axis view in the M-mode or two-dimensional echocardiography.

The cylinder and hemisphere, or bullet, method assumes a cylinder for the basilar portion of the left ventricle and a hemisphere for the apex. Left ventricular volume is calculated by summing the volumes of the cylinder and the hemisphere, in which the cross-sectional area from the short-axis mid-papillary level (A_m) and the length from a long axis view (L) are measured. Thus the left ventricular volume can be mathematically expressed as:

$$V = \frac{5}{6} A_m \cdot L. \qquad (4)$$

The left ventricular volume calculated by these methods is less accurate in the presence of regional wall motion abnormalities. The method of disks or the 'Simpson's rule' allows for more accurate and reproducible calculation of left ventricular volumes even in the presence of regional wall motion abnormalities. In this method, the left ventricle is divided into a stack of 20 disks along its long axis. The volume of each disk is calculated as the disk area multiplied by the disk length, and left ventricular

volume is calculated by summing the volumes of all disks as formulated below:

$$V = \sum_{n=20} \left[A_n \cdot \frac{L_n}{20} \right]. \qquad (5)$$

The recommended method by the American Society of Echocardiography is the modified Simpson's rule where the left ventricle is divided into three parallel disks with the cross-sectional area of A_1, A_2, and A_3 at the levels of the mitral annulus, papillary muscle, and apex, respectively. The height (h) of each disk is one-third of the long-axis length of the left ventricle. As a result, the volume can be calculated by:

$$V = (A_1 + A_2)h + \left(\frac{A_3 h}{2} \right) + \left(\frac{\pi h^3}{6} \right). \qquad (6)$$

By obtaining LV volumes at end-systole (ESV) and end-diastole (EDV), EF is calculated according to the formula:

$$EF = \frac{EDV - ESV}{EDV}. \qquad (7)$$

Most current echocardiographic imaging systems are equipped with software that uses the Simpson's rule for calculation of ventricular volumes. The technique requires identification and outline of endocardial borders in two orthogonal and four-chamber apical views at end-diastole and end-systole (**80, 81**). Thus, accurate assessment of volumes by Simpson's rule depends on clear identification of endocardial borders and on precise alignment of imaging planes through the center of the left ventricle from the apex to the base. Acoustic shadowing from ribs and papillary muscles can limit the visibility of endocardial borders.

Recently, some echocardiography platforms are equipped with three-dimensional matrix array transducers that obtain and display cardiac structures in relationship to each other in all three spatial dimensions. A 'full volume' three-dimensional data set of reflected signals from the entire left ventricle is acquired during a breath hold and over four consequent cardiac cycles. From this data set a three-dimensional image can be reconstructed. Using semi-automated endocardial tracing software, ventricular volumes can be accurately calculated. This technique requires image acquisitions through multiple cardiac cycles. Thus, a minor transducer or patient motion can result in significant loss in image quality and inaccurate measurement of ventricular volumes.

In addition to global left ventricular function, regional myocardial function is also routinely assessed by two-dimensional echocardiographic imaging. Ischemia or infarction caused by interruption of blood low in epicardial coronary arteries leads to impaired thickening and inward motion of a well defined myocardial territory. The American Society of Echocardiography has endorsed the 17-segment model recommended by the American Heart Association task force for description of regional wall motion (Lang *et al.* 2005). In this model, the left ventricle is divided into three sections: basilar, mid-ventricle, and apical. Basilar and mid-ventricular sections are each divided into six segments of anterior septum, anterior, anterior lateral, inferior lateral or posterior, inferior, and inferior septum. The apical section is divided into four segments of apical anterior, apical lateral, apical inferior, and apical septum, and a fifth segment of apex (**83**). A semi-quantitative scoring system is used to describe regional myocardial function. Wall motion is assessed in each visualized segment and a numeric score is assigned: 1 = normal, 2 = hypokinesis, 3 = akinesis, and 4 = dyskinesis. Wall motion score index is calculated by adding all segmental scores divided by the number of visualized segments. This scoring system is a useful methodology for accumulation and comparison of groups of participants, between different treatment groups in clinical trials.

Right ventricle

The normal shape of the right ventricle is complex in three dimensions. Therefore, imaging of the right ventricle can be difficult and usually requires multiple views. It wraps around and 'hugs' the left ventricle. The right ventricle can be visualized in two-dimensional echocardiographic imaging from multiple views. Namely the parasternal long-axis (**70**), short-axis (**72**), apical four-chamber (**73**), and subcostal four-chamber views (**77**). In each view, the size of the right ventricular cavity, shape, and systolic function of the right ventricular free wall can be evaluated. Moreover, information regarding the ventricular septal motion often reflects changes in the right ventricular pressure and function. The apical four-chamber and subcostal views tend to offer more complete and reliable information regarding the right ventricle. The right ventricular apex is normally closer to the base of the heart than the left ventricle. With right ventricular enlargement, the apex may be closer to or participate in forming part of the apex of the heart. The degree of right ventricular enlargement is usually estimated using the apical and subcostal views and compared to the left ventricular size, taking into account the size of the left ventricle. The degree of right ventricular enlargement is classified as mild when the right ventricle is between about three-quarters and equal to the size of the left ventricle; moderately enlarged when the right and left ventricles are approximately equal in size; and severely dilated in

83 Illustration of the 17-segment model endorsed by the American Society of Echocardiography, the American College of Cardiology, and the American Heart Association.

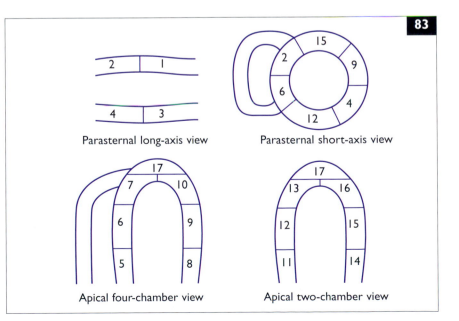

Parasternal long-axis view

Parasternal short-axis view

Apical four-chamber view

Apical two-chamber view

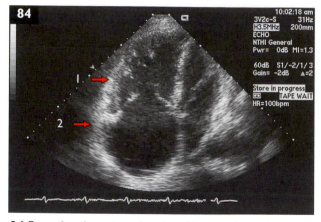

84 Four-chamber view showing dilation of the right ventricle (1) and right atrium (2).

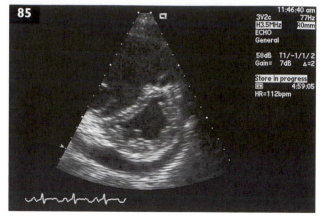

85 Parasternal short-axis view showing septal flattening ('D-shaped' septum) during diastole, consistent with right ventricular volume overload.

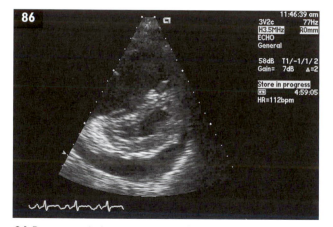

86 Parasternal short-axis view showing septal flattening ('D-shaped' septum) during systole, consistent with right ventricular pressure overload.

cases when the right ventricle is larger than the left ventricle (**84**). Pressure overload conditions, such as pulmonary hypertension, can also lead to right ventricular dilation. Hypertrophy of the right ventricular free wall can be seen in chronic pressure overload situations such as chronic pulmonary hypertension. It is usually defined as >0.5 cm thickness of the right ventricular free wall. If this finding is noted, a careful search for the etiology is certainly warranted. Other causes can be infiltrative disease such as amyloidosis, pulmonic stenosis, and hypertrophic cardiomyopathy (HCM).

The systolic function of the right ventricle is usually evaluated qualitatively as normal, mildly reduced, moderately reduced, and severely reduced.

In particular situations, such as pulmonary embolism, the right ventricular free wall can be hypokinetic with sparing of the right ventricular apex. This sign is referred to as McConnell's sign. The pattern of ventricular septal motion can be observed with two-dimensional or M-mode echocardiographic imaging. Certain cardiac disorders can alter the motion of the ventricular septum in a fairly typical manner. Perhaps most commonly, after cardiac surgery, the septum is noted to have a paradoxical motion in ventricular systole. Other conditions that can typically alter the ventricular septal motion are left and right bundle branch blocks, by altering the sequence in which the septum is activated to contract. Another common situation is the presence of right ventricular pressure and volume overload. The septum can appear flat (so called 'D-shaped') during ventricular diastole, in situations of volume overload (**85**). In this situation, the right ventricle is usually dilated. In situations of pure pressure overload, the right ventricle may not be dilated, but may demonstrate increased right ventricular wall thickness. The ventricular septum may appear flattened during systole (**86**), resulting in a leftward shift of the septum particularly at end-systole. In reality, both pressure and volume overload may be present. Pericardial disease, such as pericardial tamponade or constrictive physiology, can restrict the total cardiac volume. Changes in respiration may result in a change in ventricular septal motion, which may be a clue to the diagnosis, but is not usually diagnostic in either case.

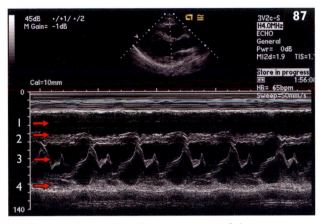

87 M-mode illustrating the movement of the mitral valve throughout the cardiac cycle. (1: right ventricle; 2: interventricular septum; 3: mitral valve; 4: posterior wall.)

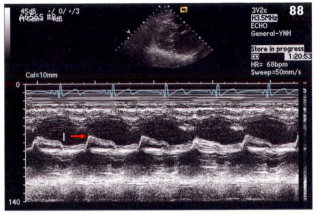

88 M-mode across the mitral valve showing thickening and delayed closure of the anterior leaflet (1), consistent with mitral stenosis.

Valves

The evaluation of valve morphology has been a valuable contribution of echocardiography from the beginning. Hemodynamic assessment of valvular function using 'spectral Doppler' will be discussed in a later section. The increased frame rate of M-mode enables assessment of subtle motion abnormalities, particularly of the mitral and aortic valve. Two-dimensional assessment of overall valve anatomy as well as leaflet thickness and mobility are standard for all four cardiac valves. The American Society of Echocardiography has published guidelines for the evaluation of valvular heart disease (Zoghbi *et al.* 2005).

The normal mitral valve consists of two leaflets, the crescent-shaped posterior leaflet and an oval-shaped anterior leaflet. The posterior leaflet is partially separated by septae into three scallops, designated P1, P2, and P3. Although no septae divide the anterior leaflet, for simplicity the corresponding sections of the anterior leaflet are designated A1, A2, and A3. The outer ring of the leaflets, the annulus, is saddle-shaped. The coaptation line of the two leaflets forms a slightly curved line and is lined on both sides with chordae that attach to the papillary muscles. The anterolateral papillary muscle provides chordae to the lateral aspect of both leaflets, and the posteromedial papillary muscle provides chordae to medial aspect of both leaflets.

M-mode evaluation of the mitral valve provides assessment of both leaflet thickness and mobility (**87**).

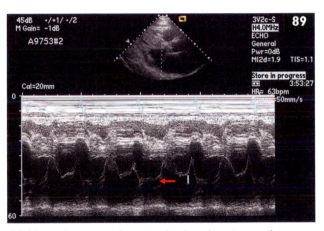

89 M-mode across the mitral valve showing prolapse (1) of the anterior leaflet.

Both mitral valve leaflets open during early ventricular diastole, begin to close during mid-diastole, and open again during late diastole. Leaflet thickening and decreased mobility of rheumatic mitral valve stenosis (**88**) can be identified by M-mode. The severity of mitral stenosis can be evaluated by M-mode; the slope of the closure of the mitral valve during early diastole is inversely correlated with severity. However, Doppler echocardiography of the mitral inflow generally provides a more accurate assessment. Mitral valve prolapse with the characteristic late systolic 'dip' of the leaflets, in particular the posterior leaflet, and the thickening of both leaflets is another pathologic finding often seen in the M-mode (**89**).

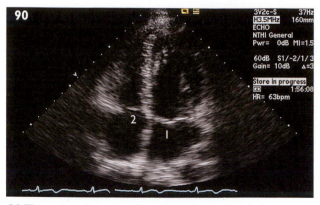

90 This apical four-chamber view shows the left and right ventricles during systole, with the mitral and tricuspid valves closed. (1: mitral valve; 2: tricuspid valve.)

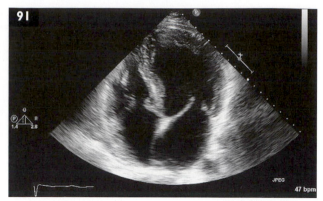

91 Apical four-chamber view during diastole, illustrating opening of the mitral and tricuspid valves.

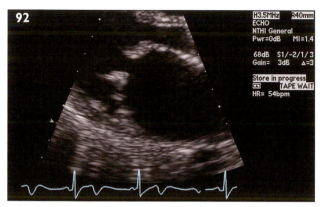

92 Parasternal long-axis view with a close-up of the mitral valve during diastole, illustrating the classic 'hockey stick' appearance of rheumatic mitral stenosis.

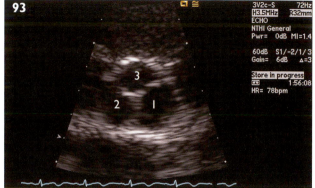

93 High parasternal short-axis view zoomed in on the aortic valve in cross-section demonstrating the three coronary cusps. (1: left coronary cusp; 2: noncoronary cusp; 3: right coronary cusp.)

Two-dimensional echocardiography provides a more thorough assessment of the mitral valve. Most importantly, the degree of flexibility of the leaflets can be seen in multiple views during systole (closed, **90**) and diastole (open, **91**). The decreased flexibility of the leaflet tips in mitral stenosis, with the classic 'hockey stick' appearance during diastole (**92**) is more completely assessed in two-dimensional echocardiography. In addition to qualitative assessment, the outline of the mitral orifice opening can be planimetered (traced) to give an estimated valve area. Suitability for percutaneous balloon valvotomy is assessed semi-quantitatively using four components seen on two-dimensional echocardiography: leaflet mobility, leaflet thickening, leaflet calcification, and subvalvular (chordal) involvement. Decreased flexibility is also seen when the leaflets are tethered toward the left ventricular apex due to remodeling after a myocardial infarction, with ischemia to a papillary muscle, or with chordal thickening. The increased flexibility of the mitral valve in mitral valve prolapse, with one of both leaflets extending into the left atrium during systole is more easily and reliably seen in two-dimensional than M-mode. Complete loss of integrity of one of the leaflets, such as with rupture of the papillary muscle, can result in a flail leaflet. In addition, mitral valve thickness and degree of calcification of the mitral annulus can be qualitatively assessed.

The normal aortic valve consists of three cusps named for the coronary artery that arises near it, the left coronary cusp, the right coronary cusp, and the noncoronary cusp (**93**). The three cusps meet at a thickened area at the mid-point of the free edge of each

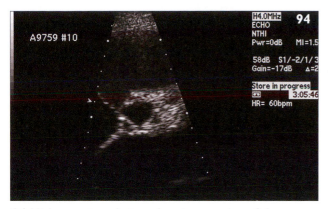

94 High parasternal view showing opening of the aortic valve.

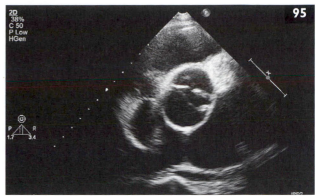

95 High parasternal short-axis view showing a bicuspid aortic valve.

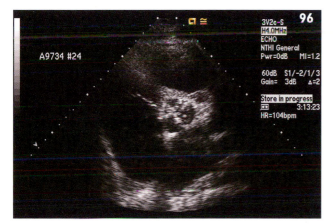

96 High parasternal short-axis view illustrating thickened aortic valve consistent with aortic stenosis.

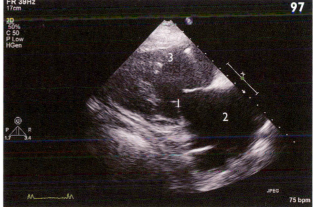

97 Parasternal 'tip-down' view showing the tricuspid valve (1), right atrium (2), and right ventricle (3) during diastole.

cusp, called the nodule of Arantius. Immediately distal to each cusp within the aorta is the sinus of Valsalva. In M-mode echocardiography, the normal motion of the aortic valve is identified with a single line during diastole and separation of the leaflets during systole. The size of the aortic root is routinely measured by M-mode.

Two-dimensional echocardiography provides good visualization of aortic valve morphology and motion. In the high short-axis view, all three cusps of the normal aortic valve can be visualized. During diastole the coaptation lines between each of the cusps forms a 'Y' shape, often referred to as an inverted 'Mercedes Benz sign' (**93**). When the valve opens during systole, the flexibility of each cusp can be visualized (**94**). Two leaflets at a time can also be seen in the parasternal long-axis view, the apical five-chamber view, and the apical three-chamber view. The relatively common congenital anomaly of bicuspid aortic valve can be

seen on two-dimensional echocardiographic imaging (**95**). The thickening and calcification as well as the decreased flexibility of the leaflets in aortic stenosis seen in two-dimensional echocardiography (**96**) provides a qualitative assessment to supplement the quantitative assessment of the hemodynamics with spectral Doppler. Tracing the opening orifice during systole in the high parasternal short-axis view may provide some insight into the degree of stenosis but has not proven reliable. Much less common than valvular aortic stenosis is supravalvular aortic stenosis or subaortic valvular stenosis.

As its name implies, the tricuspid valve has three leaflets, the larger anterior leaflet, the posterior leaflet, and the smaller septal leaflet. M-mode is rarely helpful in the assessment of the tricuspid valve, but two-dimensional echocardiography usually provides excellent visualization (**90, 97**). The tricuspid annulus

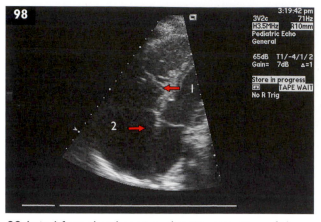

98 Apical four-chamber view showing insertion of the septal leaflet of the tricuspid valve (1) significantly more apical than the insertion of the mitral valve (2), characteristic of Ebstein's anomaly.

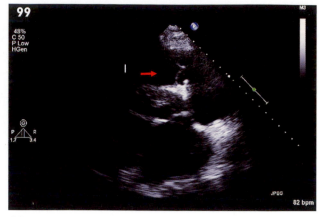

99 High parasternal short-axis view illustrating the pulmonary valve (1) during diastole.

is 0.5–1.0 cm more apical than the mitral annulus. Ebstein's anomaly is a congenital condition in which the tricuspid annulus is located more than 1 cm apical to the mitral annulus (**98**), with some right ventricular myocardium more basal to the tricuspid annulus. Tricuspid stenosis is relatively rare. However, carcinoid heart disease, an inflammatory response to an endocrine-secreting tumor, affects the tricuspid valve more often than the other valves and can cause stenosis.

The pulmonary valve also has three leaflets named the septal, anterior, and posterior leaflets. Of the four cardiac valves, the pulmonary valve is the most difficult to visualize on two-dimensional echocardiography. Usually, the valve can be seen in the short-axis view and often in the subcostal view (**99**). The short-axis view can frequently provide visualization of the bifurcation of the pulmonary artery.

Various pathologies can occur on any valve and be seen on two-dimensional echocardiography. A common indication for TTE is for the evaluation for potential bacterial endocarditis. Vegetations can be visualized on any valve, with a predilection for the upstream side of the valve (e.g. the left atrial side of the mitral valve) (**100**). They typically have echogenicity similar to that of the myocardium and are irregularly shaped. They are frequently mobile, with the motion independent of the valve leaflet. Given the resolution of TTE, the vegetations seen are generally greater than 3 mm. Increased size of the vegetation has been shown to be associated with increased mortality. Fungal vegetations tend to be larger and have poor prognosis. Although

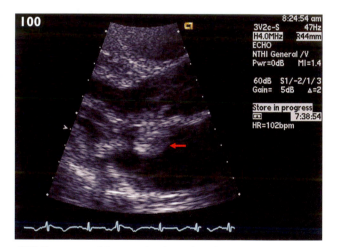

100 Parasternal long-axis view showing a vegetation (arrow) on the anterior leaflet of the mitral valve.

TTE often is insensitive and nonspecific in the setting of a prosthetic valve, vegetations can be seen. In addition to the vegetation itself, sequelae of endocarditis, such as aortic valve abscess (**101**), fistulae, emboli, or leaflet perforation (**102**), can be visualized by two-dimensional echocardiographic imaging. Identification of a vegetation on any cardiac valve argues for more careful assessment of the other valves, as multiple vegetations are frequently found. Although relatively uncommon, tumors can also be seen on cardiac valves. Most common types are fibroelastomas and papilloma. In general, the differential diagnosis of echodensities seen on cardiac valves relies heavily on the clinical situation, as differentiating them by echocardiography is difficult.

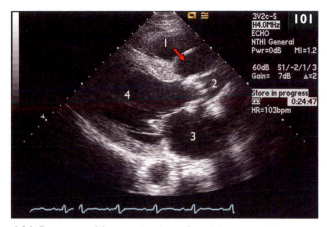

101 Parasternal long-axis view showing an aortic root abscess (1). (2: aorta; 3: left atrium; 4: left ventricle.)

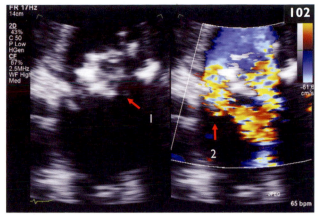

102 Split screen of the apical four-chamber view limited to the mitral valve. On the left, the two-dimensional imaging shows a vegetation (1) on the mitral valve. On the right, the color Doppler shows flow through the leaflet consistent with perforation (2).

Aorta

Evaluation of the aorta is an essential part of echocardiographic examination. Valuable diagnostic information about aortic pathology, function and competency of the aortic valve, and function of the left ventricle can be obtained in a timely fashion from a bedside study. A transthoracic echocardiogram can provide adequate visualization of the aortic root and proximal ascending aorta from parasternal long- and short-axis views (**70**). Enlargement of the aortic root with effacement of the sinuses of Valsalva, loss of sinotubular junction and dilation of the ascending aorta can be seen from the parasternal long-axis view (**103**).

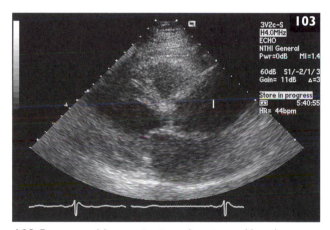

103 Parasternal long-axis view showing a dilated ascending aorta (1).

The aortic arch and portions of the descending aorta can be seen from suprasternal notch and apical two-chamber views (**78**). However, image quality is often suboptimal due to the transducer distance from the posterior aortic segments. Given the close proximity of the esophagus to the aorta, TEE provides excellent visualization of almost all segments of the thoracic aorta. High-resolution images of the aortic wall and lumen are obtained in both short- and long-axis views from the aortic valve to the level of the diaphragm.

Acute aortic dissection is one of the cardiovascular emergencies that usually occurs in the setting of pre-existing aortic wall pathology such as cystic medial necrosis or Marfan's syndrome. Dissection is usually initiated from an initial tear in the intima and entry of blood into the aortic wall with subsequent separation of the intima from the medial layers. The dissection plane can further propagate both distal and proximal to the initial intimal tear. Involvement of the proximal ascending aorta may cause acute aortic regurgitation or left ventricular ischemia from involvement of the coronary arteries. Enlargement and weakening of the aortic wall may lead to catastrophic rupture of the aorta into the pericardium or pleural space.

The aortic arch is a common site of injury with blunt chest trauma. During high-impact injury, shear forces between mobile and relatively fixed portions of the aorta can result in dissection or transection and can easily be detected with TEE. The aortic arch at the level of ligamentum arteriosum is the most common site of injury.

Atherosclerotic disease of the aorta and aortic arch is common in elderly patients with multiple risk factors. Atheromatous plaques are often seen as irregular protrusions into the aortic lumen during TEE. Complex atheromatous plaques are large plaques (>4 mm thickness) with ulceration or mobile components.

Pericardium

The pericardium consists of two layers: the visceral pericardium and the parietal pericardium. In the normal heart, these two layers are separated by approximately 15–50 mL of fluid that may be seen in some views on two-dimensional echocardiography. On echocardiography, this fluid appears as a dark space immediately exterior to the myocardium. Abnormal thickening of the pericardium may be identified in M-mode or two-dimensional echocardiography, but the sensitivity and specificity are limited. Rarely, the pericardium may be congenitally absent.

The most important application of echocardiography in evaluating pericardial disease is in identifying excess amounts of pericardial fluid (effusion) and assessing potential signs of accompanying hemodymanic changes. Usually, the fluid is free flowing within the pericardium (circumferential) and can be seen in multiple views on M-mode and two-dimensional echocardiography, with the size of pericardial effusion (small, moderate, or large) that is estimated based on the distance between the pericardial layers (**104**). Occasionally, the effusion is loculated or localized to one area, and fibrinous

material or strands can be seen within the effusion. Normal pericardial fat may appear similar to an effusion and is usually seen anteriorly.

Because the pericardium is stretched to create a fixed space containing the cardiac chambers and the pericardial effusion, pressure within the pericardium affects the passive filling pressures. Once the pressure in the pericardium exceeds the filling pressures of the cardiac chambers, the right and left atrial pressures, the right and left diastolic pressures, the pulmonary artery diastolic pressure, and the pulmonary capillary wedge pressure will equalize. This situation can cause hemodynamic compromise. M-mode and two-dimensional echocardiographic signs of pericardial effusion causing hemodynamic compromise include right ventricular diastolic collapse (**105**), right atrial diastolic collapse, and a plethoric inferior vena cava (>2.5 cm) that decreases in diameter less than 50% with inspiration. Another sign is increased respiratory variation of the mitral or tricuspid inflow velocities, which will be discussed in the Spectral Doppler section (**106**).

Echocardiography can play a key role during pericardiocentesis, or the draining of the fluid through a needle. Not only can two-dimensional echocardiography determine the size and evaluate for hemodynamic effects, it can also assist in localizing the optimal approach of the needle, usually where the fluid is the greatest, and estimate the distance from the chest wall. To ensure that the needle is in the pericardium, as opposed to having punctured a cardiac chamber such

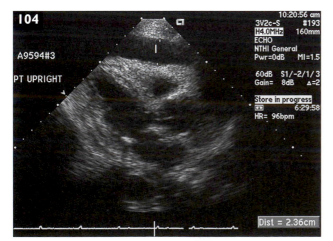

104 Parasternal long-axis view showing a large pericardial effusion (1).

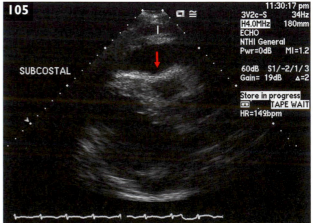

105 Parasternal long-axis view showing early diastolic right ventricular collapse (arrow).

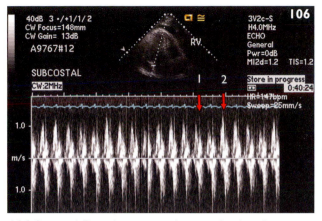

106 Spectral Doppler across the mitral valve showing increased respiratory variation of left ventricular inflow. (1: inspiration; 2: expiration.)

107 Spectral Doppler (PW) of the left ventricular outflow systolic flow (arrow) from the apical five-chamber view.

as the right ventricle, agitated saline can be injected through the needle. The echodense air filled bubbles can be easily seen within the fluid. Images taken after the procedure ensure adequate removal of the fluid. In addition, serial echocardiographic images are often obtained in the days after a pericardiocentesis to assess for reaccumulation.

SPECTRAL DOPPLER

As discussed previously, through PW Doppler and CW Doppler, the velocity of the blood can be measured and mapped over time to create a spectral Doppler image known as a time velocity integral (TVI) (**107**). Thus, various properties of flow, such as peak velocity and mean velocity, can be assessed at different locations within the heart, such as valves and shunts, throughout the cardiac cycle.

Flow rates

Volume of flow can be estimated as the TVI multiplied by the area over which it is assumed to flow. For instance, assuming a circular left ventricular outflow tract (LVOT),

$$SV = \frac{TVI_{LVOT} \times D^2_{LVOT} \times \pi}{4}, \qquad (8)$$

where SV denotes stroke volume, TVI_{LVOT} is time velocity integral of the spectral Doppler within the LVOT, and D_{LVOT} represents diameter of the LVOT. For maximal accuracy, the Doppler flow should be measured as nearly parallel as possible with the direction of flow in the LVOT, usually the apical five-chamber or three-chamber view. Cardiac output can then be estimated by multiplying the SV by the heart rate.

In addition to an overall assessment of cardiac function, the cardiac output at one site within the heart can be compared with another site. This technique can evaluate the volume of shunts. For instance, total net flow across an atrial septal defect can be estimated by subtracting the stroke volume in the LVOT from that in the right ventricular outflow tract. For clinical purposes, this assessment is usually calculated as a ratio of pulmonary flow to systemic flow (Qp/Qs).

More commonly flow rates are used to estimate aortic valve area in cases of suspected aortic stenosis using the continuity of mass principle. Essentially, this principle states that the stroke volume immediately proximal to the aortic valve is equal to the stroke volume through the aortic valve. Namely,

$$AVA = \frac{SV_{LVOT}}{TVI_{AV}}, \qquad (9)$$

where AVA denotes aortic valve area, SV_{LVOT} is stroke volume in the left ventricular outflow tract, and TVI_{AV} represents time velocity integral across the aortic valve. Thus, the area of the aortic valve can be estimated by multiplying the area of the LVOT by the TVI of the flow in the LVOT divided by the TVI of the flow across the aortic valve. While individual variation exists, generally aortic areas >1.5–2.0 cm² are associated with no significant stenosis; aortic valve areas <0.7–1.0 cm² are generally considered moderately or severely stenotic.

Echocardiographic assessment of aortic stenosis correlates well with the estimates obtained using pressure and volume measurements from cardiac catheterization, with each technique having unique limitations. The continuity of mass principle can be used to assess stenosis of the other cardiac valves. However, prevalence of these conditions is lower and assumptions of geometry around the mitral and tricuspid valves are less accurate.

Pressure gradients

Based on the law of conservation of energy, the pressure difference between two cardiac chambers can be reasonably estimated by the simplified Bernoulli equation; i.e. pressure equals four times the velocity squared ($P = 4v^2$). This technique allows for assessments of pressure gradients across valvular stenosis, of hemodynamic effects valvular disease, of estimated pulmonary pressures, and of hemodynamic significance of intracardiac shunts.

In addition to visual assessment on two-dimensional echocardiography and estimated AVA by spectral Doppler as described above, estimations of the peak and mean pressure gradients across the aortic valve by spectral Doppler are valuable clinical tools for evaluating the degree of aortic stenosis. Velocities within the LVOT are usually obtained by PW Doppler and velocities across the aortic valve are usually obtained by CW Doppler in the three-chamber and five-chamber views. Normal velocities for the LVOT are <1.4 m/s and for the aortic valve are <1.8 m/s (**107**, **108**). In aortic stenosis, the velocity of the blood increases significantly as it passes through the fixed obstruction. The degree of increase in velocity is related to the degree of obstruction. By using the simplified Bernoulli equation, peak velocity across the valve can be utilized to estimate the peak pressure gradient (**109**). Integrating the Doppler tracing (TVI) can estimate mean pressure gradients. These same principles also can be applied to stenosis of the mitral (**110**), tricuspid, and pulmonary valves.

The change in estimated pressure gradients across a valve also provides a means for estimating chamber and arterial pressures. Most commonly, the pulmonary artery systolic pressure is estimated in a multi-step process. Firstly, the right ventricular systolic pressure is estimated by measuring the peak velocity of the tricuspid regurgitant Doppler envelope (**111**). With use of the simplified Bernoulli equation ($P = 4v^2$), the peak gradient across the tricuspid valve is estimated. Secondly, the right atrial pressure is estimated, usually based on evaluation of inferior vena cava size. Normal sized inferior vena cava (<2.0 cm) and normal respiratory variation of this size with 'sniffing' (>50%

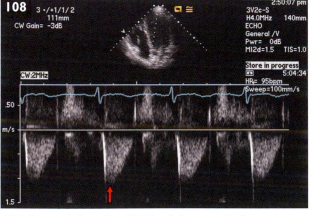

108 Spectral Doppler (CW) of the systolic flow across the aortic valve (arrow) from the apical five-chamber view.

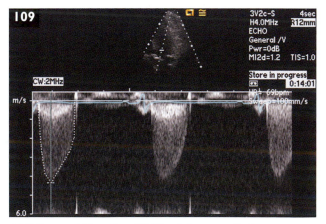

109 Spectral Doppler (CW) of the systolic flow across the aortic valve from the apical five-chamber view in a patient with severe aortic stenosis. Note the peak gradient of 75 mmHg.

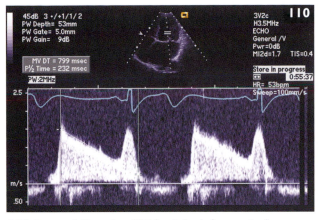

110 Spectral Doppler (PW) of the left ventricular diastolic inflow from the apical four-chamber view. ($P_{1/2}$: pressure half-time.)

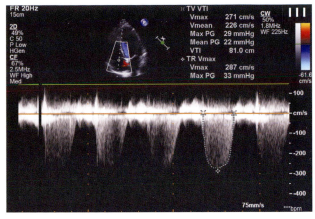

111 Spectral Doppler measuring velocity of tricuspid regurgitation which allows estimation of pulmonary artery pressures.

decrease) signifies normal right atrial pressure (<10 mmHg). Mildly increased size (2.0–2.5 cm) or decreased respiratory variation signifies mildly elevated right atrial pressure (10–15 mmHg). Dilated inferior vena cava (>2.5 cm) and decreased respiratory variation signify elevated right atrial pressure (>15 mmHg). Thirdly, assuming no significant pulmonary valvular stenosis, the pulmonary artery systolic pressure is estimated to be the sum of the estimated right atrial pressure and the estimated pressure gradient across the tricuspid valve. Often the values are reported in 5 mmHg increments. Generally, values <40 mmHg are considered normal.

In another application, the pulmonary artery diastolic pressure can be estimated in a similar fashion, if significant pulmonary regurgitation is present, as the sum of the estimated pressure gradient across the pulmonary valve from the regurgitant Doppler envelope at end-diastole. The right ventricular diastolic pressure can be estimated in the same way as right atrial pressure described above. In the setting of a ventricular septal defect, right ventricular systolic pressure can be estimated as the difference between the measured systemic systolic pressure (by sphygmography) and the pressure estimated from the peak velocity across the defect.

One method for assessing severity of aortic regurgitation is to use the slope of the regurgitant Doppler jet. From a hemodynamic perspective, insignificant aortic regurgitation will not result in significant pressure equalization between the aorta and

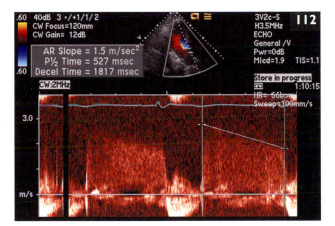

112 Spectral Doppler across the aortic valve showing aortic regurgitation (AR) and measurement of pressure half-time ($P_{1/2}$).

the left ventricle during diastole. Thus, the slope of the aortic regurgitation jet should be gradual (**112**). Usually, the degree of the slope is quantified by measuring the time taken to decrease the peak pressure in half, or pressure half-time. Pressure half-times >500 ms are consistent with mild aortic regurgitation. However, significant aortic regurgitation may lead to pressure equalization between the aorta and left ventricle during diastole with a steep Doppler slope and a pressure half-time <200 ms. Note that this method is just one of several components of assessing severity of aortic regurgitation. This method can be applied to pulmonary valvular regurgitation in a similar way.

Degree of mitral stenosis also can be assessed using the principals described above in two ways. Firstly, the mean gradient can be estimated from the CW Doppler envelop across the mitral valve, including both early (E-wave) and late (A-wave) diastolic filling if present (**110**). If a patient is in atrial fibrillation, an average of multiple (five to ten) beats should be determined. An estimate of the pressure half-time of the E-wave provides the second method of using spectral Doppler in assessing the degree of mitral stenosis. Empirically, the mitral valve (MV) area in centimeters squared is estimated to be 220 divided by the pressure half-time in milliseconds (MV area = 220/pressure half-time). Areas <1.0 cm^2 are considered severe.

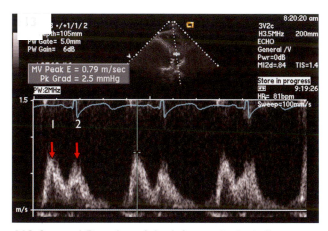

113 Spectral Doppler of the left ventricular inflow showing normal early diastolic (1) and late diastolic (2) flow.

Diastolic function

Diastolic dysfunction can be assessed by echocardiography using spectral Doppler parameters of the mitral inflow (**113**) and pulmonary vein inflow (**114**). No single parameter gives a complete assessment of diastolic function and thus reviewing multiple pieces of information is recommended. As discussed previously, in normal sinus rhythm, the mitral inflow Doppler images show an early diastolic E-wave due to left ventricular relaxation, and a late A-wave due to left atrial contraction. Diastolic function can be assessed by PW Doppler with the sample volume placed at the mitral valve tips, the point of maximal flow velocities. The major parameters assessed are the ratio of peak E-wave velocity to peak A-wave velocity (E/A) and the deceleration time (DT) of the E-wave. In normal adults the E/A ratio is usually 1.0–2.0, and the DT ranges from 140–220 ms. With a decrease in compliance of the left ventricle associated with mild diastolic dysfunction, the E/A ratio decreases below 1.0, and the DT increases above 220 ms (**115**). E/A ratios <1.0 are also seen frequently in otherwise normal people over the age of 65; whether or not this represents diastolic dysfunction or 'normal aging' is controversial. As diastolic dysfunction progresses to moderate, pressure increases in the left atrium. In response, velocities in the early filling period increase, resulting in the E/A ratio and the DT within the normal range. This stage is often called 'pseudo normal' due to a similar E/A pattern. As the left atrial pressure increases further, early diastolic filling

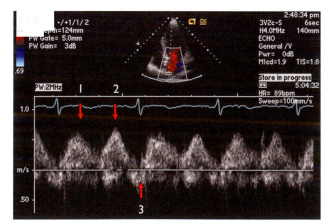

114 Spectral Doppler (pulse wave) of normal right upper pulmonary venous flow into the left atrium from the apical four-chamber view illustrating systolic (1), diastolic (2), and atrial (3) components.

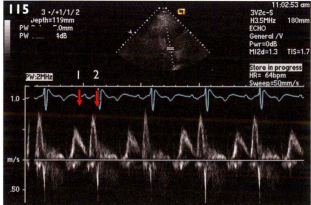

115 Spectral Doppler of the left ventricular inflow showing lower velocity early diastolic (1) flow compared with late diastolic (2) flow, consistent with mild diastolic dysfunction.

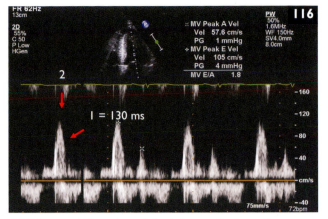

116 Spectral Doppler of the left ventricular inflow showing a short deceleration time (1) of the early diastolic (2) flow, consistent with severe diastolic dysfunction.

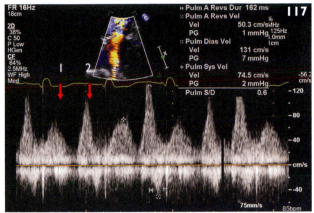

117 Spectral Doppler (PW) of right upper pulmonary venous flow into the left atrium from the apical four-chamber view illustrating diastolic dysfunction with a low systolic (1) to diastolic (2) ratio.

increases in velocity and shortens in duration, resulting in the E/A ratio increasing above 2.0 and the DT decreasing below 140 ms (**116**). This pattern represents restrictive physiology and severe diastolic dysfunction. Interestingly, decreasing left atrial filling, typically with the Valsalva maneuver, often can 'improve' diastolic filling one stage. Thus, moderate diastolic filling can look like mild and mild can look like normal. With the Valsalva maneuver, severe diastolic filling may appear moderate ('reversible') or may continue to appear severe ('irreversible').

For another parameter of diastolic function, the sample volume of the PW spectral Doppler determination is placed within the left ventricular cavity to include both mitral inflow during diastole and left ventricular outflow during systole. The time between the end of outflow and the beginning of inflow represents the isovolemic relaxation time (IVRT). Similar to the DT, the IVRT has a normal range of 60–100 ms, increases with mild diastolic dysfunction, decreases into the normal range with moderate dysfunction ('pseudo normal'), and decreases further below the normal range with severe dysfunction. The Tei index, or myocardial performance index (MPI), incorporates the isovolemic contraction time (IVCT), the IVRT, and the systolic ejection time (ET) into one assessment with the formula:

$$Tei = \frac{IVCT + IVRT}{IVCT + ET + IVRT}. \qquad (10)$$

The pulmonary vein flow also can assist in assessing diastolic function. On transthoracic echocardiography, the most reliable flow to obtain is from one of the right pulmonary veins in the apical four-chamber view. Normal spectral Doppler flow consists of a forward-flowing systolic wave (S), corresponding to left ventricular contraction and atrial relaxation; a second forward-flowing diastolic wave (D), corresponding to early mitral inflow; and a reverse-flowing late diastolic wave (A), corresponding to atrial contraction (**114**). With mild diastolic dysfunction, the D-wave decreases in velocity, similar to the decrease in the mitral inflow E-wave. With more advanced diastolic dysfunction, as ventricular compliance worsens allowing less complete atrial emptying, the velocities of the S-wave decrease and those of the D-wave increase (**117**).

Doppler tissue imaging

Blood flow within the cardiac cavities involves higher velocities and lower-intensity signals compared with tissue. Thus, for optimal spectral Doppler tracings of blood flow the ultrasound machines routinely filter out low-velocity and high-intensity signals. To obtain Doppler tracings of cardiac tissue, settings are changed to filter out high-velocity and low-intensity signals. With these filter settings changed, improved tissue Doppler imaging (TDI) can then be obtained by placing the sample volume on an area of myocardium or the mitral annulus.

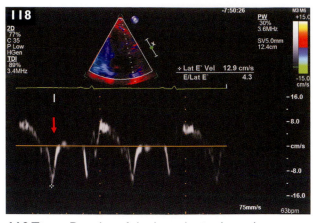

118 Tissue Doppler of the lateral mitral annulus showing normal early diastolic (1: E') excursion.

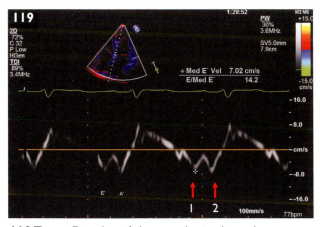

119 Tissue Doppler of the septal mitral annulus showing diastolic dysfunction with low-velocity early diastolic (1: E') excursion (2: A').

For the assessment of diastolic function, TDI is usually obtained on the septal and lateral sides of the mitral annulus in the four-chamber view. In patients with normal diastolic function, the early diastolic velocity (E') is higher than the late diastolic velocity (A') (**118**). Similar to mitral inflow, with mild diastolic dysfunction the early diastolic flow decreases below the late diastolic flow (E'/A' becomes <1.0). However, in contrast to mitral inflow, with worsening diastolic dysfunction E continues to decrease. Thus, the 'pseudo normal' mitral inflow E/A ratio of moderate diastolic dysfunction can be distinguished from normal diastolic function by a low E' (typically <8 or 9 cm/s) (**119**). In addition, a ratio of early diastolic flow velocities from mitral inflow and TDI (E/E') >10–15 can be used to identify patients with elevated pulmonary capillary wedge pressures >18–20 mmHg.

In addition to aiding in the assessment of diastolic dysfunction, TDI enables more focal assessment of systolic function. While the potential for clinical application in evaluation is broad, the area currently most developed relates to evaluating the timing of contraction at various locations within the left ventricle. Normal left ventricular activation is relatively well coordinated, leading to near simultaneous contraction throughout the left ventricle. However, patients with significant left ventricular dysfunction often display marked variation in timing of activation at different wall segments. Thus, the time interval from the QRS complex on the ECG to the peak of the systolic component of the tissue Doppler tracing can be compared at various locations within the left ventricular myocardial walls. Normal time intervals are <60 ms whereas intervals in patients with severe dyssynchrony can exceed 200 ms. Patients with significant electrical dyssynchrony are candidates for placement of biventricular pacemakers.

COLOR DOPPLER

The velocities obtained from spectral Doppler can be assigned different colors and mapped onto the two-dimensional image. Per convention, blood flow toward the transducer is displayed as red and that away from the transducer is displayed as blue, as mentioned before. The color Doppler is obtained through complex algorithms. In a normal heart, the flow across the mitral valve can be seen during diastole and that across the aortic valve can be seen during systole. However, the true value of color Doppler becomes apparent in evaluating abnormal flows such as valvular regurgitation and shunts.

Color Doppler is extremely useful in evaluating mitral regurgitation (Zoghbi *et al.* 2005). Normally, the mitral valves are reasonably competent and no or minimal blood returns from the left ventricle to the left atrium during ventricular systole. However, significant mitral regurgitation can result from many different etiologies, such as rheumatic heart disease, mitral valve prolapse, ischemic heart disease, and endocarditis. The evaluation of mitral regurgitation includes visualization of the mitral valve leaflets on two-dimensional echocardiographic images and the evaluation of the spectral Doppler envelope. However, assessment on color Doppler represents the most powerful tool and includes multiple facets.

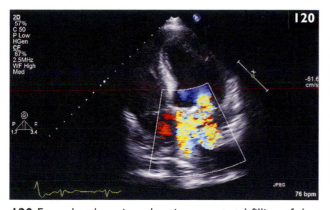

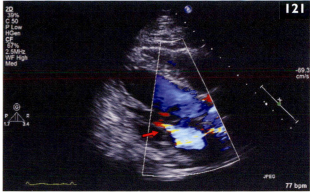

120 Four-chamber view showing near total filling of the left atrium with color Doppler during systole, consistent with severe mitral regurgitation.

121 Parasternal long-axis view showing mitral regurgitation with a vena contracta (arrow).

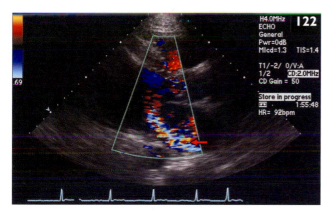

122 Parasternal long-axis view with color Doppler showing eccentric mitral regurgitation (arrow) along the posterior wall of the left atrium.

Firstly, the jet area within the left atrium can be measured and compared with the total area of the left atrium. Mild regurgitation results in jet areas <20% of left atrial areas, moderate 20–40%, and severe >40% (**120**). Secondly, in most patients the width of the mitral regurgitation jet at the level of the valve (vena contracta) can be measured, the wider the jet the more significant the regurgitation (**121**).

The third way of assessing mitral regurgitation on color Doppler is the estimation of the volumetric flow and effective regurgitant orifice by proximal isovelocity surface area (PISA). As blood in the left ventricle converges toward the mitral valve, often a 'shell' appears on color Doppler, representing the interface between red and blue created by velocities reaching the Nyquist limit. By the principle of conservation of mass (continuity equation), the blood flow across this shell is the same as the blood flow across the mitral orifice. This flow can be calculated by the formula:

$$\text{Flow rate} = 2\pi r \times \text{aliasing velocity}, \qquad (11)$$

where r is the radius of the shell. The effective regurgitant orifice (ERO) can be calculated from the formula:

$$\text{ERO} = \text{Flow rate} / V_j, \qquad (12)$$

where V_j is the velocity of the regurgitant jet obtained by spectral Doppler. The regurgitant volume (RVe) can then be calculated by:

$$\text{RVe} = \text{ERO} \times \text{TVI}_{mr}, \qquad (13)$$

where TVI_{mr} is the TVI of the regurgitant jet. Conceptually, ERO and RVe estimated by PISA are appealing. However, the questionable assumption of the blood uniformly converging toward a small flat orifice and the high potential for measurement error in the shell radius have limited routine use in most echocardiographic laboratories.

In addition to these quantitative and semi-quantitative approaches, the direction of the regurgitant jet can affect the assessment of severity of mitral regurgitation. A centrally directed jet will dislocate relatively more blood in the left atrium than an eccentric jet which may be limited by one of the left atrial walls. Since many correlation studies were performed with patients with central jets, the severity of eccentric jets may be underestimated, particularly by use of the jet area to left atrial area ratio (**122**).

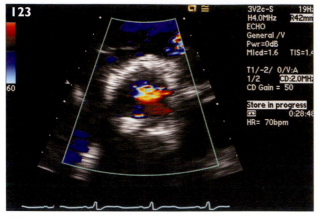

123 Color Doppler of flow across the aortic valve during diastole consistent with significant aortic regurgitation.

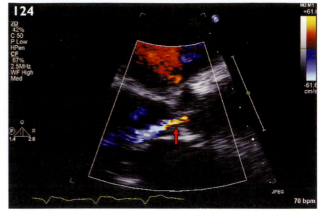

124 Color Doppler showing mild aortic regurgitation. The most narrow point of the jet is the vena contracta (arrow).

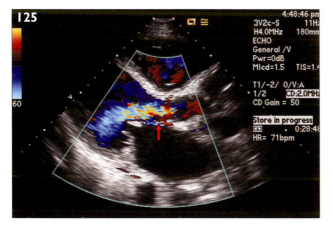

125 Color Doppler showing severe aortic regurgitation with a wide vena contracta (arrow).

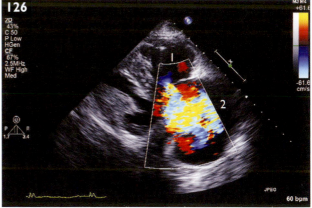

126 Color Doppler showing flow from the right ventricle (1) to the right atrium (2) during systole consistent with severe tricuspid regurgitation.

The direction of the jet also often gives clues to the etiology of the regurgitation. For instance, prolapse of the anterior leaflet of the mitral valve will usually result in a posteriorly directed regurgitant jet.

Severity of aortic regurgitation is also assessed using color Doppler. The area of regurgitant jet seen in the parasternal short-axis view correlates with severity (**123**). As the degree to which the regurgitant jet extends into the left ventricle depends considerably upon left ventricular hemodynamic parameters as well as jet direction, the area of regurgitant jet has been shown to be unreliable. However, the width of the vena contracta in the parasternal long-axis view of the regurgitant jet can be helpful in assessing severity (**124**). Widths >7 mm or ratios of jet width to left ventricular outflow width of >50% are thought to

represent severe aortic regurgitation. In the parasternal short-axis view, the area of the regurgitant jet gives two-dimensional information regarding regurgitant severity (**125**). These color Doppler techniques complement the spectral Doppler techniques discussed earlier.

The severity of tricuspid and pulmonary regurgitation has not been extensively studied. However, the general principles relating to assessing mitral regurgitation apply to tricuspid regurgitation (**126**), and those for aortic regurgitation apply to pulmonary regurgitation (**127**).

Shunts between cardiac chambers often cause significant flow and color Doppler flow. Atrial septal defects are best seen in the subcostal view, as the direction of flow most closely parallels the ultrasound wave angle. The most common secundum defects

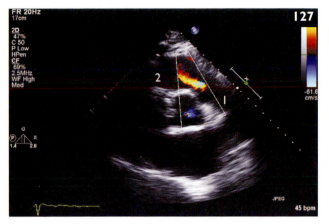

127 Color Doppler showing flow from the pulmonary artery (1) to the right ventricle (2) during diastole consistent with pulmonary regurgitation.

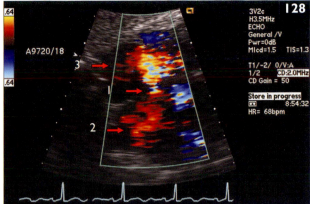

128 Color Doppler in the subcostal views showing a secundum atrial septal defect (1) with left atrial (2) to right atrial (3) flow.

result in a color Doppler flow near the center of the atrial septum (**128**). Primum defects are seen in the septum closer to the mitral and tricuspid valves. Sinus venosus defects can be seen in the septum more basally but are often missed on TTE. Patent foramen ovale is usually visualized as a small color flow in the same area as a secundum atrial septal defect. Ventricular defects are also classified based on their location. Perimembranous defects account for over 80% of congenital ventricular septal defects (**129**). Trabecular or muscular defects account for the vast majority of acquired defects, usually after a myocardial infarction, and can be multiple. Outlet defects (supracristal and infracristalis) and inlet defects are less common.

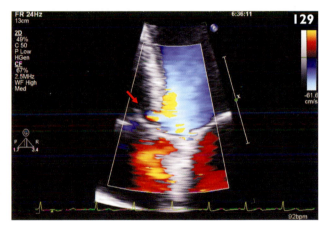

129 Apical four-chamber view showing a perimembranous ventricular septal defect (arrow).

TRANSESOPHAGEAL ECHOCARDIOGRAPHY

In TEE, an ultrasound crystal transducer is incorporated on to the tip of a directable gastroscope-like device. Using typical mouth anesthesia and conscious sedation, most individuals can swallow the probe without difficulty. Because the transducer lies in the lower esophagus in close contact with the posterior aspect of the heart, the image resolution can be improved due to increased ultrasound frequency (5–7 MHz). In addition, intervening lung and bony structures that commonly hinder transthoracic image quality are avoided. Posterior structures such as the left atrial appendage, mitral valve, pulmonary veins, and left atrium, as well as the aorta, are particularly well visualized. In addition to the semi-invasive nature, the main disadvantage of TEE is poor alignment for acquisition of Doppler velocities. In these cases, transthoracic images may be needed to supplement transesophageal assessment.

Common indications for TEE include suspected or further evaluation of endocarditis, prosthetic valve dysfunction, aortic dissection, and intracavitary thrombus (particularly in the left atrial appendage thrombus). Other potential sources of embolism can be identified on TEE such as a patent foramen ovale and aortic atherosclerosis. Intraoperative TEE is common for valvular surgery, particularly mitral valve repair and assessment of mitral regurgitation after aortic valve replacement. In addition, when transthoracic views are nondiagnostic and results may impact on the management of a patient, it is reasonable to perform a TEE.

Procedure protocol and risks

TEE should be performed by a cardiologist or anesthesiologist trained in echocardiography with adequate experience in TEE. Patients undergoing TEE should have the procedure, indications, and potential complications explained in detail. The absolute incidence of serious complications is less than 1%, which includes hypoxia, laryngospasm, transient throat pain, aspiration, and esophageal perforation. The patient should be fasted for at least 4–6 hours prior to the procedure. A history of adverse reaction to sedation and a history of esophageal injury, disease, or difficulty swallowing should be evaluated prior to commencement of the procedure.

The procedure is usually performed with the patient lying on their left side (left lateral decubitus position) or supine (particularly in intubated patients in intensive care units). The clinician performing the procedure is usually assisted by a sonographer or a trained assistant. Given the semi-invasive nature of the procedure, a registered nurse is generally preferred to monitor and document the heart rate, blood pressure, and arterial oxygenation levels properly. In addition, a nurse may be needed for suction, oxygen, and placing or replacing intravenous catheters during the procedure and in the recovery from the procedure. Local anesthesia to improve patient comfort during the procedure is accomplished through 10% lidocaine spray, applied directly to the back of the throat. Some investigators advocate using a drying agent to assist in diminishing oral secretions. However, these medications have been shown to increase heart rate. Conscious sedation is usually accomplished with a combination of intravenous fentanyl or demerol, and versed because of their short-acting nature. The total length of the procedure is approximately 30 minutes.

Once the patient is adequately sedated but not completely asleep, the TEE probe is introduced into the patient's mouth, throat, and then toward the esophagus. The probe is a modified version of the gastroscope used for endoscopy, with an ultrasound probe at the end. The probe, 10–14 mm for adults, is introduced into the esophagus and stomach. Notice that TEE can also be performed in pediatric patients, and the probe has been miniaturized to approximately 4 mm in width but with increased flexibility and decreased control. The tip of the probe is introduced slowly and smoothly, without applying pressure or force. When the probe is passed close to the esophagus, the patient will be asked to swallow. The probe can then be safely advanced into the esophagus without force. Separate rotation knobs on the handle allow for forward and backward movements of the probe as well as side-to-side movement. The newest generation of TEE probes have a multiplane transducer, which has the capacity to rotate electronically the image plane from 0° to 180°, allowing visualization of a single structure in multiple views.

Tomographic views

Tomographic images are acquired with the probe within the esophagus and the stomach. Two-dimensional as well as Doppler techniques can be employed with each view. The tip of the probe is advanced into the upper esophagus to obtain high esophageal views at different rotation angles. At this position, the probe is located posterior to the left atrium. At 0°, a four-chamber view (**130**) is obtained similar to the apical four-chamber view of the transthoracic image, except being obtained from the posterior position. Simple angulation can optimize the image in order to obtain the true left ventricular apex. However, the left ventricular apex can be foreshortened in some patients. A clear view of the atria, ventricles, anterior mitral leaflet, second posterior mitral scallop (P2), and tricuspid valve can be seen. Anterior angulation can provide a view of the LVOT, analogous to a five-chamber view on transthoracic imaging (**131**). At 30–45° of the probe, a short-axis view of the aortic

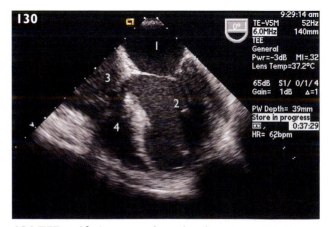

130 TEE at 0° showing a four-chamber view, with the left atrium (1), left ventricle (2), right atrium (3), and right ventricle (4).

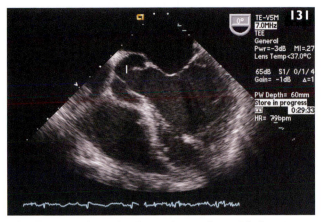

131 Transesophageal echocardiography at 0° showing a five-chamber view, with the addition of the aortic valve (1).

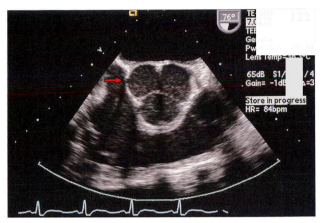

132 Transesophageal view showing the aortic valve (arrow).

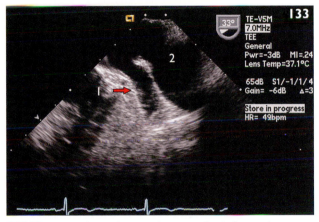

133 Transesophageal view showing the left atrial appendage (1) and left upper pulmonary vein (2).

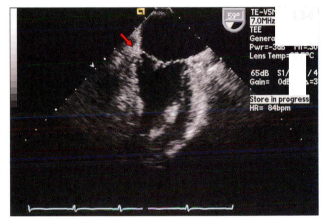

134 Transesophageal view showing the closed mitral valve (arrow).

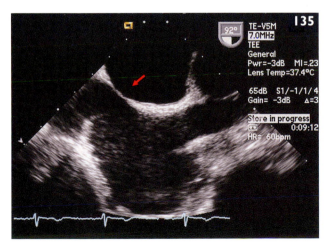

135 Transesophageal view showing the interatrial septum (arrow).

valve can be seen (**132**). The optimal angle may vary from patient to patient. The left atrial appendage can be seen in this view (**133**). By rotating the probe to 60° a two-chamber view as well as information regarding the mitral valve anatomy and function are obtained (**134**). In this view, the anterior and inferior walls of the left ventricle are seen. At 90°, another view of the left atrial appendage can be seen. In addition, the left upper pulmonary vein can be seen. With angulation of the probe, the perpendicular relationship between the aortic and pulmonic valves is appreciated. With further rotation of the probe at 90° towards the patient's right side, the interatrial septum can be visualized (**135**) in the bicaval or right atrial view. The superior and inferior vena cava can also be observed.

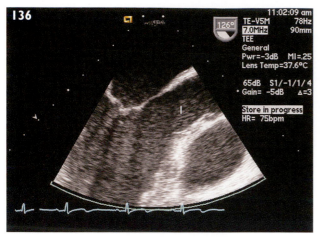

136 Transesophageal view showing the left ventricular outflow tract (I).

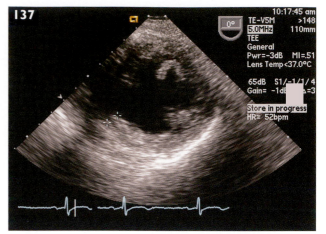

137 Transgastric view of the left ventricle in the short axis.

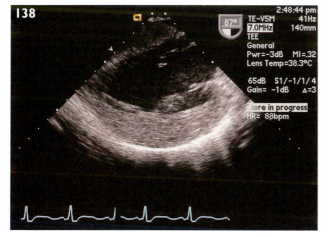

138 Transgastric view of the left ventricle in the long axis.

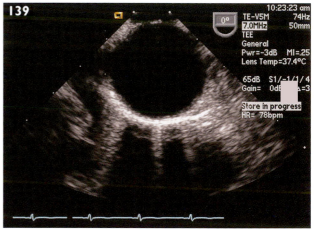

139 Transesophageal view of the descending aorta.

Images rotated to 120° will give a long-axis view of the left ventricle to include the aortic valve in the long axis, similar to a three-chamber view (**136**), in which the long axis of the proximal aorta and aortic root can be visualized. With the addition of Doppler, functional regurgitation of the aortic valve can be visualized. Moreover, the left ventricular outflow tract can be appreciated. This view can be particularly helpful with regard to aortic valve pathology such as vegetation, abscess, dissection of the ascending aorta, and congenital abnormalities.

All four pulmonary veins can be visualized as they enter the left atrium on different views as part of the standard TEE examination. Color Doppler interrogation helps in identification and characterization of certain clinical problems such as mitral regurgitation

and diastolic function. The left upper pulmonary vein is usually the easiest to identify at 0° or 90–110°. The left atrial appendage is visualized on each TEE examination as stated earlier, and is normally crescent-shaped and multi-lobed (**133**). Orthogonal views help to determine the precise anatomy and presence of pathology.

Advancement of the probe into the esophagus at 0° will yield transgastric views. At 0°, the short axis of the left and right ventricles can be appreciated (**137**). Wall motion abnormalities can be easily appreciated as well. Image rotation to 90° is usually performed and provides a view similar to the parasternal long-axis view of transthoracic imaging (**138**).

Images of the thoracic aorta from the diaphragm to the aortic arch (**139**) are obtained with excellent reliability and resolution. However, a portion of the ascending aorta can be obscured by the trachea, not permitting accurate visualization of this section of the aorta due to air. These images are usually the last part of the examination and are performed at 0°, beginning with the aorta visualized below the diaphragm and withdrawing the scope until the ascending aorta is seen. Areas in question may be viewed at 90° as well.

When interpreting TEE images, certain concepts must be kept in mind. As TEE has improved visualization of most structures, often normal structures that were not visualized on transthoracic imaging, will be seen on TEE. For example, a Eustachian valve, an embryologic remnant present in some people, may resemble a thrombus or congenital malformation. The presence of a Eustachian valve has no clinical significance. Thus, knowledge of normal structures will minimize misinterpretation of images. Images may be limited by the patient's anatomy (for example a hiatal hernia) or by mechanical valve prosthesis which can create a shadowing artifact distal to the prosthesis. In addition, imaging the apex of the heart may be difficult.

Clinical applications

In patients who have experienced a stroke or transient ischemic attack ('mini-stroke'), a cardiac source of embolization may be sought by TEE, particularly in young patients. Currently accepted definite indications for TEE in patients with suspected cerebral embolism include clinical evidence of heart disease and age under 45 years. Potential sources of embolization can be intracardiac thrombus (**140**), left-sided cardiac tumors (i.e. atrial myxoma), vegetation (**141**) on one of the cardiac valves, aorta atheroma (**142**), and paradoxical embolism from a patent foramen ovale (embryological remnant within the interatrial septum) (**143**). Other

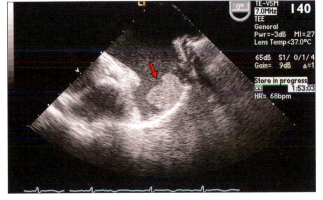

140 High resolution of the left atrial appendage with a thrombus (arrow).

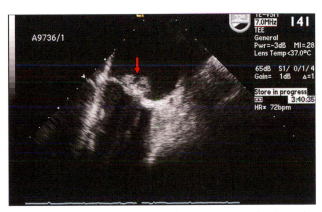

141 A vegetation (arrow) noted on the mitral valve.

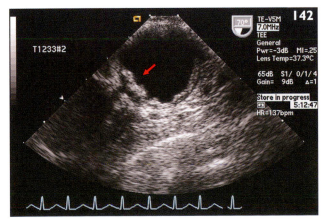

142 Transesophageal echocardiogram showing severe atherosclerotic plaque (arrow) in the aorta.

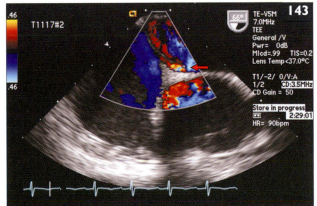

143 Color Doppler across the interatrial septum showing a patent foramen ovale (arrow).

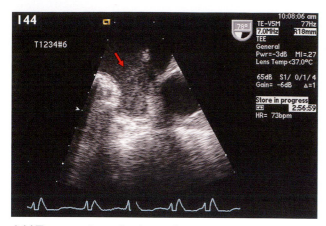

144 Transesophageal echocardiogram showing spontaneous echo contrast (arrow) or 'smoke', within the left atrial appendage.

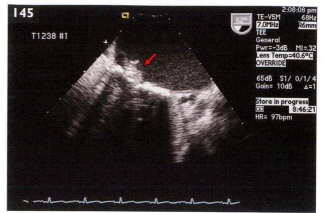

145 Transesophageal echocardiogram of the mitral valve showing a vegetation (arrow) on the atrial side of the posterior leaflet.

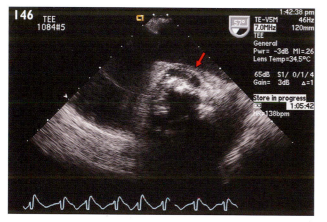

146 Transesophageal echocardiogram showing an aortic root abscess (arrow).

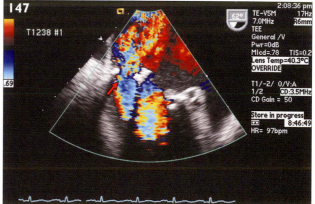

147 Color Doppler across the mitral valve during systole showing perforation (arrow) of the posterior leaflet.

common situations that may predispose to intracardiac thrombus are rheumatic mitral stenosis (in which it is more common to have atrial fibrillation as well which predisposes patients to stroke), congenital heart disease, and prosthetic heart valves (particularly mechanical rather than tissue heart valves). It should be noted that detection of thrombus after an event has occurred may be unrevealing since the thrombus may have already migrated and no longer be present. Therefore, it is important to search for conditions that predispose a patient to thrombus formation as well. Patients with atrial fibrillation who are going to undergo pharmacological or electrical cardioversion are candidates for TEE to identify thrombus in the left atrial appendage or spontaneous echocardiographic contrast ('smoke') (**144**).

Endocarditis can often be diagnosed on TTE. However, the improved resolution of valves on TEE significantly increases sensitivity. The sensitivity of TTE varies widely in the literature, from <50% to >75%. Small vegetations not well seen on TTE can be seen on TEE (**145**). Aortic root abscess (**146**) and other valvular complications (**147**) are more thoroughly evaluated on TEE. Acoustic shadowing of prosthetic valves, particularly on the atrial side of mechanical prosthetic mitral valves (**148**), substantially decreases sensitivity on TTE. Thus, TEE is often used to evaluate for endocarditis in prosthetic valves, though acoustic shadowing continues to limit sensitivity. Given the superior quality of TEE, there are some anatomic abnormalities that may mimic infective endocariditis such as artifact, thrombus, old or healed

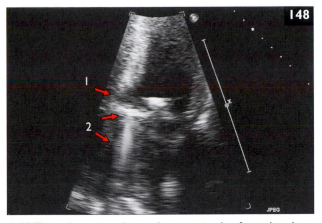

148 Transthoracic echocardiogram in the four-chamber view showing a mechanical mitral valve replacement (1) creating a shadowing (2) artifact, making assessment of the left atrium difficult.

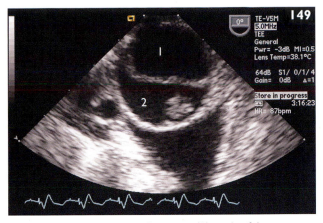

149 Aortic dissection with a true (1) and a false (2) lumen.

vegetation, inflammatory disease such as systemic lupus erythematosus that may affect cardiac valves, and other benign lesions.

Echocardiographers are frequently asked to evaluate for suspected aortic dissection. Transthoracic imaging is a good screening tool, offering imaging of the aortic root, proximal ascending aorta, and portions of the arch and descending aorta. If disease is present, the test is usually reliable. However, it is often inadequate to exclude disease completely, particularly in the aortic arch and descending aorta. TEE may be employed to visualize better more portions of the aorta. An aortic dissection flap may appear as a linear, bright, echogenic structure in the lumen of the aorta with abnormal motion compared with the normal pulsatile motion of the aorta. There can be color flow evidence of blood within the true lumen (that it has a lining of endothelium on the interior) and false lumen (the lumen created by the dissection tear) (**149**). The false lumen may contain blood clot (thrombus). With appropriate probe maneuvering to minimize nonvisualized portions of the aorta, the sensitivity of TEE can be 97% for the detection of aortic dissection. The specificity may be lower, primarily due to artifacts, such as reverberations from the left atrium. Usually, by changing probe position or angle or by use of color Doppler, artifact can be distinguished from dissection flap. In addition, nearby veins may be misdiagnosed as dissection flaps. In addition to high sensitivity and specificity, advantages of TEE

include ease of use, ability to go to the patient's bedside, expeditious nature in which it can be performed, and functional information regarding the aortic valve and hemodynamic compromise of a pericardial effusion. TEE may be used intra-operatively to assess for residual dissection after surgical repair. Other modalities, such as spiral chest CT, MRI, and contrast angiography offer different advantages and disadvantages and may be used alternatively or as complementary techniques.

INTRACARDIAC ECHOCARDIOGRAPHY

Intracardiac echocardiography (ICE) is an ultrasound technique that is used mainly during invasive procedures. During an invasive procedure, transthoracic images usually cannot offer the image quality needed for posterior structures but TEE can be employed. The invasive procedures can be lengthy, and general anesthesia may be needed. ICE can be employed to offer excellent image quality in a safe manner to guide invasive therapy. The 5–10 MHz single-plane transducer is at the tip of an 8 or 10 French, 90 cm long, disposable device that is passed from the femoral vein into the right-sided cardiac chambers (inferior vena cava, right atrium, or right ventricle). The probe has a steering capability, which allows for multiple views and directions, has two-dimensional, PW and color Doppler capabilities, and is connected to a standard ultrasound scanner.

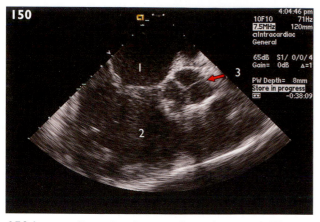

150 Intracardiac echo showing the right atrium (1), right ventricle (2), and aortic valve (3).

The procedures in which ICE can be useful are monitoring during electrophysiologic arrhythmia ablation procedures, percutaneous defect closures (for patent foramen ovale or atrial septal defect), and valvuloplasty (dilating mitral valve percutaneously). ICE images are similar to those of TEE, but with different orientations (**150**). Major limitations of the use of ICE are its invasive nature and cost (over $2,000 per probe, which is nonreusable).

STRESS ECHOCARDIOGRAPHY

As discussed in the nuclear cardiac imaging chapter of this book, exercise stress testing can be used to evaluate for significant coronary artery disease. With stress echocardiography, images are obtained at rest in four standard views:

➤ The parasternal long axis for the posterior and anteroseptal walls.
➤ The parasternal short axis for all mid-ventricular segments.
➤ The apical four-chamber for the inferoseptal and lateral walls as well as the apex.
➤ The apical two-chamber for the inferior and anterior walls of the apex.

Thus, the mid-ventricular segments of all walls are visualized in two views. The exercise component is usually treadmill exercise. However, an upright or supine bicycle can also be used. A treadmill test has the advantage of being widely available with standardized protocols. At peak exercise, the patient quickly lies down for repeat imaging of the identical four views. Images are optimally captured within 60 s of peak exercise. Images taken both at rest and post-exercise are displayed side by side for optimal comparison. With bicycle exercise, the images can be performed during the workload. However, the imaging may be technically difficult in an upright position. The supine bicycle exercise offers the potential for improving image quality, but the workload is submaximal as compared to treadmill exercise.

For patients who cannot adequately exercise, dobutamine is commonly used to increase cardiac workload. Similar to exercise echocardiography, images are acquired at rest in the four standard views outlined above. Dobutamine is infused in a standard protocol, typically at 3-minute stages of increasing doses of 5 μg/kg/min, 10 μg/kg/min, 20 μg/kg/min, 30 μg/kg/min, and 40 μg/kg/min. Atropine in doses up to 1–2 mg is often used if the heart rate response is inadequate. Dobutamine stress carries the same risks as other types of stress, but hypotension and arrhythmia are more common. With dobutamine stress echocardiography, images are taken at each stage. Typically, for the final display, rest low dose, peak stress, and post-recovery images are displayed side by side.

Segmental wall motion is graded according to a semi-quantitative scale. A score of 1 is normal wall motion, defined as normal endocardial inward motion and wall thickening in systole. A hypokinetic segment is scored as 2, and defined as a reduction in endocardial motion and wall thickening in systole. An akinetic segment is scored as 3, and is defined as the absence of inward endocardial motion or wall thickening in systole. Dyskinetic segments, scored as 4, are defined as outward motion or 'bulging' in systole.

Experienced sonographers and physicians are critical for a good-quality stress echocardiogram. Good definition of endocardial borders is also important. When imaging is suboptimal with poor endocardial definition, contrast echocardiography or another imaging modality can be used (see Contrast echocardiography). Moreover, respiratory motion after high levels of exercise can be another limitation on the acquisition of adequate images.

A normal response of the myocardium to exercise or pharmacological stress is the augmentation of myocardial thickening. Any worsening of wall motion, or failure to augment, from rest to post-exercise images are indicative of significant CAD. Overall interpretation of the stress test places the echocardiographic information in the context of the other elements of the stress test. These elements include patient history, duration of exercise, patient symptoms, heart rate and blood pressure response, ST segment changes on ECG, and occurrence of arrhythmia.

Appropriate interpretation addresses the specific indication for the test. As with the other imaging modalities that are used during stress, common indications include the detection of CAD in a patient who is previously undiagnosed, evaluation after revascularization (i.e. coronary artery bypass grafting or percutaneous angioplasty), and risk stratification after myocardial infarction. Echocardiography adds sensitivity and specificity to the exercise and electrocardiographic information obtained during a routine stress test. This increase in sensitivity and specificity is particularly important in specific patient groups such as women with chest pain syndromes. In addition to these indications that are shared with the imaging modalities, stress echocardiography is also useful in observing changes in hemodynamics with stress. For instance, echocardiography enables the measurements of valvular gradients in aortic stenosis in the setting of low cardiac output, severity of mitral regurgitation, and pulmonary hypertension. Dobutamine stress echocardiography has been proposed to be used at low doses to determine viability of myocardium. Areas of myocardium can be 'hibernating' from chronic CAD. A low dose (10 µg/kg/min) can augment myocardial thickening in patients with viability territories of myocardium. Higher doses of dobutamine, as used for stress echocardiography, would worsen ischemia and create wall motion abnormalities.

CONTRAST ECHOCARDIOGRAPHY
Overview
Contrast echocardiography is a technique of obtaining M-mode and two-dimensional echocardiographic images after intravenous injection of ultrasound contrast agent. Ultrasound contrast agents are gas-filled microbubbles that resonate with exposure to ultrasound and produce high-intensity reflections of the transmitted ultrasound signal. The reflected ultrasound signal contains the original transmitted frequency and strong harmonic frequencies (multiples of the original frequency). By processing the harmonic signals, contrast-specific images with improved signal-to-noise ratio can be

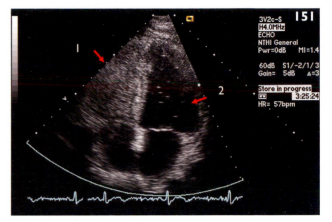

151 Apical four-chamber view showing dense opacification of the right ventricle (1) with agitated saline (bubbles) with a few bubbles seen in the left ventricle (2).

obtained. Current clinical applications of contrast echocardiography include detection of shunts, cavity opacification and endocardial border enhancement, augmentation of Doppler signals, and assessment of myocardial perfusion.

Detection of shunts
Agitated saline bubbles are created by forceful agitation of a mixture of saline solution and a small amount of air. The agitated saline is then rapidly injected intravenously. The microbubbles opacify the right heart and pulmonary arteries. Agitated saline bubbles rapidly coalesce and form larger bubbles which get trapped in the pulmonary arterioles and dissipate. Appearance of bubbles in the left heart is a sign of pathological right-to-left shunt, the location of which is determined by the timing and site of the appearance of bubbles (**151**). Early (less than three beats) appearance of bubbles in the left atrium is suggestive of right-to-left shunt at the level of the atria, such as atrial septal defect or patent foramen ovale. Delayed (greater than five beats) appearance of bubbles in the left atrium is suggestive of extracardiac shunts, such as pulmonary arteriovenous malformations.

Cavity opacification and improved border detection
The newer generation of ultrasound contrast agents consist of a shell made of albumin or synthetic phospholipid bi-layer filled with fluorocarbon gas. These bubbles are more uniform with a smaller size

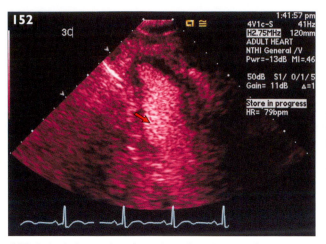

152 Apical three-chamber view showing good endocardial border definition with the use of an intracavitary contrast agent (arrow).

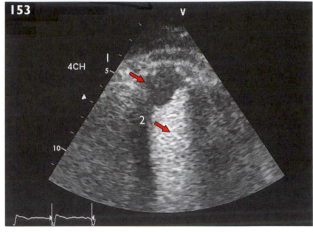

153 Apical four-chamber view showing left ventricular apical thrombus (1) with the use of intracavitray contrast (2).

allowing for passage through pulmonary capillaries. Ionic charge and reduced surface tension of the shells avoid coalescence and collapse of the bubbles, thus increasing half-life and sustained contrast effect. Continuous exposure to the ultrasound beam will cause intense resonation and ultimately destruction of the bubbles. Low mechanical index settings on the ultrasound scanner are chosen to avoid early bubble destruction and swirling.

Contrast-specific harmonic imaging will create an intense ultrasound signal in the blood pool with improved endocardial definition. One common use of intracavitary contrast agents includes improvement of endocardial border definition to evaluate regional wall motion in limited quality studies at rest or with stress echo (**152**). Another clinical use is to assess for the presence of left ventricular apical thrombus (**153**).

Contrast bubbles follow along with red blood cells in the direction of blood flow with a velocity similar to that of blood flow. However, the reflected ultrasound signal from contrast bubbles is stronger than the scattered signals from red blood cells. Contrast can therefore be used to intensify spectral Doppler signals and improve signal-to-noise ratio. This is particularly useful in instances where image quality is suboptimal or there is significant noise such as Doppler interrogation of pulmonary vein flows on transthoracic echo or enhancing spectral Doppler signals to obtain aortic flow velocity (**154**).

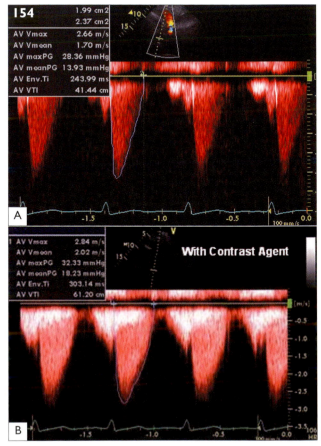

154 CW spectral Doppler across the aortic valve without (**A**) and with an intracavitary contrast agent (**B**) showing increased signal. Note that the increased flow velocity was obtained with contrast.

Myocardial perfusion contrast echocardiography

Myocardial perfusion can be detected and quantified by echocardiography. Perflurocarbon-based contrast bubbles flow with red blood cells into the coronary circulation and myocardial capillaries. After injection of a contrast bolus, reflected ultrasound from contrast bubbles in the capillaries can be detected as a bright signal in the myocardium. The intensity of the reflected signals correlates with the number of bubbles and the rate of appearance of contrast signals in the myocardium and is related to blood flow. By delivering a high-intensity (high mechanical index) ultrasound pulse one can destroy the existing bubbles in the myocardium and allow for re-accumulation in the capillaries. By repeating the high-intensity pulse in different physiological states, time–intensity curves from different myocardial regions can be obtained and compared. This technique has been shown to have good correlation with myocardial perfusion imaging in animal studies. Validation studies in humans are currently in progress. This technique has not yet been approved for clinical use by the US FDA.

THREE-DIMENSIONAL ECHOCARDIOGRAPHY

Three-dimensional echocardiography is a technique in which images of cardiac structures are obtained and displayed in all three spatial dimensions. The concept of three-dimensional echocardiography was introduced in the late 1970s, but the technology became feasible in the 1990s with development of faster computer processing.

Two approaches have been developed for obtaining three-dimensional echocardiographic images. The first approach is to create an image data set by stacking multiple parallel two-dimensional images acquired using a moving or rotating two-dimensional transducer. Each of the obtained two-dimensional images is subsequently registered with respect to the position of each imaging plane and to the timing in the cardiac and respiratory cycles. Image plane movements are usually achieved by stepwise computer-controlled rotations of TEE and TTE transducers. Ultimately, these two-dimensional images are stored and reconstructed to generate three-dimensional echocardiographic images.

The second and more popular approach is the 'volumetric' imaging described below. This technique uses a three-dimensional matrix array transducer with pyramid-shaped ultrasound beam to obtain and display real-time three-dimensional images. These probes are also capable of sending and receiving Doppler signals. The advantage of this technique is ease of use and ability to obtain three-dimensional images in real time. The major disadvantage of this technique is limited temporal and lateral resolution. Real-time volumetric images can be displayed in three-dimensions using a shade of gray levels to provide a sensation of depth (**155**). Given the time required for image processing and reconstruction, in order to preserve temporal resolution only a narrow image sector and a portion of the left ventricle can be visualized in the real-time three-dimensional images. To obtain a three-dimensional image of the entire heart, images are obtained during a breath hold over

155 Three-dimensional parasternal long-axis view showing the left atrium (1), the left ventricle (2), the proximal aorta (3), and the right ventricle (4).

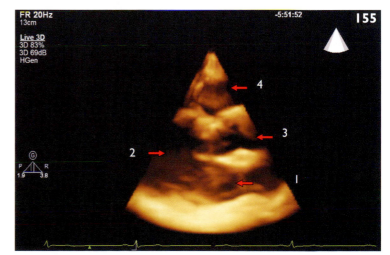

four cardiac cycles. Data from the four heart beats are combined and displayed in a full-volume three-dimensional image which can be cropped and displayed along any desired image plane (**156**). Images may also be displayed as multiple orthogonal imaging planes, known as multislice display.

Thanks to fewer geometric assumptions, three-dimensional echocardiographic imaging is more accurate and reproducible than two-dimensional echocardiographic imaging in the measurements of

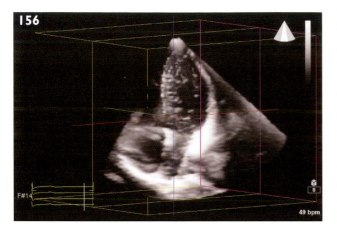

156 Three-dimensional apical view showing the potential for displaying along multiple planes.

ventricular volumes, particularly in patients with significant regional wall motion abnormalities. These measurements have shown good correlations with other imaging techniques such as CT, MRI, and radionucleotide angiography. Three-dimensional echocardiography can also provide visualization of the valvular structures in different anatomical planes. A left atrial view (surgeon's view) of the mitral valve can show the abnormalities in the leaflets and assist in understanding of mechanism and severity of mitral regurgitation. Similarly '*en face*' display of septal defects can provide better understanding of anatomical relations and provide information regarding the patient's suitability for a device for closure of septal defects. Another potential application of three-dimensional echocardiography is simultaneous acquisition of multislice images in three orthogonal planes. This will shorten the image acquisition time and potentially improve diagnostic utility.

Three-dimensional echocardiography has potential application in the assessments of left ventricular mechanics, diastolic relaxation and dysfunction, as well as myocardial strain. The current major limitations of three-dimensional echocardiographic systems are expense, lack of universal availability, and limited temporal resolution.

CLINICAL CASES

Case 1: Aortic Valve Endocarditis

Clinical history

A 44-year-old male with past medical history of intravenous drug abuse, human immunodeficiency virus (HIV) disease, and end-stage renal disease secondary to HIV nephropathy was admitted to the hospital with fevers and chills of 2 weeks' duration. The patient admitted to recent intravenous drug abuse. He was febrile to 38.2°C (100.8°F) on admission, with a normal blood pressure. He was tachycardic, and had a mild systolic ejection murmur and a diastolic murmur. There was evidence of heart failure on examination. There were no stigmata of endocarditis noted. Three sets of blood cultures were positive for Gram-positive cocci.

Imaging protocol

Transthoracic echocardiographic images revealed a thickened aortic valve without obvious mobile vegetation (**157**). Color images (not shown) demonstrated severe aortic regurgitation. These findings were suggestive, but not definitive, for endocarditis.

A transesophageal echocardiogram was obtained to determine the presence of definite vegetation and/or abscess and to plan possible surgical intervention (**158**). Aortic valve vegetation and abscess of the aortic root were noted. Moderate–severe aortic regurgitation is shown with color Doppler.

Impression

Aortic valve endocarditis and aortic root abscess.

Discussion and management

The patient was treated with intravenous antibiotics for 4 days with resolution of bacteremia. He continued to have persistent heart failure and was subsequently taken to the operating room for an aortic valve replacement. Intraoperative findings consisted of multiple valvular vegetations with an aortic root abscess extending into the mitral valve. These areas were extensively debrided and the aortic and mitral valves were replaced. He had an uneventful postoperative course and was discharged.

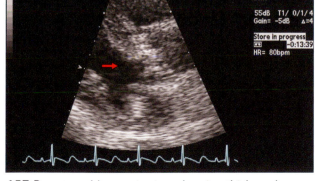

157 Parasternal long-axis view showing thickened aortic valve (arrow) without obvious mobile vegetation.

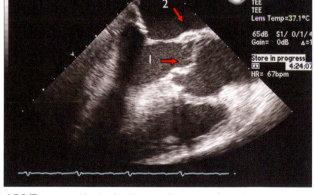

158 Transesophageal echocardiogram showing aortic valve (1) vegetation and abscess (2) of the aortic root.

Case 2: Pericardial Effusion

Clinical history

A 65-year-old male with CAD had status post coronary artery bypass grafting. He had a history of paroxysmal atrial fibrillation and took warfarin chronically. He presented to the emergency room with shortness of breath. On examination, his blood pressure was 90/60 mmHg with a pulse of 125 bpm in sinus rhythm. His jugular venous pressure was elevated, his heart sounds were distant, and his lung examination was unremarkable.

Imaging protocol

A transthoracic echocardiogram demonstrated a large pericardial effusion with fibrinous material (**159**). Echocardiographic features suggestive of tamponade physiology were seen, including right atrial collapse, right ventricular collapse, plethora of the inferior vena cava, and respiratory variation in the left ventricular inflow (**160**).

Impression

Large pericardial effusion with clinical and echocardiographic evidence of cardiac tamponade.

Discussion and management

Since a large amount of fluid was present anteriorly, a percutaneous drainage technique was attempted from a subxiphoid approach. The patient underwent successful pericardiocentesis (needle aspiration) under echocardiographic guidance. The patient recovered successfully without recurrence.

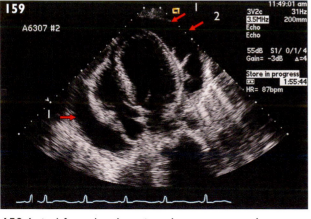

159 Apical four-chamber view demonstrates a large circumferential pericardial effusion (1) with fibrinous (2) material.

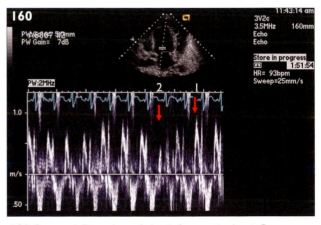

160 Spectral Doppler of the left ventricular inflow demonstrating excessive respiratory variation. (1: expiration; 2: inspiration.)

Case 3: Aortic Stenosis

Clinical history

A 60-year-old male had a past medical history of hypertension, CAD, with a prior inferoposterior myocardial infarction, and chronic renal failure secondary to hypertension. He complained of dyspnea on exertion without evidence of classic angina. On examination, he had a late-peaking systolic ejection murmur which radiated to the carotids, and an absent aortic component of the second heart sound, without a third heart sound. There was evidence of slow and delayed carotid upstroke bilaterally. He had clear lung fields without evidence of peripheral edema.

Imaging protocol

On TTE, the aortic valve was thickened and appeared to be stenotic (**161**). The LVOT diameter measured 2.2 cm (**162**). The peak instantaneous velocity across LVOT was 1.3 m/s, with a velocity time integral (VTI) of 0.251 m (**163**). The peak instantaneous velocity across aortic valve was 5.0 m/sec, with a peak instantaneous gradient of 98 mmHg, a mean gradient of 55 mmHg and a VTI of 1.11 m (**164**). The aortic valve area calculated by the continuity equation (Equation 9) was 0.9 cm^2.

Impression

These Doppler findings were consistent with the visual estimate of severe aortic stenosis.

Discussion and management

The patient underwent successful aortic valve replacement.

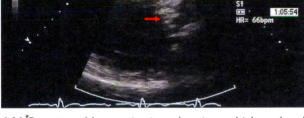

161 Parasternal long-axis view showing a thickened and stenotic aortic valve (arrow).

162 Parasternal long-axis view showing measurement of the left ventricular outflow tract diameter at end-systole.

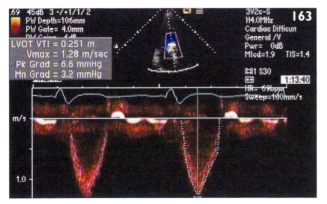

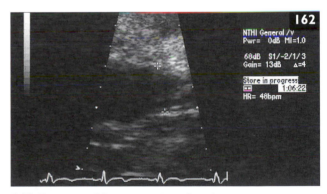

163 Spectral Doppler measuring left ventricular outflow tract velocity and velocity time integral.

164 Spectral Doppler measuring velocity and velocity time integral across the aortic valve. Note the presence of both aortic stenosis (1) and aortic regurgitation (2).

5. CARDIOVASCULAR MAGNETIC RESONANCE IMAGING

André Schmidt   Joao AC Lima

INTRODUCTION

Cardiac magnetic resonance imaging (CMRI) (Lund 2001) is a promising imaging modality with substantial clinical applications thanks to its unique diagnostic versatility. CMRI provides detailed anatomical information about the heart and also allows for the assessments of global and regional cardiac function, volumes, and mass, and the assessments of myocardial perfusion, valvular function, and tissue characterization. In this chapter various established and emerging clinical applications of CMRI will be discussed.

MRI principles

Paramagnetic substances with an odd number of protons and/or neutrons, such as ^{1}H, ^{14}N, ^{31}P, ^{13}C, and ^{23}Na, have the property of spinning (precession) around their axes and can be used for 'imaging' by MRI. When exposed to a magnetic field, these atoms will align with the magnetic field and continue to precess. Hydrogen is the atom most widely used in MRI because of its abundant presence in the human body and optimal signal strength. Therefore, unless stated otherwise, the MRI described in this chapter is referred to ^{1}H MRI.

From the basic physics it is known that a moving charged particle generates a magnetic field. When exposed to an intense magnetic field, such as that generated by MRI equipment, all individual magnetic fields are aligned and a resultant vector is obtained. Another important concept of MRI is the Larmor equation: $f = \gamma M$, where f is frequency in revolutions per second of the precessing substance, γ is the gyromagnetic ratio of the substance (e.g. hydrogen) which is a constant, and M is the strength of the magnetic field expressed in Tesla (T). According to this equation, the frequency of precession is directly proportional to the strength of the magnetic field, and since the gyromagnetic ratio is a constant being specific for each substance, the frequency of precession is unique. The strength of the magnetic field in a specific location can be manipulated to obtain information from which images can be generated.

Radiofrequency (RF) pulses are used to manipulate the strength of the magnetic field and to generate tomographic images of the body, since they can be emitted in precise dimensions. An important distinction to be made is that the continuous magnetic field in a MRI scanner is due to a direct current, while RF pulses are generated by alternating currents located in the coils inside the MRI scanner. These pulses induce an electromagnetic wave that affects the precessing, making it tip over its direction. The maximal effect is obtained when the nuclei are deflected by 90°. When the RF pulses cease, a return to its original position begins, but in order to do so, the protons have to release the energy gained from the RF pulses. By collecting this information and using a mathematical procedure called 'Fourier Transform', a computer can generate and display an accurate image with degrees of intensity (gray levels) and a precise spatial location. By using the distinct patterns of release of this energy from tissues with distinct percentages of hydrogen, a precise map of the tissues can be obtained.

CMRI (Lund 2001) has some unique characteristics. Usually, a static image can be obtained by repeating RF pulses during data acquisitions. Due to the fact that the heart is beating, electrocardiographic gating is needed to define precisely the time point in the cardiac cycle where the RF pulses are applied. This ECG-gating procedure should be repeated until the image of the particular point is completed so that image of the next point can be acquired without motion interference. Several consecutive cardiac cycles are needed to produce an image of each particular point. As such, long image acquisition time is expected for CMRI. Also, it should be understood that the patient should not breathe during the image acquisitions, since it would otherwise change the position of the heart, causing another image artifact. Thus, CMRI is an examination that requires careful monitoring in order to obtain good-quality images. Nonetheless, continuous improvements in techniques have substantially reduced the effects of cardiac and respiratory motion.

MRI scanner

MRI scanners consist of a superconducting magnet that produces a strong magnetic field, expressed in Tesla. For cardiac applications a 1.5 T MRI scanner is usually used. A uniform magnetic field can be generated and can also be manipulated with the use of gradients to produce small differences, providing spatial location. In addition, the scanner has coils to generate the specific RF pulses that resonate the specific atoms at a specific location, and antennae located in the coils will receive the signals that can be analyzed and organized by a computer to reconstruct images. The computer is also needed in order to generate the sequence of RF pulses and gradient adjustments during the examination.

MRI safety

Besides the usual precautions applicable to any MRI scan, it should be remembered that the MRI suite is a tight place, usually not suitable for emergency care. Patients who are clinically unstable should not undergo a MRI examination, unless they are supervised by trained personnel and there is emergency equipment near the MRI suite where the patients can be rapidly removed to if needed.

The main practical limitation for MRI is currently the imaging of patients with vascular clips, used for cerebral aneurysm surgery; there is a potential risk of dislodgement (Fenchel *et al.* 2005). Patients with implanted cardiac pacemakers, defibrillators, cochlear implants, and neurologic stimulators also should not undergo a MRI examination due to possible malfunctioning of these devices or the potential risk caused by the generation of currents. Recent data has shown that MRI examinations in a 1.5 T scanner are feasible and safe for most modern pacemakers and intracoronary stents, although some image artifacts occur. Prosthetic heart valves, unless they have a large amount of alloy, such as the Starr-Edwards pre-6000 series (Edwards *et al.* 2000), present no problem. Other metallic material that often exists in patients who had cardiac surgery, such as sternal wires, clips, and epicardial pacing leads, have not been reported to cause complications (Shellock & Kanal 1994).

MRI has no known effect on the fetus. Nevertheless, an MRI examination of pregnant women is usually postponed until the second trimester. Safety concerns should be balanced against the benefits expected in each individual clinical situation. Claustrophobia can occur in 1–5% of patients, but the use of light sedation, without compromising cooperation from the patient, may solve this problem. There are internet sites (e.g. www.mrisafety.com) that provide accurate and updated information on safety issues related to MRI which can be helpful in specific situations.

The increasing use of contrast agents has raised the question of intolerance and risks. Gadolinium, a rare metal, tends to accumulate in tissues due to its high affinity for membranes. It is used in the form of chelates, which are water soluble and are not nephrotoxic. Most of the injected gadolinium is excreted quickly by the kidneys. Some fecal excretion also occurs. It is rarely associated with allergic reactions (Ungkanont *et al.* 1998). Metallic taste is the most common side-effect, followed by headache, nausea, and vomiting. The side-effects are usually mild and rarely require medical intervention. Severe allergic reactions are rare (<1/300,000 in some series). For safety reasons the administration of gadolinium should be avoided in pregnant or lactating women.

CLINICAL APPLICATIONS

CMRI is an emerging diagnostic methodology. Clinical applications are expanding because of its potential for evaluating various aspects of cardiovascular diseases.

Anatomical evaluation

CMRI allows for imaging of the heart and the great vessels in any desired planes in order to explore anatomic relations and surrounding structures (**165**). Thanks to this flexibility it is possible to perform CMRI in planes that are familiar to cardiologists trained in X-ray CT and echocardiography. X-ray CT is usually used in examinations where an anatomical definition of the heart and great vessels is required, whereas echocardiography is used when the heart itself is being evaluated (Dinsmore *et al.* 1984). The accuracy of plane orientation is extreme, allowing for precise orientation and selection of the best plane to demonstrate the point of interest. Standardization of myocardial segmentation has been recommended in order to facilitate the comparison between cardio-vascular imaging modalities (Cerqueira *et al.* 2002).

Slice thickness, image resolution, and application of sequences are selected as needed to acquire the desired information. As discussed later, small structures such as the walls of coronary arteries can be defined clearly by CMRI. The use of multiple imaging planes serves well to reduce misleading information sometimes obtained from inappropriate angles of view.

Assessment of global ventricular function

Accurate and reproducible measurement of EF is of great importance in clinical cardiology. The assessments of both left and right ventricular function have

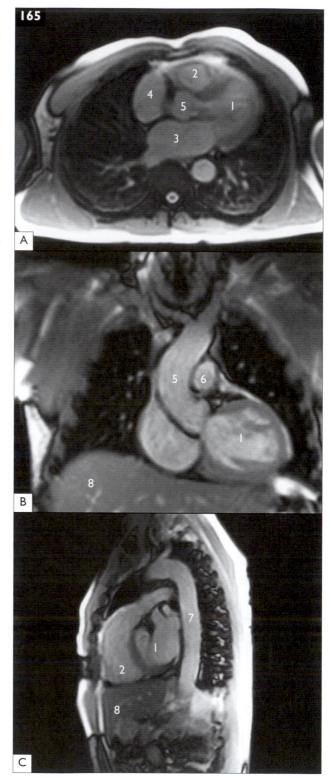

165 Cardiac MRI allows distinct planes for exploring anatomical relations between the heart and great vessels and other thoracic structures. (**A**) Axial plane. (**B**) Coronal plane. (**C**) Sagittal plane. (1: left ventricle; 2: right ventricle; 3: left atrium; 4: right atrium; 5: ascending aorta; 6: pulmonary artery; 7: descending aorta; 8: liver.)

important prognostic implications in a variety of clinical settings. CMRI has been used as the gold standard for EF calculation because of its high spatial and temporal resolution and its excellent correlation of EF with angiography (Sakuma *et al.* 1993, van Rossum *et al.* 1988a b). Endocardial borders are well defined in CMRI and multiple short-axis images can be acquired throughout the entire cardiac cycle, allowing for precise determination of multiple systolic and diastolic volumes. The development of new sequences that are faster without losing spatial and temporal resolution (Carr *et al.* 2001) has further increased the appeal of CMRI. A complete stack of short-axis slices can be obtained in 5–10 minutes. The most precise technique for calculating EF is based on the Simpson's rule which is independent of geometric assumptions. Ventricular volumes in both end-systole and end-diastole are obtained by the sum of the endocardial areas multiplied by the centers of each slice (**166**). Most commercial CMRI systems have analysis tools with automated border detection software to assist tracing the endocardium. Nevertheless, some limitations remain with excessive endocardial trabeculations and prominent papillary muscles. It is standard that the papillary muscles are excluded for the assessment of global ventricular function. In patients with heavy trabeculations, manual tracing of the endocardial borders may be needed. Because of the complex geometry of the right ventricle, it is usually preferred to trace its endocardial borders by hand. However, Simpson's rule can also be incorporated into the EF calculation for the right ventricle and good correlations can generally be obtained for the assessment of right ventricular EF (Boxt *et al.* 1992).

Assessment of ventricular mass

Myocardial mass can be estimated accurately by multiplying its volume by the specific gravity of the myocardium, 1.05 g/cm^3. The assessment of myocardial mass by MRI has been validated previously for both ventricles.

Lorenz *et al.* have published normal values for the cardiac volumes and mass that have been used widely

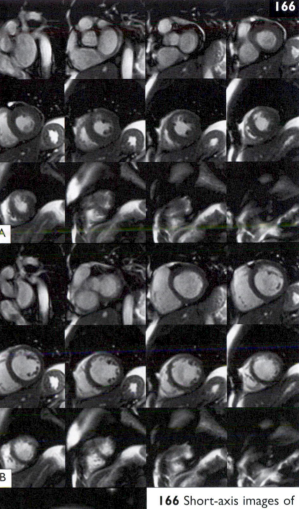

A

B

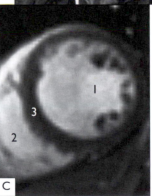

C

166 Short-axis images of the ventricles, both in systole (**A**) and diastole (**B**). Measurement of endocardial and epicardial borders in systolic and diastolic frames are used to quantify ventricular mass and volumes precisely from which ejection fraction can be calculated. Enlarged midventricular diastolic frame (**C**) shows location of the walls. Analysis of motion allows for characterization of regional wall motion abnormalities. (1: left ventricle; 2: right ventricle; 3: septum.)

as a standard reference (Lorenz *et al.* 1999, Lorenz 2000). For adults these measurements were derived from normal male and female subjects who underwent CMRI (*Table 6*), whereas the normal values for infants, children, and adolescents were extrapolated from previous echocardiographic measurements.

Assessment of regional ventricular function

Assessment of global ventricular function is of primary importance in clinical practice. However, for complete evaluation of patients with most of cardiac diseases the assessment of regional ventricular function is equally useful. For instance, the demonstration of functional recovery of injured segments in patients with ischemic heart disease is of importance as a parameter of viability and may have prognostic implications for the development or progression of left ventricular remodeling. Regional myocardial function can be estimated visually both by endocardial motion and wall thickening. Regional function is determined by measuring the velocity and amplitude of myocardial deformation of a segment submitted to a given load or stress. Most methods use endocardial motion as a

surrogate of regional function by visual analysis, a suboptimal method, although intra- and inter-observer variability is acceptable when the assessment is performed by well trained observers. Regional ventricular function can be assessed before and after an intervention with the patient serving as his/her own control.

CMRI using cine techniques has the capability of measuring endocardial motion by endocardial and epicardial border delineation in systolic and diastolic frames, but these measurements are time consuming and are subject to technical and functional limitations. Recently, most of these limitations have been overcome by the use of myocardial tagging (Zerhouni *et al.* 1988, Axel & Dougherty 1989, Moore *et al.* 2000). This technique allows for placement of virtual markers in the myocardium using selective radiofrequency excitation to saturate the magnetization in region, prior to the acquisition of images. These markers (tags) can be identified as dark lines in the myocardium on subsequent images and persist during systole and most of diastole. It is relatively easy to use this method to track the deformation of the tagged lines and to assess motion and strain in distinct myocardial regions and

Table 6 Normal values for the cardiac volumes and mass in adults according to gender. The values are expressed as mean ± SD and the 95% confidence intervals are presented in parentheses

Parameter	Males	Females
LVEDV (mL)	130 ± 30 (77–195)	96 ± 23 (52–141)
LVESV (mL)	45 ± 14 (Leung et al. 1995)	32 ± 9 (13–51)
LVEF (%)	67 ± 5 (56–78)	67 ± 5 (56–78)
LV MASS (g)	178 ± 31 (118–238)	125 ± 26 (75–175)
LVSV (mL)	92 ± 21 (51–133)	65 ± 16 (33–97)
RVEDV (mL)	157 ± 35 (88–227)	106 ± 24 (58–154)
RVESV (mL)	63 ± 20 (23–103)	40 ± 14 (12–68)
RVEF (%)	60 ± 7 (47–74)	63 ± 8 (47–80)
RVFW MASS (g)	50 ± 10 (30–70)	40 ± 8 (24–55)
RVSV (mL)	95 ± 22 (52–138)	66 ± 16 (35–98)
CO (L/min)	5.8 ± 3.0 (2.82–8.82)	4.3 ± 0.9 (2.65–5.98)

LVEDV: Left ventricle end-diastolic volume; LVESV: left ventricle end-systolic volume; LVEF: left ventricle ejection fraction; LV MASS: left ventricle mass; LVSV: left ventricle stroke volume; RVEDV: right ventricle end-diastolic volume; RVESV: right ventricle end-systolic volume; RVEF: right ventricle ejection fraction; RVFW MASS: right ventricle free wall mass; RVSV: right ventricle stroke volume; CO: cardiac output.

layers, i.e. subendocardial, mid-myocardial, and subepicardial layers (**167**). Strain analysis is more accurate and reproducible than visual estimation or thickening measurements since it takes into account the cardiac motion in all directions simultaneously. New post-processing analysis software, such as HARP (Osman & Prince 2000, Pan *et al.* 2003) and DENSE (Kim *et al.* 2004), has simplified the quantification of myocardial strain.

Myocardial tagging is a promising tool and is applied in a wide variety of clinical situations, further increasing knowledge on pathophysiological mechanisms of cardiomyopathies (Kramer *et al.* 1994, MacGowan *et al.* 1997), ischemic heart disease (Gerber *et al.* 2002), and valvular diseases (Van Der *et al.* 2002). It has also been applied to patient population studies (Fernandes *et al.* 2006). In ischemic heart disease,

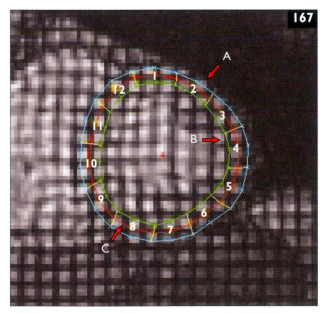

167 Tagging image of the left ventricle with HARP (harmonic phase magnetic resonance imaging) tracings for epicardial, mid-myocardial, and endocardial borders that can be used for calculating strain at any specific area. Arbitrary segmentation (in this example, 12 segments) allows for analysis of regional contractility. (A: epicardial border; B: endocardial border; C: mid-wall of the myocardium.) (Courtesy of Dr. Verônica Fernandes.)

myocardial tagging has been used in postinfarction patients to provide unique functional information about infarcted regions and compensatory changes in noninfarcted portions of the left ventricle (Kramer *et al.* 1993). It has been demonstrated that even in patients with one-vessel disease and acute myocardial infarction, circumferential shortening is affected throughout the ventricle, including remote areas that are not directly involved in the myocardial infarction (Kramer *et al.* 1996).

Stress CMRI is a promising tool in the evaluation of myocardial viability. Dobutamine CMRI is currently under intense investigation. The principle is similar to dobutamine stress echocardiography. If there is a significantly stenotic coronary artery, infusion of dobutamine will increase the demand that cannot be met adequately by increasing coronary blood flow. A motion abnormality will occur as a result of regional myocardial ischemia. Most studies have relied on visual analysis, and due to suboptimal image quality many studies could not be properly analyzed (Mankad *et al.* 2003). The published sensitivity of dobutamine CMRI varies between 83% and 96% with high specificity of 80–100%. The application of myocardial tagging may increase the sensitivity of dobutamine CMRI (Sayad *et al.* 1998, Strach *et al.* 2006).

With incorporation of recently developed post-processing techniques as described above, time involved in the analysis can be substantially shortened. It is expected that diagnosis will be improved thanks to the earlier detection of regional wall motion abnormalities.

Evaluation of ischemic heart disease

Evaluation of ischemic heart disease is currently one of the most important indications for CMRI. Some authors have proposed that CMRI is the method of choice for a complete anatomical and functional evaluation of the heart (Poon *et al.* 2002). This section will provide a brief overview of the different aspects of CMRI evaluation in ischemic heart disease.

Myocardial perfusion

Myocardial perfusion can be evaluated very effectively using a bolus injection of intravascular MRI contrast and the subsequent fast-sequence acquisition of images that record the transit of the bolus through the heart and central circulation (Schaefer *et al.* 1992). This technique is called 'dynamic first-pass imaging'.

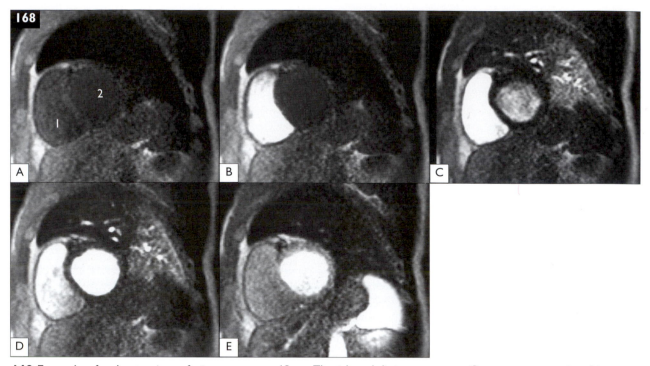

168 Example of a short-axis perfusion sequence (**A** to **E**) with gadolinium contrast. Contrast appears in white. (**A**) Initial image obtained at the start of injection in a peripheral vein. No contrast is seen. (**B**) Contrast reaches right ventricular cavity. (**C**) Left ventricular opacification begins as contrast starts to fill the cavity, but not the myocardium. (**D**) Maximum opacification of the ventricle; myocardium starts to opacify. (**E**) Uniform opacification of the myocardium. (1: right ventricle; 2: left ventricle.)

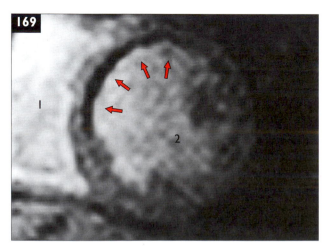

169 Example of a CMRI short-axis myocardial perfusion image in a patient with recent myocardial infarction. A subendocardial ring of hypoenhancement (arrows) appears indicating hypoperfusion in the anterior portion of the septal wall. (1: right ventricle; 2: left ventricle.)

After a peripheral injection, the contrast can be first seen in the right ventricle, subsequently in the left ventricle, and finally it opacifies the myocardium (**168**). It takes approximately ten heart beats to achieve a signal intensity that correlates with peak contrast concentration in the myocardium (Wilke *et al.* 1999, Ishida *et al.* 2003, Wu 2003).

Although it is still pending approval by the US FDA, the use of contrast permits significant collection of information. An appropriate technique and adequate dose of contrast is necessary to allow for an accurate interpretation, although inter-observer variation is high. Qualitative analysis of the signal intensity of the contrast in different regions of the heart is capable of showing the presence of hypoenhancement in the hypoperfused areas (**169**). As an alternative, one can use special software to generate signal intensity curves that will provide quantitative values in addition to the visual analysis.

The assessment of myocardial viability is one of the most important applications of CMRI for first-pass perfusion and will be explored in a later section. Another important application of CMRI perfusion imaging is in the assessment of stress perfusion. To detect significant stenoses of the epicardial coronary arteries, it is helpful to stress the patient so that a measure of the coronary flow reserve, or other similar measures such as the myocardial perfusion reserve index, can be obtained. Though technically feasible, it would be uncomfortable for a patient to perform a physical exercise stress test within the confined bore of a MR imager. Instead, a pharmaceutical agent, such as dipyridamole (typical dose: 0.56 mg/kg) or shorter-acting adenosine (typical dose: 140 µg/kg/min), can be administered to induce coronary vasodilatation. The safety profile and more consistent mechanism of action make adenosine the preferred agent for stress perfusion MRI. The safety of pharmacologic vasodilation with either dipyridamole or adenosine has been extensively documented in the nuclear cardiology literature. The presence of abnormal myocardial perfusion reserve in MRI helps distinguish patients with CAD from normal subjects (Cullen *et al.* 1999).

In a study of 104 patients, MRI had 90% sensitivity for depicting at least one coronary artery with significant stenosis and 85% specificity in the identification of patients with significant coronary artery stenoses. It has been reported that stress enhancement by dynamic MRI correlated more closely with quantitative coronary angiography results than stress enhancement of SPECT (Ishida *et al.* 2003). Findings of several studies have confirmed the sensitivity and specificity of stress perfusion MRI as equivalent or superior to those of SPECT. In the literature, sensitivity and specificity of MRI are 64–92% and 71–100%, respectively (Lauerma *et al.* 1997, Panting *et al.* 2001, Fenchel *et al.* 2005). Therefore, CMRI appears to be a reasonable alternative to SPECT for the evaluation of patients with suspected CAD, without radiation exposure and with the additional advantages of better depiction of wall motion and myocardial viability.

Post-infarct microcirculatory function and microvascular obstruction evaluations by MRI

During routine coronary angiography, it is not possible to assess adequately the microvasculature (arterioles, capillaries, and venules). Despite the recanalization of the epicardial coronary artery after acute infarction, in many instances there is persistently diminished blood flow because the microvasculature remains plugged by red blood cell stasis, myocardial edema, or endothelial cell damage from free radical formation. This is known as the 'no-reflow' phenomenon, which indicates lack of reperfusion from microvascular impairment at the core of a reperfused infarct. Using contrast-enhanced MRI (ceMRI) (Lim *et al.* 2004), in addition to hyperenhancement (see below), acutely infarcted territories often demonstrate marked heterogeneity which reflects the status of the microvasculature. In the first few minutes following a contrast bolus injection, a subset of patients develop a hypoenhanced or dark region with decreased signal intensity in the subendocardial layer of the myocardium that later enhances (Lima *et al.* 1995) (**170**). The presence of hypoenhancement correlates with an increased incidence of total coronary occlusion at initial angiography post myocardial infarction, electrocardiographic Q-waves, and greater regional dysfunction by echocardiography. However, it was also noted that half of the patients with hypoenhancement ultimately have a widely patent infarct-related artery post revascularization. Hence, it

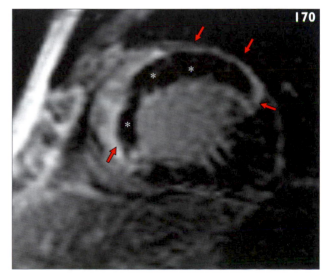

170 Delayed image (13 minutes after injection of contrast), showing a ring of hyperenhancement (arrows), indicating the area of infarction, and a large area of hypoenhancement (asterisks), indicating the region of microvascular obstruction (no-reflow).

has been postulated that these regions represent the no-reflow phenomenon or regions of microvascular obstruction as previously described in experimental and human studies.

It has been demonstrated that MRI hypoenhanced regions have microsphere-measured flow rates less than half of that in remote post-reperfusion regions and correlate in anatomical location and spatial extent to no-reflow regions as assessed by pathology (Judd *et al.* 1995). Subendocardial regions with MRI no-reflow had delayed contrast wash-in as opposed to the delayed contrast wash-out of the hyperenhanced region, which can be potentially explained by the capillary obstruction seen within the infarct. Decreased functional capillary density prolongs the time for gadolinium molecules to penetrate the infarct core, leading to the dark and low signal intensity early after a contrast bolus injection.

Microvascular obstruction (MO) following revascularization is a progressive phenomenon and, in an animal model, hypoenhancement increased three-fold during the first 48 hours post reperfusion. MRI hyperenhancement for infarct size also increased by 33% at 48 hours (Rochitte *et al.* 1998), and stabilized and disappeared by 6 months.

MO has important long-term implications (Wu *et al.* 1998). In patients with acute reperfused myocardial infarction, the presence of MO identified by ceMRI was associated with an increased rate of cardiovascular complications 16 ± 5 months post infarction (**171**). Infarct size identified by ceMRI also predicted adverse clinical outcome and MO presence was clearly associated with larger infarcts. Nonetheless, using multivariate analysis and controlling for infarct size, the presence of MO remained a significant independent prognostic factor in outcome. In patients returning for 6-month MRI follow-up, those with MO had increased end-diastolic and end-systolic volumes and increased rates of myocardial fibrous scar formation. Hence, a potential mechanism for the worse clinical prognosis associated with MO is its adverse effect on left ventricular remodeling post myocardial infarct. The explanation for this relation was elucidated by an experimental model demonstrating that increasing amounts of MO correlated significantly with altered myocardial strains both in the infarcted and adjacent noninfarcted myocardium. Interestingly, there was a time differential in the occurrence of the strain alterations with the changes occurring at 48 hours post reperfusion in the noninfarcted region versus 6 hours in

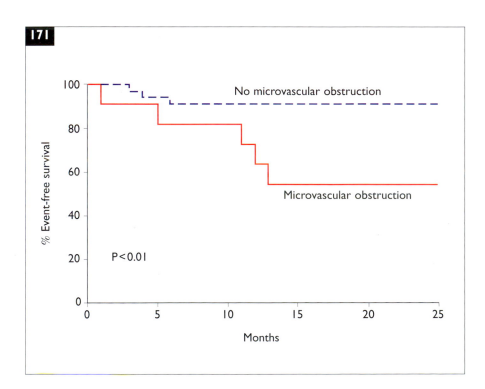

171 Long-term prognostic significance of the presence of MO. Event-free survival (clinical course without cardiovascular death, reinfarction, congestive heart failure, or stroke) for patients with or without MRI MO. Presence of MO was associated with an increased rate of cardiovascular complications. (Reprinted with permission from Wu KC, Zerhouni EA, Judd RM *et al.* Prognostic significance of microvascular obstruction by magnetic resonance imaging in patients with acute myocardial infarction. *Circulation* 1998; **97**;765–772.)

the infarcted territory. Hence, infarcted regions with widespread MO experience reduced elasticity early after reperfusion.

In summary, ceMRI is capable of identifying MO which is associated with worse prognosis and predicts the development of adverse left ventricular remodeling.

Assessment of myocardial viability

MRI has emerged as a powerful modality to assess myocardial viability, with a significant role in patients who are considered for coronary revascularization. Post-contrast myocardial delayed enhancement, detected by MRI, is the most accurate means to detect and quantify myocardial infarction. Cellular degradation in the infarcted region results in an increase in vascular permeability and enlargement of the extravascular space, and hence an increased distribution volume for the extracellular contrast agent.

Gadolinium chelate wash-out from infarcted tissue is slower than from healthy myocardium. The net result is that infarcted regions appear bright on delayed contrast-enhanced T1-weighted images. The size and location of the infarcted region, as demonstrated histochemically in animal models, correlate with the size and location of myocardial delayed enhancement. In humans, the contrast enhancement was correlated with fixed thallium defect size.

Chronic infarcts also display hyperenhancement, though the mechanisms are somewhat different. The extracellular space is increased in collagenous scars which may explain the increased volume of distribution for gadolinium in chronic infarction. Reduced capillary density in chronic scars also reduces contrast wash-out, leading to the hyperenhancement (**172**).

The accuracy of ceMRI in quantifying infarct size has been investigated and compared to histopathology. Initial studies demonstrated a strong correlation

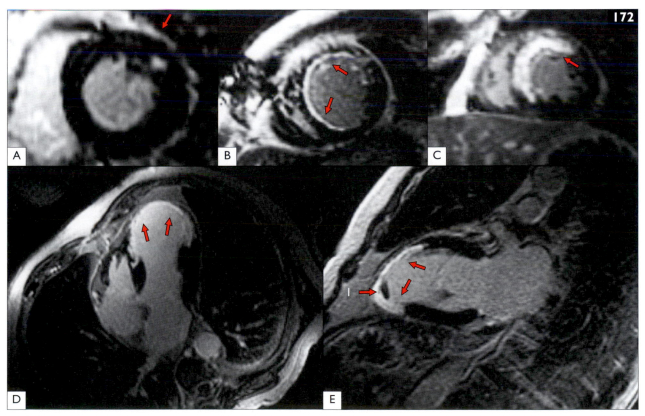

172 Contrast-enhanced images of chronic infarcts (arrows). (**A**) Small subendocardial scar located in the anterolateral wall. (**B**) Large subendocardial scar at mid-ventricular level and anteroseptal location. (**C**) Transmural anteroseptal scar. (**D**) Large transmural scar that extends from the mid-ventricular portion of the septal wall to the lateral wall, involving the apex. (**E**) Large transmural scar involving the apex. A mural thrombus (1) is seen in the apex as a hypoenhanced area.

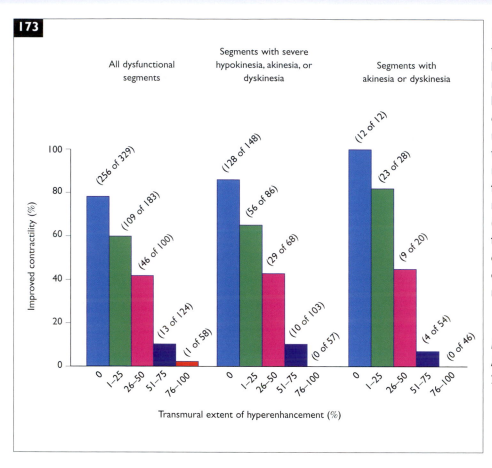

173 Relationship between transmural extent of hyperenhancement before revascularization and the likelihood of increased contractility after revascularization. The transmural extent was related with recovery of function after revascularization (Reprinted with permission from Kim RJ, Wu E, Rafael A et al. The use of contrast-enhanced magnetic resonance imaging to identify reversible myocardial dysfunction. *New England Journal of Medicine* Nov 16 2000;**343**(20):1445–1453.)

(r = 0.88–0.93) but also indicated that ceMRI overestimated infarct size by 8–15%. It has been suggested that the 'overestimation' was attributed to the partial volume effect of imaging relatively thin slices.

An early method for evaluating myocardial viability with MRI was based on end-diastolic wall thickness. End-diastolic wall thickness <5.5 mm (for defining nonviable myocardium) had 92% sensitivity in predicting functional recovery after revascularization, but specificity is not high (La Noce *et al.* 2002), making it simply an auxiliary in the diagnosis (McNamara & Higgins 1986).

MRI cine images appear to be similar to echocardiographic images for the evaluation of cardiac motion. Hence, the use of adrenergic stimulation to identify viable myocardium is performed in a similar way. CMRI has particular advantages since it permits visualization of cardiac motion with higher myocardial

border definition. It is also not affected by the limitations of poor acoustic windows. Dobutamine is infused to detect augmented contractility, indicating the presence of viable myocardium.

To visualize the major coronary territories of the heart adequately, three short-axis, one horizontal long-axis, and one vertical long-axis views of the left ventricle are acquired. Images are obtained at baseline and after dobutamine infusion. Gradient echo MRI sequences and lately steady-state free precession sequences are preferred (Hundley *et al.* 1999). Some limitations remain in this technique since visual analysis is subjective. Myocardial tagging is more accurate since it can accurately quantify local myocardial shortening at sites across the left ventricular wall thickness. Until now, only studies in small numbers of patients have been published (Geskin *et al.* 1998, Kramer *et al.* 2002), with high sensitivity and specificity (89% and 93%, respectively).

A study of 50 patients with ischemic left ventricular dysfunction has shown that the amount of delayed transmural enhancement predicts the degree of functional recovery after acute myocardial infarction. Extensive transmural myocardial delayed enhancement is highly predictive of a lack of functional improvement after revascularization. Conversely, absence of myocardial delayed enhancement correlates with a likelihood of functional recovery (Kim *et al.* 2000) (**173**).

Evaluation of valvular heart disease

CMRI has had limited application for the evaluation of valvular disease in the past years because of its high cost and the long processing time necessary to generate high-quality images comparable with those obtained with echocardiography, a cheaper and faster method with high spatial and temporal resolution. However, technical advances in the recent years have made the CMRI examination more user friendly. Due to the superior accuracy of CMRI for the quantification of cardiac function and myocardial mass as well as the capability of obtaining quantitative measurements of flow, CMRI should be considered as an alternative method in patients for whom echocardiography is not feasible.

One of the significant advantages of CMRI is that with a combination of sequences it is possible to obtain invaluable information in patients with valvular heart disease regarding chamber sizes, and regurgitant flow velocity and direction. For instance, cine MRI images allow for precise assessment of excursion of valves (and consequently valvular area) and semi-quantitative assessment of valvular regurgitation. Furthermore, it allows for the assessment of chamber size and hypertrophy. Velocity-encoded phase contrast techniques are also useful for accurate determination of regurgitant fraction/volumes, pressure gradients and valve areas (Ohnishi *et al.* 1992, Globits & Higgins 1995).

Mitral valve diseases

Mitral stenosis The main etiology of mitral stenosis is rheumatic heart disease. Thickened leaflets with reduced diastolic opening and associated enlarged left atrium can be identified by CMRI, as well as a signal-void jet beginning at the mitral valve level and extending into the cavity of the left ventricle during diastole on cine. Cine MRI can be used to quantitate mitral valve area which has been shown to correlate well with Doppler echocardiography (r = 0.86 *vs.* area by Doppler by the pressure half-time method) (Casolo *et al.* 1992). Moreover, other measurements also correlate well with echocardiography measurements, such as relative distal signal-void jet area (r = 0.77 *vs.* peak trans-valve gradient by catheterization) (Mitchell *et al.* 1989), peak trans-valve gradient (r = 0.89 *vs.* gradient by Doppler echocardiography) (Heidenreich *et al.* 1995), and using velocity-encoded technique to measure E-wave, A-wave, and pressure half-time, the results are similar to those obtained with echocardiography. The high-level reproducibility (>96%) of the data obtained from MRI has lowered the operator dependence (Lin *et al.* 2004).

Mitral regurgitation The regurgitant jet of mitral regurgitation is readily identified on cine MRI images as the signal-void systolic jet of turbulent flow extending from the mitral valve level into the left atrium (**174**). CMRI has high degree of accuracy in qualitatively identifying the regurgitant jet in comparison to Doppler color echocardiography (94–100% sensitivity

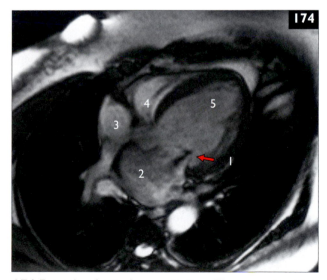

174 Example of mitral regurgitation. The regurgitant jet is readily identified on cine images as the signal-void systolic jet of turbulent flow (1) extending from the mitral valve level into the left atrium (2). (3: right atrium; 4: right ventricle; 5: left ventricle.)

and 95–100% specificity) (Wagner *et al.* 1989, Aurigemma *et al.* 1990). Besides the identification of the presence of mitral regurgitation, quantitative assessment of the regurgitant volume is of crucial importance for clinical purposes. The jet size, extension, and area are commonly measured by Doppler echocardiography. It has been shown that CMRI is well correlated with Doppler echocardiography in those measurements (e.g. r = 0.74 for distal signal-void jet size length, and r = 0.71 for absolute area) (Glogar *et al.* 1989).

Regurgitant volume/fraction evaluated by CMRI in comparison with echocardiography and ventriculography has shown even better correlation (r = 0.84–0.96). These results are promising, considering that they were obtained from selected populations some years ago (Fujita *et al.* 1994, Hundley *et al.* 1995). Recent studies with new techniques have obtained very good correlations (r = 0.91) in patients with severe regurgitation (Westenberg *et al.* 2004, 2005).

Aortic valve diseases

Aortic stenosis Concentric left ventricular hypertrophy, dilatation of the ascending aorta, and reduced aortic valve opening are well known anatomical abnormalities of aortic stenosis that can be identified by CMRI. A double-oblique cine image taken through the aortic valve plane is optimal for the visualization of the cusps and their coaptation. These images are useful for differentiating acquired aortic stenosis from congenital aortic stenosis with a bicuspid aortic valve. This sequence is also optimal for valve area evaluation and has an acceptable correlation (r = 0.75) with cardiac catheterization and Doppler echocardiography. Transvalvular gradients and peak gradients are obtained using the modified Bernoulli equation and presented excellent correlation with Doppler echocardiography (r = 0.96) (Sondergaard *et al.* 1993a, Caruthers *et al.* 2003).

Aortic regurgitation Chamber dilatation with hypertrophy is one of the main findings in aortic regurgitation that can be precisely quantified. Left ventricular function is an important determinant of prognosis. Due to its noninvasive nature, CMRI is well suited for follow-up examinations in patients with inappropriate acoustic window. The signal-void jet of

aortic regurgitation can be seen clearly on cine MRI images that show three or five chambers. Based on the identification of the jet and the analysis of the regurgitant fraction volume, CMRI has been shown to be highly accurate in comparison to echocardiography for defining the severity of aortic regurgitation (Pflugfelder *et al.* 1989, Sondergaard *et al.* 1993b).

Tricuspid and pulmonic valve diseases

The evaluation of the tricuspid valve by CMRI, although it is rarely affected by pathological conditions, is similar to that described above for the mitral valve. Ebstein's anomaly and its physiological repercussions can be assessed by CMRI. CMRI may also be useful for postoperative evaluation (Choi *et al.* 1994, Gutberlet *et al.* 2000). The pulmonic valve can be identified in sagittal views and morphologic and functional evaluations are similar to those obtained for aortic valves.

Prosthetic valves

Prosthetic valves cause limited image distortion only outside the immediate area of insertion and no patient discomfort has been reported in CMRI (**175**). Several studies demonstrated, both *in vitro* and *in vivo*, that valvular fluid profiles identified by CMRI correspond

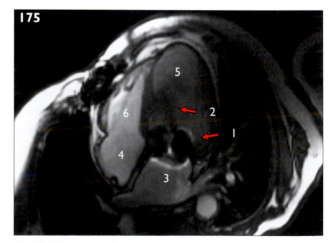

175 MRI image of prosthetic mitral valve. An artifact (1) caused by its metallic parts can be seen. However, blood flow (2) through the mitral valve can be analyzed adequately. (3: left atrium; 4: right atrium; 5: left ventricle; 6: right ventricle.)

well to those predicted. This indicates a potential new clinical application in the evaluation of patients with suspected prosthetic valvular dysfunction (Hasenkam *et al.* 1999).

Evaluation of cardiomyopathies

Cardiomyopathies, according to the World Health Organization, are diseases of the myocardium associated with cardiac dysfunction. They present with distinct morphologic, functional, and electrophysiologic characteristics. According to the classification issued by the International Society and Federation of Cardiology Task Force in 1996, cardiomyopathies are divided into dilated, restrictive, hypertrophic, and ARVD (Richardson *et al.* 1996).

CMRI, as explained earlier, provides accurate morphologic and functional evaluation of the heart, particularly of the ventricles. It is also superior in the determination of the myocardial mass. Currently CMRI is considered the 'gold standard' method for the diagnosis of cardiomyopathies. The use of contrast-enhanced images allows for the exclusion of ischemic heart disease. The differentiation between ischemic and nonischemic cardiomyopathies is frequently difficult by other imaging techniques. The presence of scar tissue identified by ceMRI techniques has also been correlated with prognosis and occurrence of arrhythmias, demonstrating a potential new frontier for CMRI.

Dilated cardiomyopathy

Dilated cardiomyopathy (DCM) is the most common form of heart muscle disease and is characterized by left ventricular or biventricular dilatation and impaired contraction (**176**). Anatomopathological findings include progressive interstitial fibrosis and relative wall thinning, especially in later stages of DCM. CMRI is capable of precise characterization of all anatomical and functional hallmarks of DCM, and also of wall stress and fiber shortening (Buser *et al.* 1989, Fujita *et al.* 1993, MacGowan *et al.* 1997). In part due to its high reproducibility and accuracy, CMRI is recognized as the preferred imaging modality to monitor effects of pharmacologic and surgical therapies on DCM (Doherty *et al.* 1992, Parga *et al.* 2001).

The etiology of DCM is unknown in approximately one-half of the cases. CMRI can help identify some obscure causes, such as hemochromatosis, a condition not readily identified by serum levels of iron but easily recognized by the increased myocardial content present in CMRI. Therefore, serial CMRI examinations can monitor deposition and early identify ventricular functional abnormalities.

CMRI has been used to evaluate patients in the acute phase of myocarditis. Hyperenhacement has been described and the signal intensity is varied according to the pulse sequence used (Friedrich *et al.* 1998, Mahrholdt *et al.* 2004). The important finding is that the hyperenhancement occurs in a typical location, usually in the epicardial portion of the

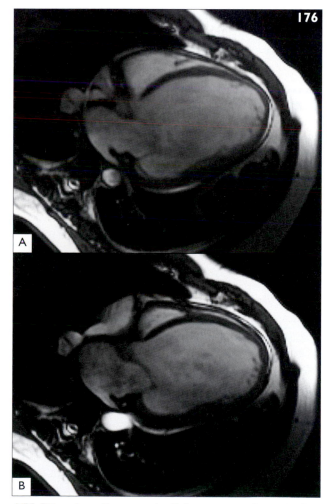

176 Dilated cardiomyopathy. Enlargement of ventricular cavities and little change between end-diastolic (**A**) and end-systolic (**B**) frames indicates low ejection fraction.

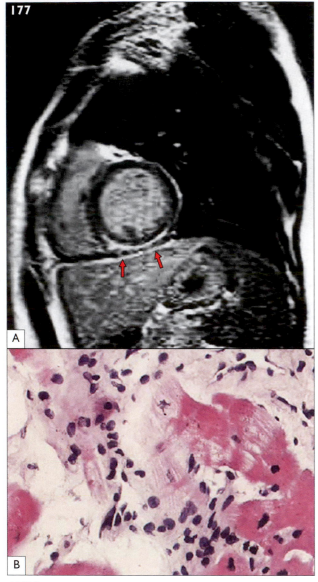

177 Patient with active myocarditis. (**A**) On the contrast-enhanced CMRI short-axis image subepicardial late-enhancement 'striae' in the posteroinferior left ventricular wall (arrows) can be appreciated. (**B**) Histology of a left ventricular endomyocardial biopsy. Clusters of lymphocyte inflammatory infiltrates associated with necrosis of adjacent myocytes (hematoxylin and eosin, original magnification ×400) can be observed. (Reprinted with permission from De Cobelli F, Pieroni M, Esposito A *et al.* Delayed gadolinium-enhanced cardiac magnetic resonance in patients with chronic myocarditis presenting with heart failure or recurrent arrhythmias. *Journal of American College of Cardiology* 2006;**47**:1649–1654.)

myocardium (**177**). In recent studies, hyperenhancement was identified in up to 70% of biopsy-proven chronic myocarditis (De Cobelli *et al.* 2006).

One of the most frequent problems that arises when evaluating patients with DCM is to discard ischemic heart disease as the etiology. Cardiac catheterization is routinely performed in those patients. The impact of this diagnosis on medical management and prognosis is well recognized. Recent studies have demonstrated that patients with DCM show myocardial scarring in a diffuse pattern, opposite to the endocardial to transmural scar as evidenced in ischemic heart disease. Good pathological correlation with the myocardial scar in DCM has also been demonstrated. The prevalence of abnormalities is variable and has achieved 41% in one series (McCrohon *et al.* 2003). Recently, the identification of scar in DCM has been related to the inducibility of ventricular tachycardia (**178**) indicating a possible prognostic value in this group of patients (Nazarian *et al.* 2005).

Hypertrophic cardiomyopathy

HCM is a genetic disorder characterized by inappropriate left ventricular myocardial hypertrophy without any obvious stimulus. Histologically, a pattern of myofibrillar disarray and areas of patchy necrosis, markers of HCM, can be found. Clinically, it manifests as heart failure, usually diastolic, but other pathophysiological abnormalities such as mitral regurgitation and LVOT obstruction can also be recognized in patients.

CMRI is highly accurate in quantifying left ventricular mass, an independent prognostic index for many cardiac diseases (Maron *et al.* 1981). In HCM the hypertrophy is predominant in the septum, making it asymmetrical, but it can also occur in any portion of the heart including the apex. Cine MRI can clearly demonstrate mitral regurgitation due to systolic anterior motion of the anterior leaflet, and acceleration at the level of the LVOT (**179**). Thanks to its high reproducibility, CMRI is considered the most reliable imaging method to evaluate post intervention by alcoholic ablation and surgery (White *et al.* 1996, Wu *et al.* 2001), since it can also identify, in gadolinium-enhanced images, the site of necrosis produced by the intervention (**180**). Current clinical

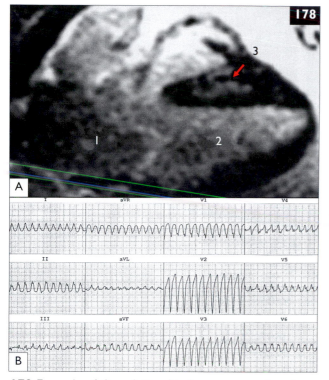

178 Example of the relationship between scar locations on delayed enhancement images and morphology of ventricular tachycardia on 12-lead ECG. (**A**) Four-chamber image of the heart, with the right atrium and right ventricle at the top of image and left atrium (1) and left ventricle (2) at the bottom. (3: midwall septal scar.) (**B**) The left bundle branch-like configuration in lead V₁ of the ventricular tachycardia ECG suggests an exit site in the right ventricle or interventricular septum and is compatible with the scar location shown in (**A**). (Reprinted with permission from Nazarian S, Bluemke DA, Lardo AC *et al.* Magnetic resonance assessment of the substrate of inducible ventricular tachycardia in nonischemic cardiomyopathy. *Circulation* 2005;112:2821–2825.)

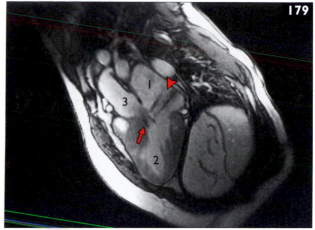

179 Obstructive hypertrophic cardiomyopathy. The systolic signal-void jet at outflow tract indicates presence of flow acceleration (arrow). Two small jets of mitral regurgitation are also seen (arrowhead). (1: left atrium; 2: left ventricle; 3: aorta.)

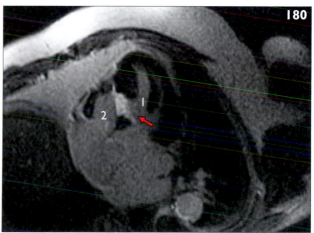

180 Delayed-enhanced image of a patient with obstructive hypertrophic cardiomyopathy who underwent alcoholic ablation through infusion in the first septal branch. A hyperenhanced region is present in the proximal septum (arrow) which is the flow area of the first septal branch of the anterior descending coronary artery. (1: left ventricle; 2: right ventricle.)

trials using MRI are evaluating prognostic implications of the extension of this necrosis. Gadolinium-enhanced images before ablation can sometimes identify areas of scar, generally present in hypertrophied regions as patchy and with multiple foci, predominantly involving the middle third of the left ventricular wall.

A relatively newer technique that relies on measurements of the effective left ventricular outflow tract area by CMRI planimetry during systole has the potential to overcome the problem of interstudy variability of the LVOT gradient due to its independence from the hemodynamic status (Schulz-Menger *et al.* 2000). There are preliminary data showing that the assessment of diastolic function utilizing MRI may be superior to conventional parameters utilizing echocardiography (Rosen *et al.* 2004), and its application for HCM is expected to occur in the near future.

Arrythmogenic right ventricular dysplasia

ARVD is characterized by a progressive degeneration of the RV, leading to enlargement and dysfunction, wall thinning, and atypical arrangement of trabecular muscles. Histologically a fibrous/fatty replacement of myocardial tissue occurs and fibromuscular bundles are separated by fatty tissues, leading to re-entry phenomena and ventricular arrhythmias, syncope, and sudden cardiac death (Corrado *et al.* 2000).

CMRI is rapidly becoming the diagnostic technique of choice for ARVD. Although echocardiography is able to show abnormalities in contractility, it is not always possible for echocardiography to obtain adequate views of the apex, especially the right ventricular apex, as well as of the right ventricular outflow tract (Kato *et al.* 2004). T1-weighted spin echo MRI images reveal an increase of signal intensity due to fatty infiltration, thinned walls, and dysplastic trabecular structures (**181**). Axial, sagittal, and short-axis views are usually recommended for optimal displays. MRI cine images reveal the characteristic of regional wall motion changes which are localized by early diastolic bulging, wall thinning, and saccular aneurismal out-pouching. *Table 7* shows the algorithms proposed by a European study group for diagnoses of this condition, based on major and minor criteria. The diagnoses can be confirmed by two major, one major and two minor, or four minor criteria in a patient.

A recent study demonstrated that high myocardial T1 signal indicative of fat is seen in 75% of the cases that fulfill the diagnostic criteria for ARVD. Dilatation of the right ventricle is also a common feature of this entity but may appear later, and serial noninvasive assessment is recommended (Tandri *et al.* 2003).

ARVD needs to be differentiated from right ventricular outflow tract tachycardia. ARVD is commonly associated with fixed focal wall thinning, regional decreased systolic wall thickening, and areas of wall motion abnormalities during systole, which is usually located above the crista supraventricularis and in the anterior and lateral right ventricular outflow

---

Table 7 Criteria for diagnosis of ARVD

Factor	Major criteria	Minor criteria
Global or regional dysfunction and structural alterations	Severe dilation and reduction of right ventricle EF; localized right ventricular aneurysms (akinetic or dyskinetic areas with diastolic bulging); severe segmental dilation of the right ventricle	Mild global dilation or EF reduction; mild segmantal dilation of the right ventricle; regional right ventricular hypokinesia
Tissue characterization of walls	Fibrofatty replacement of right ventricular myocardium (endocardial biopsy)	-
Repolarization abnormalities	-	Inverted T waves (V_2–V_3)
Depolarization or conduction abnormalities	Epsilon waves or prolonged QRS complex (>110 ms) in V_1–V_3	Late potentials
Arrhythmias	-	Ventricular tachycardia with left bundle branch block; frequent ventricular extrasystoles
Family history	Familial disease confirmed at necropsy or surgery	Familial history of premature sudden death due to unsuspected ARVD; familial history (clinical diagnosis based on present criteria)

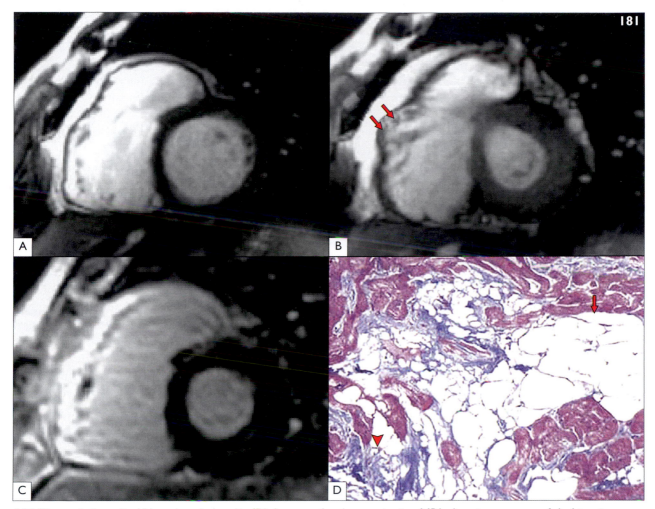

181 The end-diastolic (**A**) and end-systolic (**B**) frames of a short-axis cine MRI, showing an area of dyskinesia on right ventricular free wall characterizing a focal ventricular aneurysm (arrows). (**C**) This displays the delayed-enhanced MRI with increased signal intensity within the right ventricular myocardium, at the location of the right ventricular aneurysm. (**D**) shows the corresponding endomyocardial biopsy. Trichrome stain of right ventricular myocardium at high magnification shows marked replacement of the ventricular muscle by adipose tissue. The adipose tissue cells (arrow) are irregular in size and infiltrate the ventricular muscle. There is also abundant replacement fibrosis (arrowhead). There is no evidence of inflammation (Reprinted with permission from Tandri H, Saranathan M, Rodriguez ER *et al.* Noninvasive detection of myocardial fibrosis in arrhythmogenic right ventricular cardiomyopathy using delayed-enhancement magnetic resonance imaging. *Journal of American College of Cardiology* 2005 Jan 4;**45**(1):98–103.)

tract without fatty infiltration. ARVD in its advanced stages may not be differentiated from DCM if biventricular involvement occurs.

Restrictive cardiomyopathy

Restrictive cardiomyopathy is characterized by restrictive filling and reduced diastolic volume of either or both ventricles. Systolic function tends to be preserved. Primary infiltration of the myocardium by fibrosis may occur, or secondary forms due to infiltration of other types of tissues; these can generate the restrictive pattern of ventricular filling, atrial dilatation, and regurgitation of the atrioventricular valve of the ventricle involved. CMRI can demonstrate and quantify the abnormalities described above and the frequently required differentiation from constrictive pericarditis can be done very effectively using the T1-weighted spin echo technique.

Other cardiomyopathies

Sarcoidosis Systemic sarcoidosis (**182**) leads to cardiac involvement in 20–30% of the cases and the mortality rate related to this involvement is up to 50% of the cases. CMRI can demonstrate infiltrates as high-intensity areas in T2-weighted contrast-enhanced scans; these areas are associated with myocardial perfusion defects and reduction of regional wall motion (Tadamura *et al.* 2005). Sensitivity of ceMRI was 100% and specificity was 78% in a recent study of 58 patients with biopsy-proven sarcoidosis, indicating the increased value for the use of CMRI in diagnosis of this condition (Smedema *et al.* 2005).

Amyloidosis Infiltration of the heart by amyloid deposits is found in almost all cases of primary amyloidosis and in 25% of familial amyloidosis. CMRI can be useful for the detections of amyloidosis and thickening (>6 mm) of the right atrial posterior wall or interatrial septal wall. Recent evidence of contrast-enhanced images revealed a diffuse subtle enhancement in some cases, suggesting that tissue characterization is probably helpful for diagnostic purposes (Sueyoshi *et al.* 2006, vanden Driesen *t al.* 2006).

Chagas' disease Chagas' disease is caused by infection by the parasitic protozoan *Trypanosoma cruzi*. The chronic form of the disease can affect the heart since the protozoan, in cystic form, causes an inflammatory reaction of the myocardium, leading to dilated chambers and low EF. This reaction causes destruction of myofibrillar elements, explaining the clinical manifestations described above. Also, fibrosis replaces the heart muscle, further aggravating dysfunction.

CMRI is a promising tool for the evaluation and stratification of Chagas' patients. ceMRI can identify the areas of fibrosis especially in the apex, a distinctive pattern of this condition (Kalil & de Albuquerque 1995) (**183**). Due to the fibrous tissue, ventricular arrhythmias are also a common feature and can lead to sudden death. A recent study has demonstrated that the extension of fibrosis is related to the occurrence of ventricular tachycardia, suggesting a prognostic value of CMRI in Chagas' disease (Rochitte *et al.* 2005).

Endomyocardial fibrosis Cardiac involvement of the hypereosinophilic syndrome, also known as endomyocardial fibrosis or Loeffler's endocarditis, is not uncommon. Usual CMRI features show wall thickening, followed by extensive subendocardial fibrosis, apical thrombus secondary to reduction in contractility in the affected area, and progressive obliteration of both apices leading to diastolic dysfunction and reduced stroke volume. The morphological and functional features of endomyocardial fibrosis, and the mitral and tricuspid insufficiencies that can be associated with this condition, are well quantified by CMRI. The fibrosis may be visible as a dark thick apical rim in bright blood gradient echo sequences.

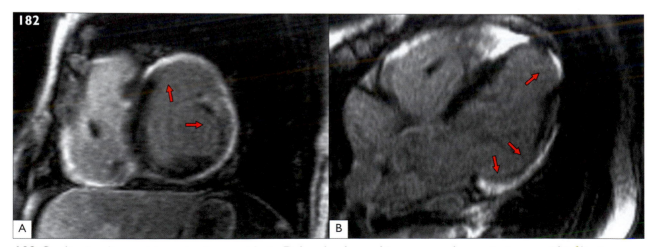

182 Cardiac involvement in systemic sarcoidosis. Delayed-enhanced images can demonstrate sarcoid infiltrates as high intensity areas (arrows) that correlate with motion abnormalities in cine images. (**A**) Short-axis image. (**B**) Four-chamber view.

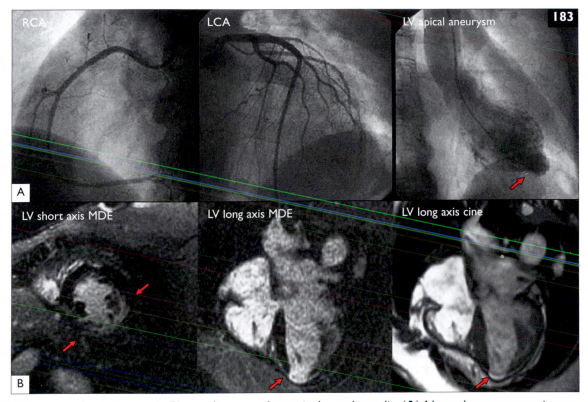

183 MRI images of a patient with Chagas disease and ventricular tachycardia. (**A**) Normal coronary angiograms in the left and middle panel. The right panel shows the LV ventriculogram. The arrow points to the apical aneurysm, a typical feature of the cardiac involvement in Chagas' heart disease. (**B**) Delayed-enhanced MRI images showing apical and inferolateral hyperenhanced pattern typical of this disease (arrows). (Reprinted with permission from Rochitte CE, Oliveira PF, Andrade JM *et al*. Myocardial delayed enhancement (MDE) by magnetic resonance imaging in patients with Chagas' disease. *Journal of American College of Cardiology* 2005;**46**:1553–1558.) (MDE: myocardial delayed enchancement; RCA: right coronary artery; LCA: left coronary artery; LV: left ventricle.)

Evaluation of pericardial disease

The pericardium is currently best evaluated by echocardiography which provides both morphologic and functional details such as volumes, filling velocities, and chamber distortions. However, the limitations of acoustic window in echocardiography and/or localized alterations in the pericardium (e.g. post thoracotomy) make this imaging modality suboptimal. CMRI can overcome those limitations and provide more accurate detailed morphologic information by evaluating the surrounding structures of the pericardium.

The pericardium is usually seen in spin echo sequences as a thin low signal (hypointense) layer located between the epicardium and mediastinal fat, both with high intensity signals. The normal amount of fluid in the pericardium (15–50 mL) has low protein content, contributing to the low signal intensity. The normal thickness of the pericardium is

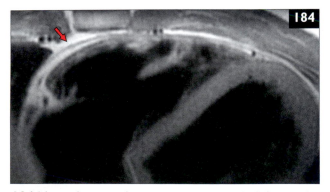

184 Normal pericardium presenting as a dark line with a thickness of 2–3 mm (arrow). This pattern is due to dephasing of moving fluid.

usually 1–2 mm, while the values of 4 mm or below are also considered normal (**184**). The pericardium is not often visualized surrounding the heart and the thickness may vary depending on the region. The pericardium located in the right ventricle is commonly well visualized. On the contrary, it is seldom seen over the lateral wall of the left ventricle because the lung parenchyma restricts its visualization (Sechtem *et al.* 1986b). Thickening of the pericardium can be attributed to distinct pathological conditions, which is easily identified by CMRI, even if it is focal, an advantage over other imaging techniques (Sechtem *et al.* 1986a).

Another unspecific reaction to pericardial injury is the fluid accumulation. According to the specific pathological condition, the effusion may have low or high protein content which affects the signal intensity in some imaging sequences and thus further increases the diagnostic capability of CMRI.

Congenital pericardial abnormalities

Pericardial cysts resulting from incomplete coalescence of lacunae are present during fetal life and are usually not symptomatic unless compression of the surrounding structures occurs. CMRI can readily identify those cysts by their morphology (rounded with regular margins) and location (most on the cardiophrenic angles). Since they are not pathological, fluid with low protein content is present in variable amounts. MRI images of the cysts are not enhanced with the administration of gadolinium chelates (White 1995). Congenital absence of pericardium is a rare condition and is usually partial. It is often associated with other congenital abnormalities, such as patent ductus arteriosus, atrial septal defects, or tetralogy of Fallot.

Acquired pericardial abnormalities

Acute pericarditis frequently results in pericardial effusion of variable volumes, as a consequence of the lymphatic or venous obstruction of the normal drainage from the heart, and pericardial thickening (**185**). CMRI is indicated when a complex effusion not adequately evaluated by echocardiography is suspected, such as pleural effusions that can sometimes mimic pericardial effusion. As mentioned above, since the appearance of the fluid on spin echo and gradient recalled echo cine MRI images is different dependent on its protein content, CMRI may also have etiological capability. If volume quantitation is desired, Simpson's rule can be applied to the short-axis images. Thickening can be confirmed if the pericardium measures >4 mm,

and is the result of inflammatory processes from distinct etiologies, i.e. tuberculosis, sarcoidosis, viral infections, rheumatic heart disease or other autoimmune conditions, and trauma. It is important to recognize that pericarditis can also occur without thickening or constriction, but enhancement of the pericardium after the administration of gadolinium-based contrast material suggests inflammation.

Constrictive pericarditis and restrictive cardiomyopathy are two distinct diseases which are not easily differentiated by clinical evaluation. However, precise diagnosis is essential since treatment of the first condition is curative. CMRI provides crucial information for the differential diagnosis of constrictive pericarditis *vs.* restrictive cardiomyopathy. Abnormal thickening when accompanied by the clinical findings of heart failure, is highly suggestive of constrictive pericarditis. MRI has an accuracy of 93% for differentiation between constrictive pericarditis and restrictive cardiomyopathy on the basis of depiction of thickened pericardium (4 mm) (Masui *et al.* 1992, Srichai & Axel 2005). The central cardiovascular structures may show a characteristic morphology in constrictive pericarditis. The right ventricle tends to have a narrow tubular configuration. In some patients, a sigmoid-shaped ventricular septum or prominent leftward convexity in the septum can be observed. Thanks to the higher temporal resolution provided by cine MRI, the late diastolic filling of the ventricles due to the abnormally thickened and confining pericardium in constrictive pericarditis is distinguishable from the delayed diastolic filling patterns of the ventricles due to restrictive

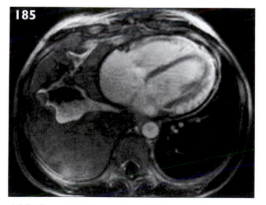

185 Constrictive pericarditis secondary to tuberculosis. The pericardium is thickened all around the cardiac cavities.

cardiomyopathy in the absence of significant pericardial thickening.

Neoplasms and hematomas are the most common diagnosed pericardial masses. Primary neoplasms of the pericardium are rare. However, metastatic involvement is more frequent in neoplasms, especially from breast and lung cancers, although melanoma, lymphoma, and metastasis from renal tumors can also occur. Hematogenic, lymphatic, and contiguous dissemination are common pathways of spread. Tumors that have invaded the pericardium may be recognized by focal obliteration of the pericardial line and the presence of pericardial effusion. Another suggestive feature is the irregularity or modularity of the pericardium. Most neoplasms have low signal intensity on T1-weighted images and high signal intensity on T2-weighted images. Contrast-enhanced MR images usually demonstrate high signal intensity of metastatic lesions and hypointense MR images may be suggestive of thrombus (Chiles *et al.* 2001).

Hematomas reflect peculiar signal intensity on T1-weighted and T2-weighted MR images. Acute hematomas demonstrate homogeneous high signal intensity, whereas subacute hematomas that are older (1–4 weeks) typically show heterogeneous signal intensity with areas of high signal intensity on both T1-weighted and T2-weighted images (Seelos *et al.* 1992, Meleca & Hoit 1995, Vilacosta *et al.* 1995). Coronary or ventricular pseudo aneurysms or neoplasms may resemble hematomas on MR images, but contrast-enhanced MR images allow for the differentiation of these entities because the intensity is not enhanced for hematomas.

Evaluation of aortic disease

CMRI has evolved in recent years as a noninvasive tool capable of providing accurate evaluation of the thoracic aorta. Together with TEE and X-ray CT, CMRI has relegated X-ray CT-based contrast angiography to a secondary role for the diagnostic evaluation of the aorta (Link *et al.* 1993), as well as for the detection of postoperative complications following thoracic aortic surgery (Auffermann *et al.* 1987, White & Higgins 1989). Complete evaluation of the thoracic aorta by CMRI typically requires a combination of static and cine images, along with contrast MRI angiography. Proper evaluation of the extension of aortic involvement and of surrounding structures that are potentially affected is mandatory. A complete examination should start at the level of the aortic valve and continue until the diaphragm is reached. Any suspicion of intra-abdominal aortic involvement indicates the need for further exploration.

Aortic root

Discrete aneurysms involving one or more sinuses of Valsalva occur below the sino-tubular ridge. In a nonacute setting, MRI may be used to visualize the aneurysm, the donor sinus, and recipient chamber of a small fistula. Bright blood techniques are particularly well suited for these evaluations. Cine MRI might be useful in demonstrating a fistula (Ho *et al.* 1995).

Congenital disease can also affect the aortic root, for instance in Marfan's syndrome (Banki *et al.* 1992, Roman *et al.* 1993). The characteristically pear-shaped dilatation of the aortic root can be well demonstrated with MRI and allows for accurate measurement of its diameter, an important criterion in surgical decision making (**186**). Associated dissection can be detected and aortic valve incompetence can be quantified with MRI as well.

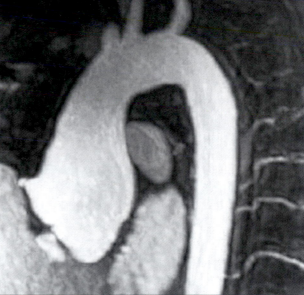

186 Aneurysm of the aortic root. The dimension of the aneurysm can be precisely evaluated, an important criterion for surgical indication. (Reprinted with permission from Russo V, Buttazzi K, Renzulli M, Fattori R. Acquired diseases of the thoracic aorta: role of MRI and MRA. *European Journal of Radiology* 2006;**16**:852–865.)

Ascending aorta

The ascending thoracic aorta extends from the sino-tubular ridge to immediately proximal to the innominate artery origin. Aortic dissection, a potentially life-threatening condition, may be fatal if it extends proximally into the aortic root, the aortic valve, and the coronary arteries, which potentially results in intrapericardial hemorrhage/cardiac tamponade, acute aortic insufficiency, and myocardial ischemia, respectively. The DeBakey and Stanford criteria divide aortic dissections into those that involve the ascending aorta or aortic arch (Stanford type A or DeBakey I and II) and into those that are delimited to only the descending thoracic aorta beyond the left subclavian artery origin (Stanford type B or DeBakey III). The first category indicates surgical intervention since the life-threatening complications described above are more prone to occur (**187**).

MRI is a highly sensitive and specific technique for the detection of aortic dissection that has proven to be superior to conventional angiography, X-ray CT, and TTE (Nienaber *et al*. 1993). As compared to TEE, both X-ray CT and MRI techniques have demonstrated a similar high sensitivity (98–100%), whereas MRI has a significantly higher specificity (98–100%) than TEE (68–77%) in high-risk populations.

The entity of noncommunicating dissecting intramural hematoma is considered to be a precursor lesion that can evolve to aortic dissection. Technically, this may be described as dissection of the aortic wall without intimal rupture or tear. The etiology is unknown, but presumably is related to weakening of the media. Clinically, the presentation of hematoma is almost always similar to that of aortic dissection. The diagnosis of an intramural hematoma should be entertained, once a communicating aortic dissection has been excluded. On MRI designed to exclude communicating aortic dissection, an intramural hematoma is identified as a smooth crescentic to circumferential area of thickened aortic wall without the evidence of blood flow in the false channel. Depending on the age of the hematoma, the area of thickening may be isointense or hyperintense relative to skeletal muscle on spin echo MRI. The signal intensity is relatively isointense in the acute phase and thus becomes greatest in the subacute stage (Murray *et al*. 1997).

It is important to locate the most proximal area of a dissecting aneurysm as well as the extension of the intimal flap. This is necessary in order to recognize the risk in occlusion of the aortic arch vessels which may produce cerebral ischemia or infarction, another critical complication though not necessarily life-threatening. Subacute hemorrhage presents as a typical image with crescentic or lentiform high intramural signal due to the appearance of methemoglobin. Eventually chronic cases will show images of organized thrombus in the false channel (Link *et al*. 1993, Nienaber *et al*. 1993), or in a re-entry channel if it is present. Signs that have been

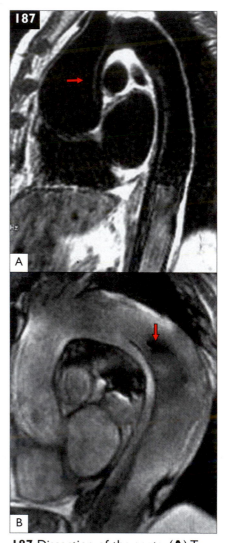

187 Dissection of the aorta. (**A**) Type A dissection with intimal flap visible as a subtle linear image (arrow) in the ascending and descending aorta. (**B**) Type B dissection with signal void (arrow) in the descending aorta indicating the entry site.

reported to be more consistent with a diagnosis of thrombosed false channel associated with dissection are a compressed or eccentric patent channel and extensive thrombus with associated wall thickening over a length >7 cm. These signs are easily appreciated by MRI (Flamm *et al.* 1996).

Chronic aortic aneurysms (Prince *et al.* 1996, Krinsky *et al.* 1997) are diagnosed by measuring the diameter of the aorta in perpendicular position. Normal diameters of aortic root, mid-ascending aorta, aortic arch, and descending aorta are 3.3 cm, 3.0 cm, 2.7 cm, and 2.4 cm, respectively. A true aneurysm is considered present if all three mural layers of the aortic wall are involved, otherwise it is considered to be a pseudo-aneurysm. Aneurysms >5 cm, that are associated with symptoms and/or are expanding rapidly, need surgical correction. The etiology of aneurysms can sometimes be defined easily. Valvular aortic stenosis usually causes aneurismal dilation being limited to the mid ascending aorta where poststenotic flow effects are most prominent. Aortic regurgitation aneurysms can involve the ascending aorta but extend into the transverse arch because of the 'water hammer' effect and, in long-standing cases, also may involve the descending thoracic aorta. Mycotic aneurysms are resulted from the weakening of the aortic wall by infection. Pseudo-aneurysms are typically caused by trauma (e.g. automobile accidents) and occur most commonly at the level of the ligamentum arteriosum.

Aortic arch

CMRI can identify anatomical variations that commonly occur in the aortic arch, such as the common origin of the innominate and left common carotid arteries. Another significant variant is the separate origin of the left vertebral artery from the arch.

Congenital diseases can be manifest clinically if the primitive aortic arches fail to fuse or regress, resulting in vascular rings that can encircle the trachea or esophagus, and also resulting in stridor, wheezing, or dysphagia (Bisset *et al.* 1987). The most common vascular rings are a left aortic arch with an aberrant right subclavian artery, a right aortic arch with an aberrant left subclavian artery, and a double aortic arch. Vascular rings are usually well demonstrated without MR angiography. When a surgical correction is intended MRI can be very helpful in designing the surgical approach.

Descending aorta

The descending thoracic aorta extends from the ligamentum to the aortic hiatus of the diaphragm. Atherosclerotic aneurysms occur most typically in the descending thoracic aorta and may be fusiform or saccular in morphology. A penetrating aortic ulcer is another entity that tends to present in the descending aorta where the bulk of atherosclerosis occurs. There is no consensus on the natural history of penetrating atherosclerotic ulcers. They must be differentiated from focal saccular aneurysm and intramural hematoma (Welch *et al.* 1990).

Evaluation of thrombi and masses

CMRI can contribute in the evaluation of patients with masses in the cardiovascular system, especially for planning therapy. It also allows for evaluation of the mediastinum and lungs, frequent sites of metastatic lesions for the heart, with excellent spatial resolution. CMRI provides superb soft-tissue contrast resolution, clearly favoring depiction of the morphologic details of a mass, including its extent, site of origin, and secondary effects on adjacent structures. MRI is capable of differentiating adipose from soft tissue, and both from cystic fluid collections. Dynamic MRI (cine and tagging) also has the ability to provide functional images of the heart that can be used to study the pathophysiological consequences of cardiac masses. Contrast-enhanced MR images and perfusion MR images are becoming routinely used to evaluate vascularization of the masses and differentiating them from thrombi. Myocardial tumors may be infiltrative and it can be difficult to visualize them adequately. Contrast-enhanced CMRI increases the sensitivity of tumor detection due to appreciation of vascularized areas in the areas of malignancy. As a general rule malignant tumors are visualized more intensely than the surrounding myocardium (Niwa *et al.* 1989), but this can not be used as the rule of thumb since the patterns of enhancement are varied. A significant limitation of CMRI is its inability to detect calcification.

Primary cardiac tumors are rare and three-quarters of the cases are benign (Luna *et al.* 2005). CMRI cannot differentiate benign from malignant tumors, but some findings, if present, may suggest malignancy, such as involvement of the right side of the heart, infiltrative masses, and associated hemopericardium. On the other hand, benign tumors tend to occur on the left side of the heart along the interatrial septum and they rarely cause pericardial effusion.

Myxomas

Myxomas are responsible for 50% of all benign tumors. They are usually located within the cavity of the left atrium attached to the interatrial septum in the majority of cases. In CMRI, variability in the appearance of myxomas may reflect their variable composition of water-rich myxomatous tissue *vs.* fibrous tissue and calcification. Cine MR images can show mobility of the tumor and its pedunculate appearance in some cases.

Lipomas

Lipomas are the second most common benign tumor of the heart and have variable location. Subendocardial location is the most common, usually in the interatrial septum. Eventually large epicardial lipomas may cause extrinsic compression of surrounding structures. The high fat content of this tumor makes it very bright with well defined borders on T1-weighted images. A decrease in signal intensity using a fat presaturation technique confirms the diagnosis (**188**). Lipomatous lesions are not encapsulated, unlike lipomas, and are not quite homogeneous.

Rhabdomyomas

Rhabdomyomas nearly always involve the myocardium or the ventricles, affecting both ventricles with an equal frequency, and are the most common cardiac tumors of infants and children. They can be large enough to cause obstruction of a valve or cardiac chamber. In CMRI, a rhabdomyoma may be slightly hypointense to slightly hyperintense in the myocardium on T1-weighted images, and slightly hyperintense on T2-weighted images.

Fibromas

Fibromas are benign tumors primarily affecting older children (>10 years old). They are usually in the myocardium which can cause blood-flow obstruction, ventricular dysfunction, or conduction abnormalities. In CMRI, fibromas are hypointense to slightly hyperintense on T1-weighted images as compared to skeletal muscle, but they have lower signal intensity than the myocardium on T2-weighted images. This is attributed to their fibrous nature or deposits of calcium related to necrosis.

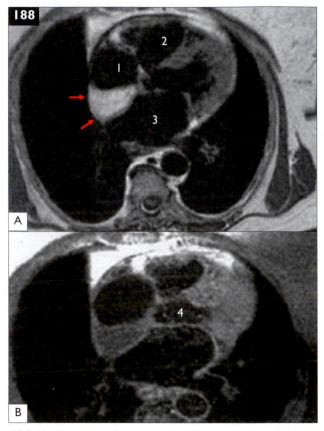

188 Lipomatous infiltration of the interatrial septum (arrows). (**A**) Notice that signal intensity of the mass is similar to that of subcutaneous and mediastinal fat. (**B**) Fat suppressed image of the same mass. (1: right atrium; 2: right ventricle; 3: left ventricle; 4: aorta.) (Reprinted with permission from Sparrow PJ, Kurian JB, Jones TR, Sivanathan MU. MR imaging of cardiac tumors. *Radiographics* 2005; **25**(5):1255.)

Thrombi

Thrombi are frequent findings in CMRI. Their preferential location is in the left atrium especially in patients with atrial fibrillation, or in the left ventricle especially in patients with regional myocardial dysfunction, notably in the apex. The signal intensity of a thrombus depends on its age. Recent thrombi have higher signal intensity than the subjacent myocardium. However, as time goes by, variation on signal intensity will occur and chronic organized thrombi are of low signal because of loss of water and protons. Gadolinium-enhanced images will not turn the signal to hyperintense since it is not vascularized (**172E**). Combining analysis of static MR images and cine MR images to observe contractility of the subjacent myocardium will be helpful for diagnosis.

Malignant tumors

Among malignant tumors of the heart, the most common are angiosarcomas, rhabdomyosarcomas, and fibrosarcomas.

Angiosarcomas Angiosarcomas occur generally in the right side of the heart, and are polymorphic in appearance with distinct levels of signal intensity. Since the tumor is vascularized, gadolinium administration will enhance nonhomogeneously in the periphery of the mass. Angiosarcomas also have a propensity to involve the pericardium, resulting in hemopericardium. Metastases occur in 66–89% of cases, with the lungs being the most frequent site of spread.

Rhabdomyosarcomas Rhabdomyosarcomas are the most common malignant tumors of infants and children, although they account for only 4–7% of all cardiac sarcomas. Frequently rhabdomyosarcomas extend beyond the myocardium, causing a polypoid extension into a chamber cavity, simulating a myxoma (**189**). While some reports suggest a predisposition for right-sided cavities, rhabdomyosarcomas have no strong predilection for a specific chamber, and multiple locations are frequently found (60%). A rhabdomyosarcoma is more likely than other sarcomas to involve or arise from cardiac valves. Pericardial involvement is also frequent. MRI signal intensity is intermediate on precontrast T1-weighted images, similar to that of adjacent myocardial tissue, but shows enhancement of the lesion after administration of contrast (Mader *et al.* 1997).

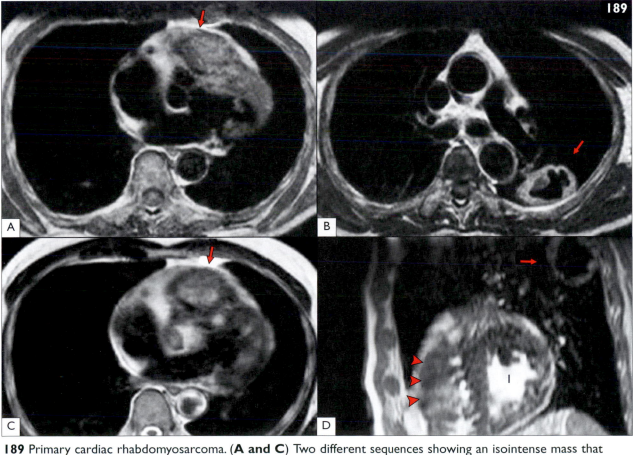

189 Primary cardiac rhabdomyosarcoma. (**A and C**) Two different sequences showing an isointense mass that arises from myocardial wall of the right ventricular outflow tract (arrows). (**B**) Cavitating metastasis in the left lower lobe (arrow). (**D**) A short axis image showing the obliteration of the right ventricle (arrowheads) (Reprinted with permission from Sparrow PJ Kurian JB, Jones TR, Sivanathan MU. MR imaging of cardiac tumors. *Radiographics* 2005; **25**(5):1255.) (I: left ventricle.)

Metastases

Metastases usually involve the pericardium and myocardium, while they rarely involve the valves and the endocardium. In addition, the right side of the heart is more frequently involved than the left side of the heart. Metastases may involve the heart via direct extension, hematogeneous dissemination, or lymphatic spread. Bronchogenic carcinoma is the most frequent primary malignancy that metastasizes to the heart followed by breast carcinoma, malignant melanoma, lymphoma, and leukemia.

Evaluation of congenital heart disease

Cardiac MRI is particularly useful in the evaluation of complex congenital cardiac conditions since it provides excellent anatomical and physiological information (both pre- and postinterventions, either corrective or palliative). The myriad of conditions and association of defects requires that a physician with expertise in congenital heart disease (cardiovascular radiologist or cardiologist) be present in the MRI suite in order to explore its multiplanar nature by tailoring the examination based on previous clinical and imaging information.

Sequential analysis is the most successful approach for morphologic description of a congenital cardiac malformation by any imaging modality. The first step in this approach is the determination of atrioviseral situs by reviewing the localization of inferior vena cava, abdominal aorta, liver, spleen, and stomach, and the morphology of the atrial appendages and mainstem bronchi. This is followed by the determination of ventricular morphology using the muscular outflow tract and the moderator band as landmarks of the anatomical right ventricle. The aortic arch and the pulmonary bifurcation identify with the great vessels. Atrioventricular and ventriculoarterial connections are assessed to be either concordant or discordant. A concordant atrioventricular connection means that the anatomical left atrium is connected to an anatomical left ventricle. A discordant ventriculo-arterial connection means that the anatomical right ventricle is connected to the ascending aorta, as in the classic D transposition of the great arteries (TGA). Combined atrioventricular and ventriculoarterial discordance is the hallmark L-transposition. Associated lesions, such as septal defects or aortic arch coarctation, can be evaluated. The evaluation of the main abnormalities is described below.

Atrial and ventricular morphology

The right atrium receives both superior and inferior venae cavae and the coronary sinus. Morphologically, the right atrium is characterized by the right atrial appendage (triangular shape) and the crista terminalis located in the lateral wall. The left atrium is connected to the left atrial appendage that is long and has a narrower connection with the left atrium than the connection of the right atrial appendage to the right atrium. Atrial situs is determined by their morphology.

Shape, trabecular appearance, and the relation with semilunar valves define the ventricles. The endocardial surface of the right ventricle presents trabeculations and the moderator band, a muscular trabeculation that connects the interventricular septum and the free wall near the apical portion. Papillary muscles in the right ventricle originate from both the interventricular septum and the free wall. The left ventricular papillary muscles do not originate from the septum. The semilunar valves present a fibrous continuity with the mitral valve, but in the right ventricle the infundibulum separates the tricuspid valve from the semilunar ones.

Aortic anomalies

Coarctation of the aorta (CoAo) is clearly defined by CMRI (**190**). Anatomically, the focal narrowing of the proximal descending aorta, most commonly at the junction of the ductus arteriosus and aorta, and the resultant hypoplasia of the distal aortic arch, as well as the arterial collateralization (dilatation of the internal mammary and intercostal arteries) can be precisely measured by MRI. The relation of the CoAo and the left subclavian artery is also an important anatomical definition. CMRI allows for the detection of CoAo severity (Nielsen *et al.* 2005). The noninvasive nature of CMRI is especially relevant in the follow-up of recently diagnosed cases to identify early aneurismal dilatation. It is also important in the postoperative evaluation of surgical or balloon interventions for the detection of residual stenosis and its hemodynamic effect as the patient grows, if correction is performed at a young age (Cowley *et al.* 2005, Vriend & Mulder 2005).

Pulmonary artery anomalies

Anatomical characterization of the pulmonary artery is one hallmark of CMRI when echocardiography is technically limited, allowing for characterization of its origin, dimensions, and eventual obstructions in any possible regions from infundibulum to secondary branches. Right ventricular hypertrophy secondary to pulmonary hypertension or pulmonary artery obstruction can also be easily determined by CMRI (Bouchard *et al.* 1985; Boxt 1996).

Intracardiac and extracardiac shunts

CMRI not only can visualize the anatomy of the intracardiac defect, but also is capable of defining its hemodynamic repercussion by showing chamber dilatation and hypertrophy. This is useful for estimation of the severity of the shunt and ultimately prognosis. Calculation of shunt fraction is generally performed using the volume–flow analysis of great artery flow with velocity mapping. Quantitation of shunt size can be obtained by measuring the net blood flow volumes within the main pulmonary artery and ascending aorta over a cardiac cycle. If the relation Qp/Qs (ratio of pulmonary flow to systemic flow) is positive, then the shunt is left to right. In contrast, a negative value of Qp/Qs indicates a right-to-left shunt. The correlation between the MRI shunt measurements and those obtained from the catheterization room are very good.

Atrial septal defect Precise anatomical definition of atrial septal defect (ASD) type is accomplished with CMRI based on anatomical definition of each defect (**191**). The overall sensitivity and specificity is approximately 97% and 90%, respectively (Diethelm *et al.* 1987; Kersting-Sommerhoff *et al.* 1989). Commonly associated defects such as anomalous pulmonary venous return are seen well in CMRI (Beerbaum *et al.* 2003).

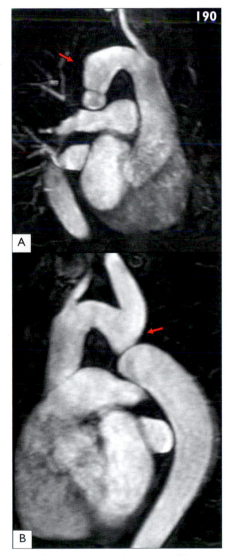

190 Coarctation of the aorta. Abrupt narrowing in the descending aorta after the emergence of left subclavian artery (arrows). (**A**) Posterior view. (**B**) Lateral view

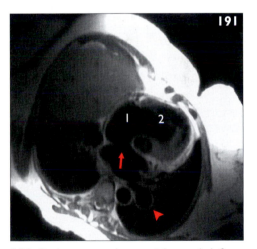

191 Ostium secundum atrial septal defect. The right atrium (1) and right ventricle (2) are enlarged. The discontinuity of the interatrial septum (arrow) is clearly seen. Incidentally, notice the dilated descending left pulmonary artery (arrowhead). (Reprinted with permission from Boxt LM. Magnetic resonance and computed tomographic evaluation of congenital heart disease. *Journal of Magnetic Resonance Imaging* 2004;19:827–847.)

One of the most interesting new applications of CMRI is its use to measure and guide transcatheter closure of ASD. Clinical studies for establishing the size and rim morphology of the ASD have demonstrated excellent correlation with echocardiography (Durongpisitkul *et al.* 2004). Promising results in experimental settings were achieved using real-time CMRI to guide ASD closure (Rickers *et al.* 2003; Schalla *et al.* 2005).

Ventricular septal defect The high spatial resolution of CMRI allows for the demonstration of the presence and the size of ventricular septal defects (VSDs). The multiplanar capability of CMRI facilities the determination of the exact location of subaortic and membranous VSDs. Cine MRI identifies the direction of the shunts. Atrioventricular septal defects (endocardial cushion defects) involve the atrioventricular septum and primum portion of the interatrial septum and may also involve the anterior mitral and septal tricuspid leaflets as well as the membranous interventricular septum. MRI can be used to determine the size of the ventricular component of the defects and the presence of ventricular hypoplasia (Parsons *et al.* 1990; Yoo *et al.* 1991).

Patent ductus arteriosus The ductus arteriosus may be difficult to visualize in infants because of its small size. If an aneurysm is present, it can be seen in a regular MR image. Although a comprehensive approach to the utility of CMRI in the evaluation of patent ductus arteriosus (PDA) is lacking, CMRI may be a useful method for shunting evaluation.

Evaluation of complex congenital malformations

Tetralogy of Fallot Tetralogy of Fallot is the most common cyanotic form of congenital heart disease, and surgical correction in early infancy has significantly improved survival. CMRI can identify all defects described in this syndrome, and can readily identify residual defects or sequelae after repair. Recent evidence suggests that long-term prognosis is related to the presence of right ventricular dilatation, pulmonary regurgitation, and right ventricle and/or left ventricle low EF. Nowadays a growing population of patients is achieving advanced age, and thus repeated imaging evaluation is needed. CMRI can

provide qualitative and quantitative analysis of residual defects and the severity of pulmonary regurgitation and residual shunts (Geva *et al.* 2004, Chowdhury *et al.* 2006, Norton *et al.* 2006).

Another important feature after Fallot repair, for instance after previous Blalock–Taussig anastomosis, patients often suffer from pulmonary artery branch stenosis which can be well visualized by CMRI (Greenberg *et al.* 1997).

Functional univentricular hearts: tricuspid atresia and double inlet left ventricle Patients with tricuspid atresia have the atrioventricular ring replaced by fat, and thus the continuity between the right chambers no longer exists. Due to absence of flow to the right ventricular chamber, the right atrium is enlarged and is usually hypoplastic. An ASD is mandatory and has to be large. CMRI can identify those alterations and also detect others such as VSDs and dimensions of the pulmonary artery. Functionally the heart behaves as a univentricular heart.

Univentricular heart is described as rudimentary ventricle, either right or left according to its morphology as described above, and a double inlet or a common atrioventricular valve. If the ventricular chamber cannot be defined morphologically it will be named as the ventricular chamber. Several surgical options have been developed to redirect the systemic venous blood to the pulmonary arteries. The Fontan procedure and all its variants have had a major impact on the treatment of single ventricle, but the long-term outcome remains uncertain. The classic Fontan operation consisted of a conduit from the right atrium to the central pulmonary arteries. Sometimes the conduit is only connected to the left pulmonary artery in combination with a Glenn procedure and a separate anastomosis of the superior vena cava to the right pulmonary artery. MRI flow studies have demonstrated that the success of RV incorporation could not be reliably determined on the basis of flow velocity measurements alone. Volumetric flow also had to be taken into account. Furthermore, the ratio of left-to-right pulmonary artery flow was found to be reversed after Fontan surgery (Rebergen *et al.* 1993).

Pulmonary artery size and confluence of the central pulmonary artery branches are crucial determinants of outcome after Fontan surgery, and

MRI was shown to be superior to echocardiography in evaluating these parameters (Fogel *et al.* 1994). Recent studies have demonstrated tagging techniques in the evaluations of strain and ventricular motion, and of flow direction during ventricular filling with blood pool tagging (Fogel *et al.* 1997, 1999). It was recently suggested that CMRI could be the single examination before correction by Fontan procedure (Fogel 2005).

Transposition of the great arteries: postoperative evaluation

Patients with D-type TGA (Duro *et al.* 2000) have to be separated into those who have been treated with the older, and nowadays mostly abandoned, techniques that redirect blood at the atrial level (Mustard or Senning operation) and those who have been treated with the arterial switch (Jatene) operation. The latter category is generally younger, the majority now reaching adulthood. Both categories are significantly different in the nature of the postoperative residua and sequelae. The Mustard or Senning procedure leaves the anatomical right ventricle in the systemic position. It is known that this is at the base of a range of problems, with late sudden right ventricle failure and death at the end of the spectrum. Other hemodynamic problems often encountered are arrhythmias, (baffle) obstruction to pulmonary or systemic venous return, pulmonary hypertension, and tricuspid regurgitation. The post-Mustard anatomy and the stent placement for baffle obstruction have been successfully demonstrated with MRI (Sampson *et al.* 1994, Ward *et al.* 1995). The function of the anatomical right ventricle in the systemic circulation appears to be of particular interest. Late cardiac failure is a serious matter of concern in these patients and diastolic dysfunction may be an early sign of cardiac failure. After Mustard or Senning repair, cine MRI techniques are usually used to quantify right ventricular hypertrophy when right ventricle volumes and EF are normal. Phase contrast techniques have been used to study diastolic characteristics by measuring tricuspid flow in Mustard or Senning patients and demonstrate differences with normal volunteers (Rebergen *et al.* 1995). After the arterial switch procedure, common complications include right ventricular outflow tract obstruction and pulmonary artery stenosis, either at the supravalvular or branch level. The postoperative status of the great vessels can be adequately assessed with spin echo MRI.

Marfan's syndrome

The characteristically pear-shaped dilatation of the aortic root is well demonstrated with MRI, and its diameter can be accurately measured using conventional spin echo techniques. The aortic root diameter is an important criterion in surgical decision-making. Associated dissection can be detected and aortic valve incompetence can be quantified with MRI. Furthermore, previous MRI studies have investigated the compliance of the aortic wall, either using conventional pulse sequences or by measuring the velocity of the flow wave along the descending aorta. This can potentially be used to monitor the effect of beta-blocker medication that may slow down the loss of elasticity in Marfan patients. Very recently, MRI was reported to demonstrate dual ectasia, one of the rare diagnostic criteria, occurring in 92% of Marfan patients.

EMERGING APPLICATIONS OF CARDIOVASCULAR MRI
Atherosclerosis imaging

Atherosclerosis is a lifelong process that begins early in life as a thickening of the arterial wall, initially with an exocentric deposition (positive arterial remodeling) without affecting blood flow until the later stages of disease. Most acute clinical events from atherosclerosis occur with mild to moderate stenoses in patients who have little or no clinical signs of the disease. Prevention and early diagnosis of subclinical atherosclerosis is extremely critical since a significant percentage of first events result in high morbidity and mortality. The characterization of the different stages of atherosclerosis from early positive arterial remodelling to overt atherosclerosis can be detected by MRI.

MRI has emerged as a powerful modality to assess subclinical and overt atherosclerotic changes in different vascular beds thanks to its high image resolution, three-dimensional capabilities, truly noninvasive nature, and the capacity for soft tissue characterization (Choudhury *et al.* 2002, Desai & Bluemke 2005).

MRI of carotid atherosclerosis

The carotid artery is the vessel of choice for MRI of atherosclerosis because of the excellent image quality. Also, it has been validated by comparison with other noninvasive imaging techniques such as carotid ultrasonography and by the correlation with anatomopathological specimens obtained surgically. MRI can clearly demonstrate the state of carotid plaque substructure, including the unstable fibrous cap, lipid core, hemorrhage, and calcification (Yuan *et al.* 2002, Mitsumori *et al.* 2003). Previous studies have demonstrated the ability of MRI to detect longitudinal changes in plaque size after aggressive therapeutic intervention using statins. A recent study also demonstrated the effects of aggressive and conventional lipid lowering by two different dosages of simvastatin on early human atherosclerotic lesions using serial carotid and aortic MRI (Corti *et al.* 2005). *Post-hoc* analysis showed that patients reaching mean on-treatment low-density lipoprotein cholesterol ≤2.59 mmol/L had larger decreases in plaque size. The ability of using MRI to show the correlation between cholesterol subfractions and atherosclerotic plaque components of the carotid artery has also been demonstrated (Desai *et al.* 2005).

MRI of aortic atherosclerosis

Aortic atherosclerosis can be accurately detected using surface MRI when compared to histopathology and TEE for the assessment of plaque thickness, extent, and composition (Correia *et al.* 1997, Fayad *et al.* 2000). MRI of the aorta has demonstrated that lipid-lowering therapy can be a treatment for aortic plaque regression. A new technique of transesophageal MRI (TEMRI) using a loopless antenna coil has been developed to improve aortic MRI. The feasibility and utility of this technique have been demonstrated in patients with aortic atherosclerosis (Shunk *et al.* 2001).

Interventional cardiovascular MRI

In recent years, stimulated by the need for high-definition images and low-radiation procedures especially for the youth population, new MRI scanners and new sequences with the improvements in medical technology have been developed to allow for real-time MRI. In parallel, developments of miniature MR-compatible internal catheters, guidewires, and ablation catheters also turn the field of interventional and therapeutic MRI into reality.

Real-time MRI

The advancement of the MR gradient hardware has made it possible to encode the spatial information of image data rapidly to generate a 256 × 256 image of 24 cm field of view with 1 mm spatial resolution in approximately 120 ms. If the spatial resolution is reduced to 128 × 128, the processing time can be further reduced to 50 ms (20 frames/s). The next important development in this field is the ability to perform real-time interactive manipulations of the image data utilizing a user interface in conjunction with a short-bore cardiovascular scanner and fast spiral imaging. Such developments lead to:

➤ Rapid data acquisition, data transfer, image reconstruction, and real time display.
➤ Interactive real-time control of the image slice.
➤ High-quality images without cardiac or respiratory gating.

The real time MR hardware platform consists of a workstation and a bus adapter and can be adapted into the conventional scanner at reasonable cost.

Accurate visualization and positioning of the interventional devices in relation to the surrounding anatomy is critical for a successful and safe image-guided interventional procedure. There are primarily two methods that have evolved over the years to aid in endovascular navigation of the interventional devices: passive MR tracking and active MR tracking (Leung *et al.* 1995, Bakker *et al.* 1997). Passive MR tracking techniques are based on visualization of the signal void and susceptibility artifacts caused by the interventional instruments themselves due to displacement of the protons. This form of tracking constitutes the normal imaging process and does not require any extra post-processing or hardware. The artifact generated by a particular material is dependent upon a multitude of factors, such as the magnetic field strength, spatial orientation of the device with respect to the magnetic field, physical cross-section of the device, pulse sequence, and imaging parameters. Active tracking requires the creation of a signal that is actively detected or emitted by the device to identify its location. This can be achieved by visualizing a signal from a miniature RF coil which is incorporated into the commercially available interventional devices, such as embolization catheters and balloon catheters (Wildermuth *et al.* 1998). The miniature coils are connected, through a fully insulated coaxial cable embedded in the catheter wall, on to the surface coil reception port for signal reception. A coil-tipped catheter is made by winding the miniature coil, a copper wire spiral, for 16–20 turns around the tips of interventional devices to identify actively their position. In the active tracking technique, the position of the device is derived from the signal received by a miniature RF coil that is attached to the instrument itself (Wendt *et al.* 1998). Three-dimensional coordinates of the coil can be tracked in real time at a rate of 20 frames/s with a spatial resolution of 1 mm. The position of the coil is used to control the motion of a cursor over a scout (roadmap) image. Another technique in active tracking utilizes the loopless antenna made from a coaxial cable consisting of a conducting wire that is an extended inner conductor from the coaxial cable. Loopless antennae are particularly useful because they provide a superior field of view compared to the internal coils. In this regard, they have been adapted to support TEMRI (Shunk *et al.* 1999) and subsequently to the entire development of MR-guided electrophysiology (Lardo *et al.* 2000). The entire body of the loopless antenna can be observed under MRI. This antenna can be either directly inserted into small or tortuous vessels, or placed into the central channel of interventional devices. These advances are being tested in therapeutic procedures such as baloonangioplasty, stent placement, and electrophysiological studies.

In vivo MRI of vascular gene therapy

Gene therapy is rapidly emerging as a viable modality and has shown a tremendous potential in the treatment of atherosclerotic diseases. Recently, MRI has been evaluated for monitoring and guiding vascular gene delivery, tracking vascular gene expression, and enhancing vascular gene transfection/transduction (Yang *et al.* 2001). Gene transfer into a target-specific cell is a major challenge in this field for which the current success rate is very low (1%). It is known that gene transfection or expression can be significantly enhanced one- to four-fold with heating. Local heat generation at the target site using an easily placed internal heating source could be a logical way to improve success. A MRI-guidewire, called MR imaging-heating-guidewire can be used to deliver external thermal energy into the targeted vessels, and has the following functions:

➤ As a receiver antenna to generate intravascular high-resolution MR images of atherosclerotic plaques of the vessel wall.

➤ As a conventional guidewire to guide endovascular interventions under MRI.

➤ As an intravascular heating source to deliver external thermal energy into the target vessel wall during MRI of vascular gene delivery, and thereby enhance vascular gene transfection.

Tracking gene expression requires sophisticated imaging methods to assess gene function by detecting functional transgene-encoding proteins (referred to as 'imaging downstream') at the targets over time. MRI can be used to track over-expression of the transferring gene which produces a cell-surface transferrin receptor. The transferrin receptor is then probed specifically by a superparamagnetic transferrin that can be subsequently detected using MRI (Weissleder *et al.* 2000).

Evaluation of coronary arteries

X-ray coronary angiography is an invasive procedure, exposing patients and operators to ionizing radiation, in which a small but finite risk of serious complications exists. A cost-effective, noninvasive, and patient-friendly imaging modality, such as coronary magnetic resonance angiography, may address some of these issues. For successful coronary MRI, a series of major obstacles has to be overcome. The heart is subject to intrinsic and extrinsic motion due to its natural periodic contraction and breathing. Both of these motion components exceed the coronary artery dimensions and therefore coronary MR data acquisition in the sub-millimeter range is technically challenging and efficient motion suppression strategies need to be applied. In addition, enhanced contrast between the coronary lumen and the surrounding tissue is crucial for successful visualization of both coronary lumen and the coronary vessel wall. The cardiac and respiratory motion compensations have to be taken into account. While recent progress has been made on motion suppression, MRI hardware, software, scanning protocols, and contrast agents, the spatial resolution obtained by MRI needs to be further improved so that it can be comparable to that of X-ray coronary angiography of which the resolution is less than 300 μm).

CLINICAL CASES

Case 1: Mass in the Apex of the Left Ventricle

Clinical history
A 15-year-old boy without clinical symptoms was found to have an abnormal resting ECG in the course of evaluation for a high-school football team. The ECG was suggestive of a mass located in the apex of the left ventricle.

Imaging protocol
A cardiac MRI was performed.

Impression
The resting ECG shows deep inverted T waves in leads V_4 to V_6 (**192A**). The cardiac MR image shows an ill defined mass in the apex of the left ventricle that extends into the lateral wall (arrows, **192B**). A contrast-enhanced MR image shows a very well circumscribed region of hyperenhancement at the apex surrounded by normal muscle (arrow, **192C**). Cine MR images (not shown) revealed normal wall movement in the regions not involved with the mass.

Discussion
The patient was appropriately referred for cardiac MRI. MRI is well suited to define further the probable etiology of the apical mass. Delayed ceMRI showed hyperenhancement, indicating poor vascularization in the affected area and presence of fibrosis.

Management
Based on these results, the patient was referred for cardiac surgery suspected of having a cardiac fibroma. Although this is a benign tumor, it may cause arrhythmias and sudden cardiac death. The fibroma was confirmed by anatomopathological examination of the surgical specimen. The cardiac MR images were helpful in establishing a tentative diagnosis and in further management.

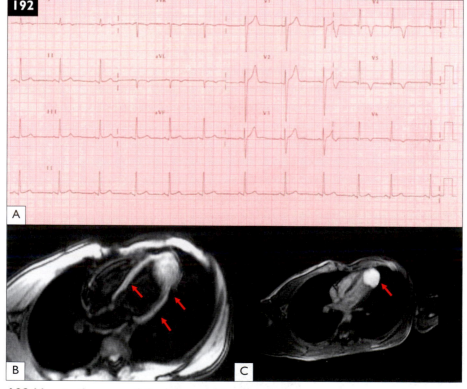

192 Mass in the apex of the left ventricle.

Case 2: Large Anterior Myocardial Infarction

Clinical history

A 57-year-old male was admitted to the emergency room with a typical acute chest pain which started 6 hours prior to the admission. The ECG revealed a large evolving anterior myocardial infarction. Coronary angiography showed a proximal occlusion of the LAD. During a percutaneous coronary intervention, patency of the artery was achieved by angioplasty.

Imaging protocol

The patient was subsequently evaluated by cardiac MRI to define the extent of myocardial infarction since he had an episode of acute heart failure before the intervention and also had a suspected intracavitary thrombus during echocardiographic examination. A set of contrast-enhanced delayed images are shown in **193**. Two-chamber (**193A**) and four-chamber (**193B**) views of the left ventricle show the extension of fibrosis (arrows) and a mural thrombus (arrowheads). **193C–F** show the short-axis views of the left ventricle. The transmural extension of the myocardial infarction can be appreciated.

Impression

The MRI cine images showed severe left ventricle systolic dysfunction with akinesis of anteroseptal and anterior walls. The apex was completely dyskinetic. The left ventricle end-diastolic volume was at the upper limit of normal and the left ventricle end-systolic volume was increased. EF was 34%. On delayed enhancement images, there was a medium to large region of delayed enhancement (infarction/scar) measuring 36% of the total left ventricular mass, involving the septal wall from mid-ventricle to apex (arrows, **193C** and **D**), and the anterior wall from mid-ventricle to apex, which was completely involved including the inferior apical wall. The extent of the myocardial infarction from mid-ventricular to apical regions was transmural (>75% of the left ventricle wall thickness) suggesting absence of residual viability. In the basal septal region it was mainly subendocardial, suggesting presence of viability. There was evidence of a mural left ventricle apical thrombus.

Discussion

The ability of cardiac MRI to define a mural thrombus and its accuracy is demonstrated in this patient. The large apical thrombus was easily identified and measured. In addition, left ventricle EF and infarct size can be measured precisely. These parameters both have important prognostic value.

Management

Based on these results, the patient was referred for oral anticoagulation. He had medications optimized in order to control incipient signs of heart failure.

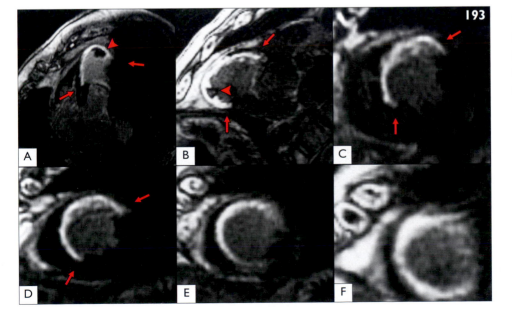

193 Large anterior myocardial infarction. (arrowheads: mural thrombus; arrows: extension of fibrosis)

Case 3: Microvascular Obstruction

Clinical history

A 49-year-old male with acute chest pain was admitted to the emergency room. The chest pain started 8 hours prior to the admission. An anterior myocardial infarction was confirmed by ECG and elevation of cardiac enzymes.

Imaging protocol

The patient received thrombolytics and a cardiac MRI was ordered 2 days after admission for the evaluation of the extent of the myocardial infarction.

Impression

The MRI perfusion images (**194**) showed a large nonperfused area apparently related to MO. A large hypodense area can be appreciated in the septal and anterior walls at the mid-ventricle level (arrows, **194A**). MO was related to a posterior fibrotic area as seen in the delayed contrast-enhanced image (**194B**). This was present in the acute phase of myocardial infarction, but disappeared after a few weeks. In this case, the delayed images demonstrated that the contrast was not diffused into the MO area, indicating a severely ischemic region.

Discussion

MO is usually limited to the subendocardial region. Subendocardial regions with MRI no-reflow had delayed contrast wash-in as opposed to the delayed contrast wash-out of the hyperenhanced region, potentially explained by the capillary obstruction seen within the infarct. Decreased functional capillary density prolongs the time for gadolinium molecules to penetrate the infarct core leading to the dark, low signal intensity early after a contrast bolus injection. In this particular patient the usual contrast-enhanced signals, expected to be present in the delayed images using inversion recovery sequence, were not seen due to the slow inflow of contrast to the necrotic region.

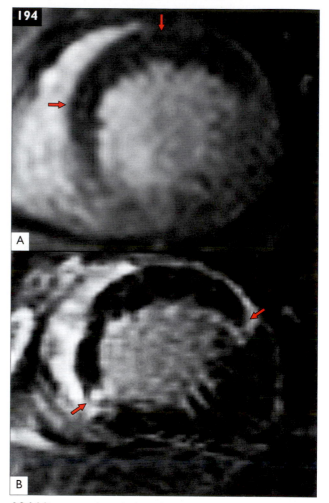

194 Microvascular obstruction.

As such, the hyperenhanced signals are restricted to the border zones (arrows, **194B**).

Management

The presence of a large area of MO has prognostic implications and the patient was placed in a high-risk management group.

Case 4: Dilated Cardiomyopathy

Clinical history

The patient was a 35-year-old male with known DCM and symptoms of heart failure. The etiology was unclear. He was referred for the implantation of an ICD as a precaution against sudden cardiac death.

Imaging protocol

Cardiac MRI was performed to assess left ventricular EF more precisely. Echocardiographic examination in this patient was of limited value due to the poor acoustic window.

Impression

The end-diastolic and end-systolic MRI images are shown in **195A** and **B**, respectively. Left ventricular end-systolic volume was increased (102 mL), whereas the left ventricular mass was within the normal limit. The left ventricular function was reduced due to diffuse moderate hypokinesia (EF = 40%). As can be appreciated from the delayed postcontrast-enhanced images (Figures **195C–F**), no myocardial scar was noticed.

Discussion

When evaluating a patient with DCM it is important to rule out ischemic heart disease as the etiology. Cardiac MRI is a noninvasive imaging technique, well suited for the detection of myocardial scar when a silent or unrecognized myocardial infarction is suspected. Scars due to myocardial infarction occur usually in the subendocardial regions and may extend transmurally throughout the myocardium. In contrast, scars in idiopathic DCM tend to be subepicardial and often show a diffuse pattern.

Management

The presence of a myocardial scar may have prognostic implications in DCM patients. Arrhythmias are more inducible in patients presenting with myocardial scars. The patient presented in this case did not have myocardial scars. His left ventricular EF was reduced but not severely enough to justify the implantation of an I

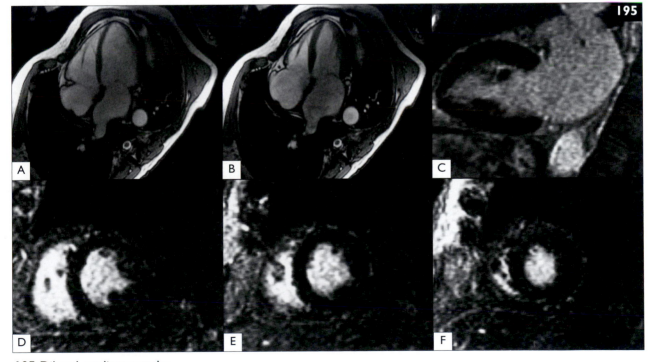

195 Dilated cardiomyopathy.

Case 5: Hypertrophic Obstructive Cardiomyopathy

Clinical history

The patient was a 35-year-old male with a history of hypertrophic obstructive cardiomyopathy.

Imaging protocol

A cardiac MRI was performed 48 hours after selective alcoholic septal ablation to verify the extension and location of the affected myocardium.

Impression

A transmural scar was seen in the proximal portion of the septum (arrows, **196**). These images demonstrated that the alcoholic ablation had been successful. Note that hypodense areas were also seen, suggesting MO within the scar tissue.

Discussion

A precise selection of the septal artery that irrigates the basal portion of the septum is mandatory for a successful ablation procedure. Concomitant contrast echocardiography during catheterization may be helpful to guide the procedure. Subsequently, it is important to verify the transmural extent of the ablation, since residual viable myocardium in the ablated area may represent hypertrophic myocardium and result in persistent obstruction.

Management

Complete healing of the scar tissue usually takes about 3 months. Thus follow-up MRI imaging at this time is required to assess the final scarring of the septum and verify the absence of outflow obstruction.

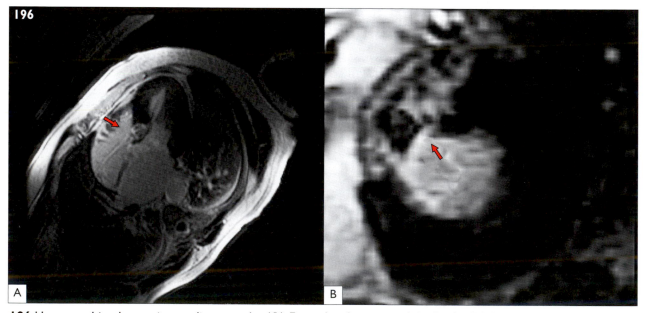

196 Hypertrophic obstructive cardiomyopathy. (**A**) Four chamber view of the heart. (**B**) Short axis view of the left ventricle. A transmural scar is seen in the proximal portion of the septum (arrows)

6. FUTURE PROSPECTS OF CARDIOVASCULAR IMAGING

Albert J. Sinusas

INTRODUCTION

The diagnosis and management of patients with cardiovascular disease has become expensive. Part of the increasing expense is associated with the development and application of advanced imaging technology. To control the escalating costs of healthcare there has been a shift in emphasis from treatment to the prevention of disease. However, the prevention of disease necessitates risk stratification and early detection, which may depend on genotyping, or assessment of circulating biomarkers, as well as noninvasive imaging. This presents new challenges to basic research and clinical practice, and involves technologic adaptations and integration of existing diagnostic approaches. In the past, the prognostication and evaluation of cardiovascular disease or therapeutic interventions were assessed by studying physiological consequences expressed in changes in flow, function, and/or metabolism. Future strategies should involve use of targeted markers of biological processes for early detection. The development of biologically targeted markers has become possible with recent molecular biological advances, including genomics and proteomics. The application of targeted molecular imaging based on these novel markers may provide additional unique molecular and pathophysiological insights that will allow a more personalized approach to evaluation and management of cardiovascular disease. The effective application of these technologic advances will require the establishment of multidisciplinary teams, with a wide range of expertise. Targeted cardiovascular molecular imaging is expected to play a key role in this interdisciplinary approach to understand origins, pathogenesis, and progress of diseases and to evaluate therapeutic interventions. Each of the imaging modalities has the potential to observe a component of *in vivo* complex system functions at the molecular, cellular, organ, as well as whole body level. The future of cardiovascular imaging rests on integration of these technologies in a comprehensive and cost-effective strategy.

MOLECULAR IMAGING

The concept and practice of molecular imaging is defined as the visualization, characterization, and measurement of biological processes at the molecular and cellular levels in humans and other living systems. Molecular imaging typically includes two- or three-dimensional imaging as well as quantification over time. Molecular imaging has been around for decades and originated with targeted nuclear imaging. However, other molecular imaging techniques include MRI, magnetic resonance spectroscopy, optical imaging, and ultrasound imaging, along with other developing imaging technologies. Targeted imaging can be defined in terms of a probe–target interaction, whereas the probe localization and magnitude are directly related to the interaction with the target epitope or peptide. Molecular imaging agents can include both endogenous molecules and exogenous probes. Nuclear medicine is particularly suited for targeted *in vivo* molecular imaging because of the relatively high sensitivity of the nuclear imaging approaches. The nuclear approaches include the use of monoclonal antibody targeting of a particular cell membrane epitope, targeted imaging of a receptor with radiolabeled peptides or peptidomimetics, imaging the activity of a particular enzyme, or even a transporter-specific probe.

Historical perspective

Imaging cell-specific surface antigens or epitopes with radiolabeled monoclonal antibodies constitutes some of the earliest molecular imaging applications that are still used in experimental studies and clinical nuclear medicine. Initial studies involved tumor imaging with radiolabeled native antibodies (i.e. IgG) (Brumley & Kuhn 1995). The introduction of genetic engineering provided a powerful tool to design recombinant fragments that retained high affinity for target antigens, providing rapid targeting and concomitant clearance from normal tissues. More recently, the imaging of various cell surface receptors using radiolabeled regulatory peptides has provided an alternative strategy for targeted imaging. These peptides are small, readily diffusible molecules that induce a broad range of receptor-mediated actions. These high-affinity receptors are over-expressed in many pathological states and represent molecular targets for diagnosis and assessment of the therapy. A host of radiolabeled peptidomimetics have been created based on the structure of natural peptides that target the same receptors, although they may have improved uptake and clearance kinetics for targeted imaging of selected biological processes or tissues.

The most widely used radiolabeled agent for molecular imaging in clinical practice is FDG. Imaging of glucose utilization with this agent provides an *in vivo* assay of enzymatic activity. This imaging approach is based on an enzyme-specific radiolabeled probe and an enzyme-metabolic trapping mechanism that provides an amplification of the signal in target tissue, facilitating *in vivo* imaging. While ^{18}F-FDG PET imaging has been used for imaging of cardiac metabolism for many years, the use of this agent has become far more prevalent for detection of a wide range of tumors that demonstrate increased glucose metabolism, and for tracking response to cancer therapy.

Another classic targeted molecular imaging approach involves the imaging of cardiac neuroreceptors in the heart. Most of this work has focused on imaging of the sympathetic nervous system. Important alterations in pre- and postsynaptic cardiac sympathetic function occur in several cardiovascular diseases, including ischemic heart disease. Presynaptic function can be measured using ^{11}C-meta-hydroxyephedrine (mHED), a PET radiotracer, or ^{123}I-meta-iodobenzylguanidine (MIBG) a SPECT radiotracer. Postsynaptic function can be assessed with ^{11}C-CGP12177, a radiolabeled beta-blocker for PET imaging. This topic is the focus of several excellent reviews (Tseng *et al.* 2001, Link *et al.* 2003).

Newer applications

Recent progress in the knowledge of the molecular–genetic mechanisms as well as technologic development of new imaging strategies has led to the application of new molecular-based approaches. Methods are actively being developed for controlled gene delivery to various tissues using novel gene constructs. Moreover, gene expression can be controlled and imaged using cell-specific, drug-controlled expression systems. New molecular-based imaging strategies have been developed and successfully employed in both basic and clinical research studies. For example, radiolabeled thymidine analogues, such as 5-iodo-2'-deoxy-uridine ([123]IdU, [124]IdU, and [131]IdU) and 5-bromo-2'-deoxy-uridine ([76]BrdU), have been used to image cell proliferation and DNA synthesis.

More complex indirect molecular imaging strategies have also been developed involving multiple components. Reporter gene/probe imaging is an example of an indirect imaging strategy. This approach employs both a reporter gene and a reporter probe, the mechanism of which was detailed in a recent review (Chang *et al.* 2006). Reporter gene imaging involves construction of a DNA sequence coding a specific reporter, which is carried into a target cell by a vector delivery system. When the transfected cell is exposed to the corresponding reporter probes, the expression of the reporter gene product catalyzes an enzymatic reaction, which 'turns on' the imaging signal in the probe and entraps activated probe inside the cells. The imaging signal may be a radiolabeled or optical probe and is detected by the corresponding imaging devices. This approach is particularly helpful in imaging cell-based therapies, since accumulation of the reporter probe requires cell viability and ongoing expression of the reporter gene product. Because the reporter gene becomes integrated into the cellular chromosomes and is passed on from mother to daughter cells, this approach allows for tracking of cell proliferation. In addition, multiple reporter genes can be combined for multimodality visualization or can be combined with specific promoters for analyses of molecular pathways or differentiation processes (Barbash *et al.* 2003, Chen *et al.* 2004). Another advantage of this approach is the enzymatic amplification of the probe signal that facilitates imaging the magnitude and location of reporter gene expression.

A major goal of molecular imaging involves the imaging of molecular markers and biological pathways that give insight into the pathogenesis and progress of diseases and assessment of therapeutic intervention. These include novel imaging strategies for heart failure, thrombosis, apoptosis, atherosclerosis, and angiogenesis. Some of these approaches will be discussed in detail below.

Imaging technology

There have been tremendous technologic advances in instrumentation for cardiovascular imaging. These advances, including a whole host of imaging systems dedicated for small animal imaging, have facilitated the growth of molecular imaging. Each imaging methodology has unique advantages as well as practical limitations. The relative strengths and weaknesses of each of the imaging modalities relative to their potential for molecular imaging are summarized in *Table 8*, (overleaf) and the relative value of each modality for imaging anatomical structure, physiology, metabolism, and molecular events is illustrated in **197**.

The optical and nuclear imaging approaches offer relatively high sensitivity, an important issue for detection and imaging of localized molecular or cellular processes. However, due to their relatively poor spatial resolution, the application of these approaches for imaging anatomical structure is somewhat limited. In contrast, techniques such as X-ray CT, ultrasound-based approaches, or MRI offer much better spatial resolution, although provide much lower sensitivity for evaluation of specific molecular processes. Consequently, many investigators and commercial vendors have developed hybrid imaging systems that facilitate optimization of imaging for small animals as well as for patients. The introduction of hybrid systems for imaging of small animals (microSPECT/CT and microPET/CT) greatly enhanced the performance and accuracy of nuclear imaging. The CT component could be used for anatomical localization, attenuation correction, and correction of partial volume errors.

MicroSPECT imaging offers several advantages over microPET imaging in small animals, and these include availability of a host of targeted radiotracers with a longer half-life, improved spatial resolution (<1 mm), and greater availability and affordability of the SPECT technology. The inherent resolution of PET radiotracers is fundamentally limited by physical behavior of positron decay (1–3 mm), associated with the significant movement of positron prior to annihilation, and deviation from exact 180° angular separation. SPECT imaging approaches also allow for simultaneous multiple-isotope imaging capability. On the other hand, microPET technology offers several

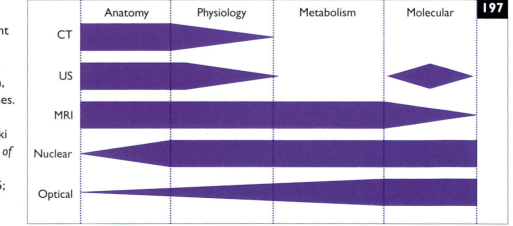

197 Illustration of relative value of current imaging modalities for evaluation of anatomy, physiology, metabolism, and molecular processes. (Reprinted with permission of Dobrucki WL, Sinusas AJ. *Journal of Nuclear Medicine and Molecular Imaging* 2005; **49**:106–115.)

Table 8 Selected operational parameters for different imaging modalities and the potential advantages and disadvantages

Modality	Spatial resolution	Temporal resolution	Penetration depth	Sensitivity (mol/l)	Advantages	Disadvantages
PET	1–3 mm	Sec to min	No limitation	10^{-11}–10^{-12}	Very high sensitivity ^{11}C, ^{18}F imaging Attenuation correction	Limited resolution of anatomical information Expensive
SPECT	0.5–1.5 mm	Min	No limitation	10^{-10}–10^{-11}	High sensitivity High resolution Multiple isotope imaging Availability of tracers and instruments	Limited attenuation correction Larger sized probes
Optical: biolumine- scence	3–5 mm	Sec to min	1–2 mm	10^{-15}–10^{-17}	Superior sensitivity High throughput	Very low penetration depth
Optical: fluorescence	2–3 mm	Sec to min	<1 mm	10^{-9}–10^{-12}	Superior sensitivity	Lack of anatomical information
MRI	25–100 μm	Min to hrs	No limitation	10^{-3}–10^{-5}	Superior spatial resolution Anatomical imaging	Lack of targeted probes Low sensitivity Expensive
CT	25–200 μm	Min	No limitation		Superior spatial resolution Anatomical imaging	Use of X-radiation Lack of targeted probes
Ultrasound	50–500 μm	Sec to min	mm–cm		Availability Anatomical imaging	Lack of targeted probes Low penetration depth

unique advantages over microSPECT imaging. The clear advantages of PET imaging include:

➤ Higher sensitivity, enabling dynamic imaging.
➤ Creation of radiolabeled probes with natural radioisotopes such as ^{11}C that do not alter chemical behavior.
➤ Well established approach for attenuation correction.
➤ A greater potential for absolute image quantification.

Advances have also been made regarding ultrasound imaging in small animals. Ultrasound imaging systems are available with small-profile high-frequency transducers that facilitate imaging in small animals, including transgenic mice and even transcutaneous imaging of intrauterine fetuses. However, the major advance regarding molecular imaging with ultrasound has been associated with the development of targeted ultrasound contrast agents (Morawski *et al.* 2005, Behm & Lindner 2006).

MRI is also emerging as a technique for molecular imaging. MRI provides high spatial resolution and the unique capability to elicit both anatomical and physiological information simultaneously (Lanza *et al.* 2004, Wickline *et al.* 2006). The MR signal is created through the interaction of the total water signal (proton density) and the magnetic properties of the tissues being imaged. This provides an opportunity for the development of contrast agents that can be used for both positive ('hot spot') and negative ('cold spot') enhancement (Morawski *et al.* 2005). The most commonly used nonspecific contrast agents are gadolinium based which provide an increase in signal. More recently, superparamagnetic iron oxide particles have been developed that create signal voids on MR images. While MRI generally offers much lower sensitivity than optical or radiotracer-based approaches for targeted molecular imaging, novel approaches are now being applied to increase the contrast payload of MR targeted contrast agents, making molecular imaging with MRI systems feasible.

Microscopic bioluminescent and fluorescent optical imaging has been used for decades by molecular biologists, but only recently have these technologies been applied for *in vivo* molecular imaging of living animals (Choy *et al.* 2003). The application of optical imaging has been primarily limited to small animals because of issues related to tissue penetration, although recently intravascular fiberoptic catheters and probes have been applied in larger animals or even humans for *in vivo* imaging.

Image quantification

Quantification of molecular imaging refers to the determination of regional concentrations of molecular imaging agents and biological parameters. This quantification is a key element of molecular imaging data and image analysis, especially for inter- and intrasubject comparisons. The accuracy of microSPECT imaging is fundamentally limited by the attenuation of the low-energy photons by body tissues. This introduces an error in relating the density of detected photons to the concentration of the radiopharmaceutical in an organ. Moreover, the presence of photon scatter limits spatial resolution. The microPET imaging systems generally provide better attenuation correction. However, most state-of-the-art microSPECT and microPET imaging systems are fused with microCT, which can facilitate accurate attenuation correction.

SPECIFIC CARDIOVASCULAR APPLICATIONS OF MOLECULAR IMAGING

The following sections will review several specific applications for cardiovascular molecular imaging, including the imaging of angiogenesis, atherosclerosis or vascular injury, postinfarction remodeling, and apoptosis. The emphasis will be on the use of radiolabeled SPECT tracers, although other molecular imaging approaches will be briefly discussed.

Imaging of angiogenesis

Angiogenesis represents the formation of new capillaries by cellular outgrowth from existing microvessels (Battegay 1995), and occurs as part of the natural healing process following ischemic injury. The process of angiogenesis includes local proliferation and migration of vascular smooth muscle and endothelial cells and is modulated by circulating inflammatory and stem cells. Hypoxia, inflammation, and shear stress are the principal stimuli for angiogenesis. A large number of other local and circulating angiogenic factors are involved in the angiogenic process, including vascular endothelial growth factor (VEGF), angiopoietins, basic fibroblast growth factor (bFGF), and transforming growth factor (TGF)-β. The angiogenic response is also modulated by the extracellular matrix (ECM) and intercellular adhesions, including integrins (Brooks *et al.* 1994a, 1994b). Integrins are a family of cell surface receptors capable of mediating an array of cellular processes, including cell adhesion, migration, proliferation, differentiation, and survival (Schwartz *et al.* 1995). The specific αvβ3 integrin has been identified as a critical modulator of angiogenesis (Brooks *et al.* 1994a). Thus, the angiogenic process is a complex multistep phenomenon that involves many stimuli, growth factors, and interactions between multiple cell types (Haas & Madri 1999), all of which could be targets for identification of angiogenesis at the molecular or cellular level. Approaches for the targeted imaging of angiogenesis have been previously reviewed (Sinusas 2004). Only the most established approaches for targeted imaging of angiogenesis will be highlighted in this chapter, and include the evaluation of VEGF receptors and the αvβ3 integrin.

Imaging of VEGF and receptors

The expression of VEGF is induced by hypoxia, and is a key natural mediator of angiogenesis in response to ischemia. VEGF mediates many cellular functions, including release of other growth factors, cell proliferation, migration, survival, and angiogenesis (Ferrara *et al.* 2003). Indium-111(^{111}In)-labeled VEGF$_{121}$ has been used for the noninvasive detection of angiogenesis in a rabbit model of unilateral hindlimb ischemia, and the *in vivo* imaging results were validated with tissue counting of radioactivity and immunohistochemic analyses (Lu *et al.* 2003). This preclinical study supports the feasibility of imaging ischemia-induced angiogenesis using a naturally occurring growth factor as the imaging probe for evaluation of the upregulation of an angiogenic receptor. VEGF receptor imaging could provide complementary information to routinely available clinical assessments of flow by imparting physiological information on hypoxic stress within viable tissue (Cerqueira & Udelson 2003). VEGF receptor imaging could also be potentially useful in the evaluation of therapeutic angiogenic strategies. Further studies in more clinically relevant models will be required to validate the concept of angiogenic receptor labeling as a clinically useful imaging approach.

Imaging of αvβ3 integrin

As outlined above, the αvβ3 integrin is expressed in angiogenic vessels and is known to modulate angiogenesis, and therefore represents another potential novel target for imaging angiogenesis (Sipkins *et al.* 1998, Haubner *et al.* 1999). Haubner *et al.* reported the synthesis and characterization of a series of radiolabeled αvβ3 antagonists, reporting

kinetics in both *in vitro* and *in vivo* preparations (Haubner *et al.* 1999, 2001a, 2001b). Harris *et al.* reported the high affinity and selectivity of an ^{111}In-labeled quinolone (^{111}In-RP748, Bristol Myers-Squibb) for the αvβ3 integrin using assays of integrin-mediated adhesion (Harris *et al.* 2003). Meoli *et al.* were the first to report the potential of ^{111}In-RP748 for *in vivo* imaging of myocardial angiogenesis (Meoli *et al.* 2004). The specificity of ^{111}In-RP748 for targeted imaging of the αvβ3 integrin was confirmed by nonimaging studies employing a rat model of injury-induced myocardial angiogenesis, and a nonspecific isomeric negative control compound (Meoli *et al.* 2004). These rat studies of nontransmural infarction demonstrated that only ^{111}In-RP748 was selectively retained in regions of injury-induced angiogenesis. In follow-up imaging studies using a large animal model of myocardial infarction, ^{111}In-RP748 demonstrated favorable kinetics for imaging of ischemia-induced angiogenesis in the heart. *In vivo* and *ex vivo* dual isotope SPECT short-axis ^{111}In-RP748 and ^{99m}Tc-sestamibi images are shown following myocardial infarction in a model of ischemia-induced angiogenesis (**198**).

Additional studies have demonstrated the value of a ^{99m}Tc-labeled peptide (NC100692, GE Healthcare, UK) for targeted imaging of the αvβ3 integrin in rodent models of hindlimb ischemia and models of myocardial infarction, using high-resolution planar and microSPECT/CT imaging (Su *et al.* 2003, Hua *et al.* 2005, Lindsey *et al.* 2006). In the initial validation studies employing a model of hindlimb ischemia, mice were sacrificed after NC100692 imaging at different time points post ischemia for gamma well counting and immunohistologic analysis of muscle tissue distal to the vascular occlusion (Hua *et al.* 2005). A significant increase in NC100692 activity was observed in the ischemic limb at 3 and 7 days after the occlusion which normalized by 14 days post occlusion. Immunohistochemical staining for lectin, an endothelial cell marker, confirmed a progressive increase in capillary density in the ischemic hindlimb at these time points. The observed changes in regional NC100692 uptake in the ischemic tissue derived from quantification of the noninvasive imaging were confirmed by gamma well counting of tissue. However, the imaging approach tended to underestimate the relative increases of tissue NC100692 uptake. These differences probably reflect

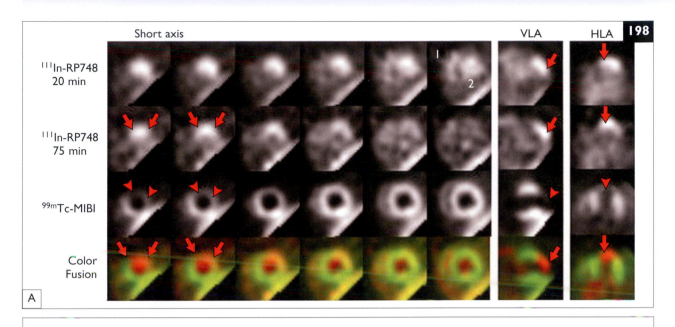

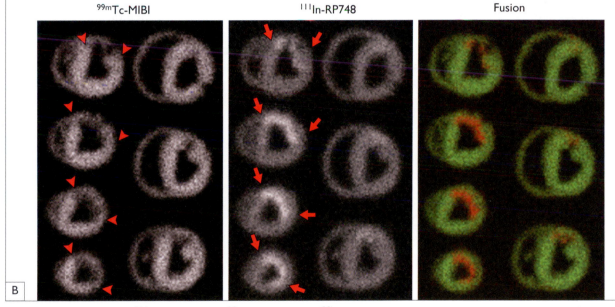

198 *In vivo* and *ex vivo* ^{111}In-RP748 and ^{99m}Tc-sestamibi (^{99m}Tc-MIBI) images from dogs with chronic infarction. (**A**) Serial *in vivo* ^{111}In-RP748 SPECT short-axis, vertical long-axis (VLA), and horizontal long-axis (HLA) images in a dog with 3 weeks following LAD occlusion at 20 minutes and 75 minutes post injection in standard format. ^{111}In-RP748 SPECT images were registered with ^{99m}Tc-MIBI perfusion images (third row). The 75 minutes ^{111}In-RP748 SPECT images were colored red and fused with ^{99m}Tc-sestamibi (MIBI) images (green) to demonstrate better localization of ^{111}In-RP748 activity within the heart (color fusion, bottom row). Right ventricular (1) and left ventricular (2) blood pool activity are seen at 20 minutes. Arrows indicate a region of increased ^{111}In-RP748 uptake in anterior wall. This corresponds to the anteroapical ^{99m}Tc-sestamibi perfusion defect (arrowhead). (**B**) *Ex vivo* ^{99m}Tc-sestamibi (left) and ^{111}In-RP748 (center) images of myocardial slices from a dog with 3 weeks post LAD occlusion, with color fusion image on the right. Short-axis slices are oriented with anterior wall on the top, right ventricle on the left. Arrowheads indicate anterior location of nontransmural perfusion defect region, and arrows indicate corresponding area of increased ^{111}In-RP748 uptake. (Reprinted with permission from Meoli DF, Sadeghi MM, Krassilnikova S *et al.* Noninvasive imaging of myocardial angiogenesis following experimental myocardial infarction. *Journal of Clinical Investigation* 2004;**113**:1684–1691.)

errors due to the attenuation and partial volume effects associated with imaging. Representative *in vivo* NC100692 images from this study are shown in **199** (Hua *et al.* 2005). Another group of investigators has also demonstrated the value of a ^{123}I-labeled peptide for *in vivo* imaging of angiogenesis using a similar murine model of hindlimb ischemia (Lee *et al.* 2005). Using an analogous ^{125}I-labeled peptide they also observed maximal uptake of the αv targeted compound at 3 days post ischemia.

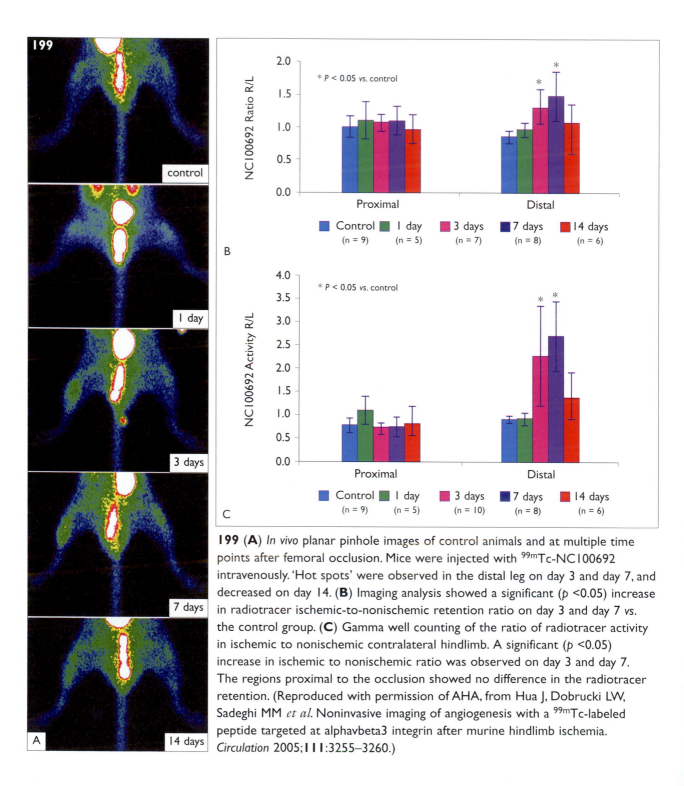

199 (A) *In vivo* planar pinhole images of control animals and at multiple time points after femoral occlusion. Mice were injected with ^{99m}Tc-NC100692 intravenously. 'Hot spots' were observed in the distal leg on day 3 and day 7, and decreased on day 14. **(B)** Imaging analysis showed a significant (p <0.05) increase in radiotracer ischemic-to-nonischemic retention ratio on day 3 and day 7 *vs.* the control group. **(C)** Gamma well counting of the ratio of radiotracer activity in ischemic to nonischemic contralateral hindlimb. A significant (p <0.05) increase in ischemic to nonischemic ratio was observed on day 3 and day 7. The regions proximal to the occlusion showed no difference in the radiotracer retention. (Reproduced with permission of AHA, from Hua J, Dobrucki LW, Sadeghi MM *et al.* Noninvasive imaging of angiogenesis with a ^{99m}Tc-labeled peptide targeted at alphavbeta3 integrin after murine hindlimb ischemia. *Circulation* 2005;111:3255–3260.)

Leong-Poi *et al.* recently demonstrated that targeted contrast-enhanced ultrasound (CEU) and microbubbles targeted to endothelial integrins could be used to assess noninvasively early angiogenic responses to ischemia and growth factor therapy (Leong-Poi *et al.* 2003). Hindlimb ischemia was produced in rats by ligation of an iliac artery. Half of the animals received intramuscular sustained-release fibroblast growth factor-2 (FGF-2). Immediately after ligation and at subsequent intervals from 4–28 days, blood flow in the proximal adductor muscles was measured by CEU perfusion imaging. Targeted CEU imaging of $\alpha v\beta 3$ and $\alpha 5\beta 1$ integrin expression was performed with microbubbles bearing the disintegrin echistatin. Signal from integrin-targeted microbubbles was intense and peaked before flow increase (days 4–7). FGF-2-treated muscle had a greater rate and extent of blood flow recovery and greater signal intensity from integrin-targeted microbubbles (**200**). These results suggest that molecular imaging of integrin expression may be useful for evaluating proangiogenic therapies.

These experimental studies suggest that radiolabeled and microbubbles targeted agents at integrins may be valuable noninvasive markers of angiogenesis following ischemic injury. Additional experimental studies will be required to define the duration of integrin expression/activation following ischemic injury or following stimulated angiogenesis. The changes in expression/activation of integrins will also need to be related to changes in more functional parameters, such as myocardial perfusion, regional mechanical function, permeability, and regional hypoxia. The potential for targeted imaging of other integrins, e.g. $\alpha v\beta 5$, must also be considered.

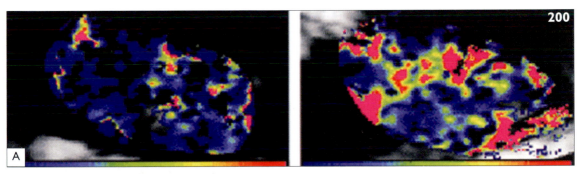

Control　　　　　　　　　　　Ischemic

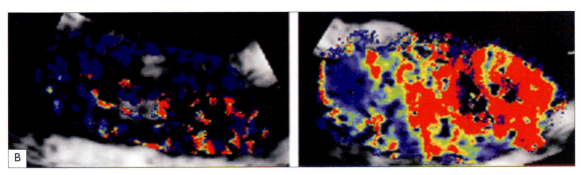

Control　　　　　　　　　　　Ischemic

200 Examples of color-coded CEU images reflecting retention fraction of integrin-targeted microbubbles in control and ischemic proximal hindlimb adductor muscles from untreated (**A**) and FGF-2-treated (**B**) rat 4 days after iliac artery ligation. Color scales appear at bottom. (Reproduced with permission of AHA, from Leong-Poi H, Christiansen J, Klibanov AL *et al.* Noninvasive assessment of angiogenesis by ultrasound and microbubbles targeted to [alpha]v-integrins. *Circulation* 2003;**107**:455–460.)

Imaging of atherosclerosis and vascular injury

Integrins, particularly αvβ3, have also emerged as a promising target for imaging injury-induced vascular remodeling/proliferative process (Sadeghi & Bender 2007). Sadeghi *et al.* have demonstrated that novel ^{111}In-labeled αvβ3 integrin-specific molecules, RP748 and its homologs, bind preferentially to activated αvβ3 on endothelial cells *in vitro* and exhibit

favorable binding characteristics for *in vivo* imaging (Sadeghi *et al.* 2004). These investigators demonstrated that RP748 uptake can track the proliferative process associated with carotid artery injury by targeting activated αvβ3 integrin expression *in vivo* in apolipoprotein E-negative mice (**201**). Similarly, Winter *et al.* employed the use of paramagnetic nanoparticles targeted to αvβ3 integrin, demonstrating the feasibility of MR molecular

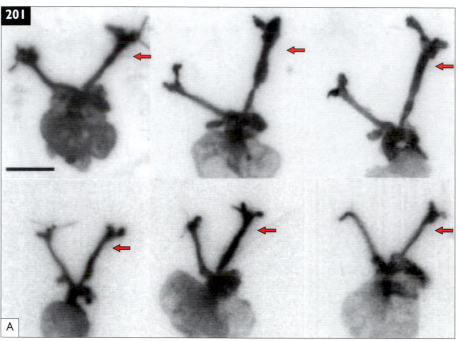

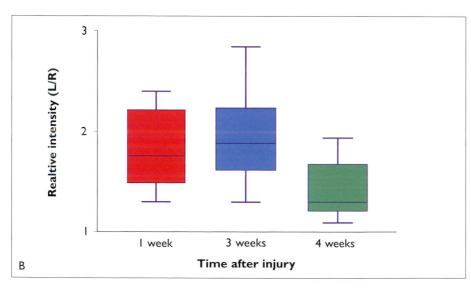

201 Autoradiographic analysis of RP748 uptake after left carotid injury.
(**A**) Examples of carotid autoradiographs at 1, 3, and 4 weeks after left carotid injury. Arrows point to sites of injury.
(**B**) Range and quartiles of relative autographic intensity (left/right). Box extends from 25th to 75th percentile, with a line at median. Whiskers show highest and lowest values. N = 9 at each time point. (Reproduced with permission of AHA, from Sadeghi MM, Krassilnikova S, Zhang J et al. Detection of injury-induced vascular remodeling by targeting activated [alpha]v[beta]3 integrin *in vivo. Circulation* 2004;110:84–90.)

imaging of expanded vasa vasorum in atherosclerotic lesions in cholesterol-fed rabbits (**202**) (Winter *et al.* 2003). In contrast, rabbits on a control diet exhibited no increased signal and background was minimal. Expression of αvβ3 integrins in the adventitial layer and beyond was confirmed by histologic staining of αvβ3 integrin and an endothelial marker. These targeted αvβ3 integrin imaging approaches may potentially lead to the development of noninvasive imaging strategies for identification of atherosclerosis, and vascular cell proliferation-associated states, whether focal (i.e. postangioplasty restenosis) or diffuse (i.e. pulmonary hypertension).

Schäfers *et al.* investigated the feasibility of scintigraphic imaging of matrix metalloproteinases (MMPs) *in vivo* using a radiolabeled broad-spectrum MMP inhibitor (CGS27023A) in an established animal model of arterial remodeling and lesion development where MMPs are induced and activated (Schafers *et al.* 2004). The MMPs constitute a large family of proteolytic enzymes responsible for degradation of myocardial ECM that is associated with vascular remodeling.

Other investigators have focused on the imaging

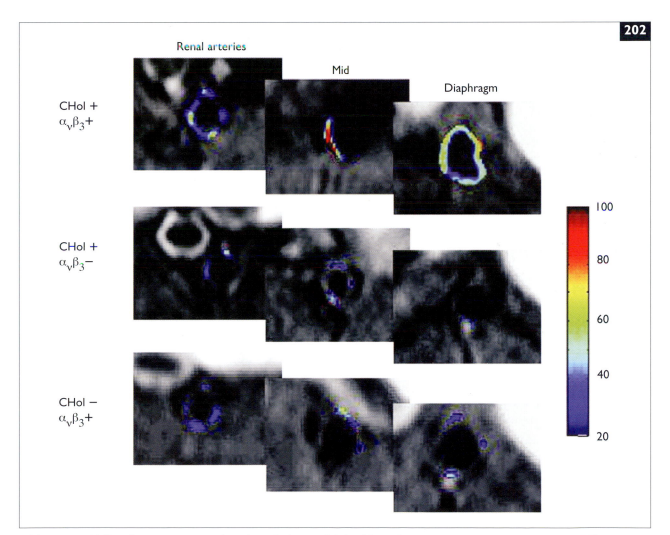

202 Targeted MRI of angiogenesis induced in cholesterol-fed rabbits. Aortic cross-sections imaged at 1.5 T with nanoparticles targeted at αvβ3 integrin from the level of the renal arteries to diaphragm. Note heterogeneous distribution in aortic cross-sections (false colored contrast enhancement), but little enhancement in nontargeted rabbits (αvβ3-) or rabbits on a standard diet (Chol-). (Reproduced with permission of AHA, from Wickline SA, Neubauer AM, Winter P *et al.* Applications of nanotechnology to atherosclerosis, thrombosis, and vascular biology. *Arteriosclerosis, Thrombosis, and Vascular Biology* 2006;**26**:435–441.)

of vascular smooth muscle cell proliferation (Narula, *et al.* 1997) and apoptosis of these cells or macrophages within the vessel wall (Kolodgie *et al.* 2003). One useful marker of smooth muscle cell proliferation is the negative charge-modified Z2D3 antibody which has been used for immunoscintigraphic targeted imaging of atherosclerosis (Narula *et al.* 1997).

Targeted radiotracer imaging of atherosclerosis or vascular remodeling presents a unique problem, in that the target lesion has a very low mass and may be located deep in the body. Existing PET and SPECT instrumentation may be insufficiently sensitive to detect these small deep lesions. Accordingly, several groups of investigators are developing intravascular scintillation catheters that can be used to detect local uptake of radiotracers targeted to components of the atherosclerotic or unstable vascular plaque (Zhu *et al.* 2003, Piao *et al.* 2005, Strauss *et al.* 2006). Most of these intravascular detectors employ plastic scintillators linked to fiberoptics which may transmit signal down a flexible catheter system.

Imaging of postinfarction remodeling

Left ventricular remodeling refers to the adverse changes in the structure, geometry, and, eventually, function of the left ventricle that occur following myocardial infarction, and has been shown to be an important independent risk factor following myocardial infarction.

A number of clinical parameters have been predictive of postmyocardial infarction remodeling; these include infarct size, transmurality of myocardial injury, patency of the infarct related artery, and degree of microvascular obstruction. Cardiac catheterization, echocardiography, nuclear imaging, cardiac MRI, and X-ray CT have all been used to follow and predict postmyocardial infarction left ventricular remodeling. Most of these techniques have been used to evaluate anatomical features or the physiological consequences of remodeling. However, recently molecular approaches have been used for early detection, risk stratification, and monitoring of the remodeling process following myocardial infarction.

Several investigators have focused on the role of MMPs. MMPs are a family of zinc-dependent enzymes that are responsible for degradation of the myocardial ECM and are associated with the postmyocardial infarction left ventricular myocardial remodeling that

often leads to heart failure. A clear cause–effect relationship between MMPs and the left ventricular remodeling process has been demonstrated using a host of preclinical animal models of postmyocardial infarction remodeling and heart failure. The importance of detecting and quantifying MMP activity *in vivo* during the evolution of post-myocardial infarction remodeling has provided the impetus to develop a noninvasive method that will help to translate these basic preclinical observations to clinical applicability.

The measurement of MMP and tissue inhibitors of MMPs (TIMP) levels in tissue and plasma can provide important insights into a critical determinant of MMP activity. However, due to the multiple post-translational steps regulating MMP activity, several approaches have been developed to quantify directly MMP activity *in situ* and even *in vivo*. The *in situ* approaches include zymography or the use of fluorogenic-labeled peptide substrates. However, these peptide constructs are unstable in plasma, bound by nonspecific proteins, and have a limited half-life, all of which limit the *in vivo* clinical applicability. Recent effort has been placed in developing nonpeptide markers for MMP activity based around the structural configuration of pharmacologic MMP inhibitors. Bristol-Myers-Squibb has developed MMP-targeted SPECT radiotracers which demonstrate selective binding kinetics to the active MMP catalytic domain. Binding of these radiotracers to the exposed catalytic domain of active MMPs provides a means to detect and image MMP activation *in vivo* using a conventional gamma camera.

Su *et al.* demonstrated the feasibility of noninvasive MMP imaging using an ^{111}In-labeled nonspecific MMP inhibitor (^{111}In-RP782) to evaluate temporal changes in MMP activation in a murine model of myocardial infarction (Su *et al.* 2005). Gamma well counting revealed a significant increase in ^{111}In-RP782 activity in myocardial infarction regions of the postmyocardial infarction group compared with the control group. ^{111}In-RP782 retention correlated well with MMP activity defined by *in situ* zymography. Additional imaging studies in rodent, porcine, and canine models of myocardial infarction have been performed using a ^{99m}Tc-labeled analog of ^{111}In-RP782 (^{99m}Tc-RP805) confirming feasibility of this approach for *in vivo* imaging of MMP activation (McAteer *et al.* 2005, Su *et al.*

2005). Representative, *in vivo* MMP-targeted microSPECT/CT images in mice post infarction are shown in **203**. Using ^{99m}Tc-RP-805 in a porcine model of chronic myocardial infarction, the temporal and spatial variation of MMP activity postmyocardial infarction was defined relative to ^{201}Tl perfusion with dual isotope SPECT/CT imaging (McAteer *et al.* 2005). The serial MMP targeted images demonstrated that myocardial MMP activity was highest in all regions of the heart at 1 and 2 weeks following myocardial infarction and declined by 4 weeks. The temporal and spatial changes in MMP activity observed with serial imaging were confirmed using postmortem well counting of the myocardium.

The myocardial activity was expressed as a percentage of the injected dose in order to define absolute changes in MMP activity in infarcted and remote regions of the heart. As previously observed in the murine models of myocardial infarction, myocardial MMP activity was greatest in the infarct region, with lesser increases in the peri-infarct and remote regions relative to noninfarcted control animals (McAteer *et al.* 2005, Sahul *et al.* 2006).

Traditionally risk stratification of patients following myocardial infarction and evaluation of the left ventricular remodeling process has been restricted to imaging of changes in left ventricular geometry and function. However, with the advent of targeted

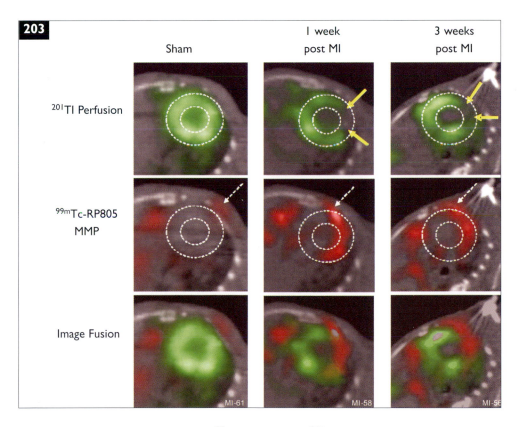

203 *In vivo* hybrid microSPECT/CT ^{99m}Tc-RP805 and ^{201}Tl images from sham mouse (left), and mice 1 week (middle) and 3 weeks (right) post myocardial infarction. *In vivo* ^{201}Tl (green) microSPECT/CT (first row) and ^{99m}Tc-RP805 (red) microSPECT/CT (second row) short-axis images. ^{99m}Tc-RP805 images were co-registered with ^{201}Tl perfusion images (third row). Yellow arrows in the first row indicate ^{201}Tl perfusion defect that corresponds to the area of increased ^{99m}Tc-RP805 uptake. ^{99m}Tc-RP805 uptake is also seen in chest wall (white arrows) at the thoracotomy site. (Reprinted with permission of AHA, Su H, Spinale FG, Dobrucki LW *et al.* Noninvasive targeted imaging of matrix metalloproteinase activation in a murine model of postinfarction remodeling. *Circulation* 2005;112: 3157–3167.)

molecular imaging the pathophysiological changes can be related to the underlying molecular and cellular events, and tracked noninvasively with novel hybrid imaging approaches.

Imaging of apoptosis

Apoptosis, or programmed cell death, occurs in association with many cardiovascular diseases. This pre-programmed cell death often occurs in combination with cell death by necrosis. Cells undergoing apoptosis express on their cell membrane phosphatidyl serine (PS), a constitutive plasma membrane anionic phospholipid, which is not expressed in normal cells, thus it presents a favorable target for imaging of apoptotic processes. Annexin-V is a medium-sized physiological human protein with a high, Ca^{2+}-dependent affinity toward the PS on the outer leaflet of the cell membrane. Annexin-V has been labeled with either fluorescent or radionuclide agents and used in apoptosis imaging.

Recently, a novel real-time imaging model to visualize apoptotic membrane changes of single cardiomyocytes in the injured heart of a living mouse has been reported using fluorescent labeled Annexin-V (Dumont *et al.* 2001). Others have used Annexin-V labeled with a radionuclide agent to image apoptotic cell death *in vivo* (Strauss *et al.* 2000). Recently, ^{99m}Tc-labeled Annexin-V has been used to track heart transplant rejection process. In fact, apoptosis has been noninvasively identified in an animal model of heart transplant rejection (Blankenberg *et al.* 1998) and allograft rejection in rat liver transplantation. Others investigated the clinical role of imaging with Annexin-V for the detection of apoptosis in cardiac allograft recipients (Narula *et al.* 2001). These studies have demonstrated the usefulness of radionuclide imaging with Annexin-V in human subjects who had undergone heart transplantation. Endomyocardial biopsies were performed within the first 4 days following imaging to confirm imaging data by histology. Patients with focal ^{99m}Tc-Annexin-V uptake had histologically verified transplant rejection (grade ≥2). If a correlation between the biopsies and imaging results can be confirmed in larger studies, Annexin-V imaging should help obviate the need for highly invasive serial endomyocardial biopsies. Thus, apoptosis imaging could be used for monitoring of a host of cardiovascular diseases, and potentially for evaluation of the efficacy of interventions directed toward inhibition of apoptosis.

MULTIDISCIPLINARY CARDIOVASCULAR IMAGING PROGRAMS

In order to translate molecular imaging to clinical practice effectively, changes in the usual clinical imaging paradigm are needed. As originally proposed in a joint statement from the European Association of Echocardiography, the Working Groups on Cardiovascular Magnetic Resonance, Computers in

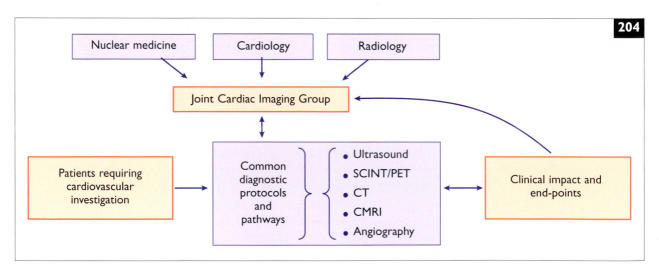

204 Suggested organization of joint, multidisciplinary diagnostic imaging services. (Modified with permission of The European Society of Cardiology, Fraser AG, Buser P, Bax JJ *et al.* The future of cardiovascular imaging and noninvasive diagnosis. *European Journal of Echocardiography* 2006;**7**:268–273.)

Cardiology, and Nuclear Cardiology of the European Society of Cardiology, the European Association of Nuclear Medicine, and the Association for European Pediatric Cardiology, the clinical use of diagnostic cardiovascular imaging technologies should be coordinated through a multidisciplinary collaborative service (**204**). While these working groups focused on the organizational structure for the most effective application of advanced cardiac imaging, a similar structure certainly would be needed for translation of cardiovascular molecular imaging to clinical practice. The physical coalition of cardiovascular imaging services is ideal, although it is not necessary as long as the patients referred to any component of the cardiovascular imaging program follow common clinical investigative pathways that are agreed upon. A common contact for processing requests for sophisticated cardiovascular diagnostic tests is preferred, since it allows recommendation or selection by experts of the most appropriate test in any specific circumstance. If direct access to diagnostic services is offered to noncardiovascular specialists or to primary care physicians, then patients should be referred to the multidisciplinary diagnostic team. Ideally, reports should be issued jointly by cardiologists and radiologists, but in principle a study can be performed and interpreted by any appropriately trained specialist.

SUMMARY

The recent introduction of novel gene therapies for treatment of cardiac and noncardiac diseases has caused a remarkable need for noninvasive imaging approaches to evaluate and track the progress of these therapies. In the past we have relied on the evaluation of the physiological consequences of therapeutic interventions, although with advances in targeted molecular imaging we now have the ability to evaluate early molecular effects of these therapies. The development of dedicated high-resolution small animal imaging systems and the establishment of transgenic animal models has enhanced understanding of cardiovascular disease and has expedited the development of new gene therapies. Noninvasive targeted molecular imaging will allow direct tracking of biochemical processes and signaling events that precede the pathophysiological changes.

The examples of targeted molecular imaging outlined in this chapter provide some insight into the bright and growing future of cardiovascular molecular imaging. The success of this new field rests on the development of targeted biological markers of molecular and physiological processes, development of new instruments with improved sensitivity and resolution, and the establishment of multidisciplinary teams of experimental and clinical investigators with a wide range of expertise. Molecular imaging already plays a critical role in the experimental laboratory. We expect that in the near future, targeted molecular imaging will be routinely used in clinical cardiovascular imaging laboratories in conjunction with existing imaging modalities for both diagnostic and prognostic purposes, as well as for evaluation of new genetic-based therapeutic strategies.

REFERENCES

CHAPTER I

Bacharach SL, Bax JJ, Case J *et al*. (2003) PET myocardial glucose metabolism and perfusion imaging, American Society of Nuclear Cardiology Practice Guidelines. *Journal of Nuclear Cardiology* **10**:543–554.

Beller GA (2006) A proposal for an advanced cardiovascular imaging training track. *Journal of the American College of Cardiology* **48**:1299–1303.

Bonow RO (1993) Radionuclide angiography for risk stratification of patients with coronary artery disease. *American Journal of Cardiology* **72**:735–739.

Brindis RG, Douglas PS, Hendel RC *et al*. (2005) ACCF/ASNC appropriateness criteria for single photon emission computed tomography myocardial perfusion imaging (SPECT MPI): a report of the American College of Cardiology Foundation Quality Strategic Directions Committee Appropriateness Criteria Working Group and the American Society of Nuclear Cardiology. *Journal of American College of Cardiology* **46**:1587–1605.

DePuey EG, Garcia EV (2001) Updated imaging guidelines for nuclear cardiology procedures Part 1. *Journal of Nuclear Cardiology* **8**:G1–G58.

Diamond GA, Forrester JS (1979) Analysis of probability as an aid in the clinical diagnosis of coronary artery disease. *New England Journal of Medicine* **300**:1350–1358.

Elhendy A, Schinkel A, Bax JJ *et al*. (2003) Long term prognosis after a normal exercise stress Tc-99m Sestamibi SPECT study. *Journal of Nuclear Cardiology* **10**:261–266.

Faber TL, Cooke CD, Peifer JW *et al*. (1995) Three-dimensional displays of left ventricular epicardial surface from standard cardiac SPECT perfusion quantification techniques. *Journal of Nuclear Medicine* **36**:697–704.

Faber TL, Cooke CD, Folks RD *et al*. (1999) Left ventricular function and perfusion from gated SPECT perfusion images: an integrated method. *Journal of Nuclear Medicine* **40**:650–659.

Framingham Score: http://www.nhlbi.nih.gov/about/framingham/riskabs.htm

Gardin JM, Adams DB, Douglas PS *et al*. (2001) American Society of Echocardiography: http://www.asecho.org/freepdf/Standardized_Echo_Report_Rev1.pdf

Germano G, Kiat H, Kavanagh PB *et al*. (1995) Automatic quantification of ejection fraction from gated myocardial perfusion SPECT. *Journal of Nuclear Medicine* **36**:2138–2147.

Germano G, Kavanagh PB, Waechter P *et al*. (2000) A new algorithm for the quantitation of myocardial perfusion SPECT. I: technical principles and reproducibility. *Journal of Nuclear Medicine* **41**:712–719.

Gibbons RJ, Baldy GJ, Bricker JT *et al*. (2002) ACC/AHA 2002 guideline update for exercise testing: summary article: a report of the American College of Cardiology/American Heart Association Task Force on Practice Guidelines (Committee to Update the 1997 Exercise Testing Guidelines). *Circulation* **106**:1883–1892.

Hachamovitch R, Berman DS, Kiat H *et al*. (1996) Exercise myocardial perfusion SPECT in patients without known coronary artery disease: incremental prognostic value and impact on subsequent patient management. *Circulation* **93**:905–914.

Hendel RC, Wackers FJ Th, Berman DS *et al*. (2003) Reporting of radionuclide myocardial perfusion imaging studies. *Journal of Nuclear Cardiology* **10**:705–708.

Khorsand A, Graf S, Frank H *et al*. (2003) Model-based analysis of electrocardiography-gated cardiac ^{18}FDG PET images to assess left ventricular geometry and contractile function. *Journal of Nuclear Medicine* **44**:1741–1746.

Klocke FJ, Baird MG, Bateman TM *et al*. (2003) ACC/AHA/ASNC guidelines for the clinical use of cardiac radionuclide imaging: a report of the American College of Cardiology/American Heart Association Task Force on Practice Guidelines (ACC/AHA/ASNC Committee to Revise the 1995 Guidelines for the Clinical Use of Cardiac Radionuclide Imaging). *Circulation* **108**:1404–1418.

Lang RM, Bierig M, Devereaux RB *et al*. (2005) Recommendation for chamber quantification: a report from the American Society of Echocardiography's Guidelines and Standards Committee and the Chamber Quantification Writing Group, developed in conjunction with the European Association of Echocardiography, a branch of the European Society of Echocardiography. *Journal of American Society of Echocardiography* **18**:1440–1463.

Lee FA, Fetterman RC, Zaret BL, Wackers FJT (1985) Rapid radionuclide-derived systolic and diastolic cardiac function using cycle-dependent background correction and Fourier analysis. *Proceeding of Computer in Cardiology IEEE Computer Society* 443–446.

Liu YH, Sinusas AJ, DeMan P *et al*. (1999) Quantification of single-photon emission computed tomographic myocardial perfusion images: methodology and validation of the Yale-CQ method. *Journal of Nuclear Cardiology* **6**:190–203.

Liu YH, Sinusas AJ, Khaimov D *et al*. (2005) New hybrid

count and geometry-based method for quantification of left ventricular volumes and ejection fraction from ECG-gated SPECT: methodology and validation. *Journal of Nuclear Cardiology* **12**:55–65.

Port SC (1999) Imaging guidelines for nuclear cardiology procedures Part 2. *Journal of Nuclear Cardiology* **6**:G48–G84.

Pryor DB, Harell FE, Lee KL *et al.* (1983) Estimating the likelihood of significant coronary artery disease. *American Journal of Medicine* **75**:771–780.

The 1st National SHAPE Guideline. Association for Eradication of Heart Attacks: http://www.aeha.org

CHAPTER 2

Achenbach S, Ulzheimer S, Baum U (2000) Noninvasive coronary angiography by retrospectively ECG-gated multislice spiral CT. *Circulation* **102**(23):2823–2828.

Achenbach S, Giesler T, Ropers D (2001) Detection of coronary artery stenoses by contrast-enhanced, retrospectively electrocardiographically-gated, multislice spiral computed tomography. *Circulation* **103**(21):2535–2538.

Achenbach S, Moselewski F, Ropers D (2004). Detection of calcified and noncalcified coronary atherosclerotic plaque by contrast-enhanced, submillimeter multidetector spiral computed tomography: a segment-based comparison with intravascular ultrasound. *Circulation* **109**(1):14–17.

Agatston AS, Janowitz WR, Hildner FJ *et al.* (1990). Quantification of coronary artery calcium using ultrafast computed tomography. *Journal of American College of Cardiology* **15**(4):827–832.

Alkadhi H, Wildermuth S, Bettex DA (2006). Mitral regurgitation: quantification with 16-detector row CT – initial experience. *Radiology* **238**(2):454–463.

Anders K, Baum U, Schmid M (2006) Coronary artery bypass graft (CABG) patency: Assessment with high-resolution submillimeter 16-slice multidetector-row computed tomography (MDCT) versus coronary angiography. *European Journal of Radiology* **57**(3):336–344.

Arad Y, Spadaro LA, Goodman K *et al.* (2000) Prediction of coronary events with electron beam computed tomography. *Journal of American College of Cardiology* **36**(4):1253–1260.

Bateman TM (1995) Coronary angiographic rates after stress single-photon emission computed tomographic scintigraphy. *Journal of Nuclear Cardiology* **2**(3):217–223.

Baumert B, Plass A, Bettex D (2005) Dynamic cine mode imaging of the normal aortic valve using 16-channel multidetector row computed tomography. *Investigative Radiology* **40**(10):637–647.

Bell MR, Lerman LO, Rumberger JA (1999) Validation of minimally invasive measurement of myocardial perfusion using electron beam computed tomography and application in human volunteers. *Heart* **81**(6):628–635.

Blankenhorn DH, Stern D (1959) Calcification of the coronary arteries. *American Journal of Roentgenology, Radium Therapy, and Nuclear Medicine* **81**(5):772–777.

Canty JM Jr, Judd RM, Brody AS *et al.* (1991) First-pass entry of nonionic contrast agent into the myocardial extravascular space. Effects on radiographic estimates of transit time and blood volume. *Circulation* **84**(5):2071–2078.

Caussin C, Ohanessian A, Lancelin B (2003) Coronary plaque burden detected by multislice computed tomography after acute myocardial infarction with near-normal coronary arteries by angiography. *American Journal of Cardiology* **92**(7):849–852.

Dambrin G, Wartski M, Toussaint M (2004) [Anomalies in myocardial contrast uptake revealed by multislice cardiac CT during acute myocarditis]. *Archives des Maladies du Moeur et des Maisseaux* **97**(10):1031–1034.

de la Pena-Almaguer E, Azpiri Lopez JR, Gonzalez-Camid Fde J *et al.* (2005) [Evaluation of left ventricular function with a 16-slice multidetector tomograph (MDCT-16): correlation with cardiovascular magnetic resonance imaging]. *Archivos de Cardiología de México* **75**(1):55–60.

Dery R, Lipton MJ, Garrett JS *et al.* (1986) Cine-computed tomography of arrhythmogenic right ventricular dysplasia. *Journal of Computer Assisted Tomography* **10**(1):120–123.

Detrano RC, Anderson M, Nelson J (2005) Coronary calcium measurements: effect of CT scanner type and calcium measure on rescan reproducibility – MESA study. *Radiology* **236**(2):477–484.

Frink RJ, Achor RW, Brown AL, Jr *et al.* (1970) Significance of calcification of the coronary arteries. *American Journal of Cardiology* **26**(3):241–247.

Funabashi N, Toyozaki T, Matsumoto Y (2003) Images in cardiovascular medicine. Myocardial fibrosis in Fabry disease demonstrated by multislice computed tomography: comparison with biopsy findings. *Circulation* **107**(19):2519–2520.

George RT, Cordeiro MA, Silva C *et al.* (2005) Multi-detector computed tomography quantifies myocardial perfusion during adenosine stress. *Circulation* **112**(17):(Supplement) II-465.

George RT, Resar J, Silva C *et al.* (2006a) Combined computed tomography coronary angiography and perfusion imaging accurately detects the physiological significance of coronary stenoses in patients with chest pain. *Circulation* **114**:(Supplement) II-691.

George RT, Silva C, Cordeiro MA *et al.* (2006b) Multidetector computed tomography myocardial perfusion imaging during adenosine stress. *Journal of American College of Cardiology* **48**:153–160.

George RT, Jerosch-Herold M, Silva C *et al.* (2007) Quantification of myocardial perfusion using dynamic 64-detector computed tomography. *Investigative Radiology* **42**(12):815–822.

Gerber BL, Garot J, Bluemke DA *et al.* (2002) Accuracy of contrast-enhanced magnetic resonance imaging in predicting improvement of regional myocardial function in patients after acute myocardial infarction. *Circulation* **106**(9):1083–1089.

Giesler T, Baum U, Ropers D (2002) Noninvasive visualization of coronary arteries using contrast-enhanced multidetector CT: influence of heart rate on image quality and stenosis detection. *American Journal of Roentgenology* **179**(4):911–916.

Haberl R, Becker A, Leber A (2001) Correlation of coronary calcification and angiographically documented stenoses in patients with suspected coronary artery disease: results of 1,764 patients. *Journal of American College of Cardiology* **37**(2):451–457.

Haller S (2006) Coronary artery imaging with contrast-enhanced MDCT: extracardiac findings. *American Journal of Roentgenology* **187**:105–110.

Hoffmann U, Millea R, Enzweiler C (2004a) Acute myocardial infarction: contrast-enhanced multi-detector row CT in a porcine model. *Radiology* **231**(3):697–701.

Hoffmann U, Moselewski F, Cury RC (2004b) Predictive value of 16-slice multidetector spiral computed tomography to detect significant obstructive coronary artery disease in patients at high risk for coronary artery disease: patient versus segment-based analysis. *Circulation* **110**(17):2638–2643.

Ingkanisorn WP, Rhoads KL, Aletras AH *et al.* (2004) Gadolinium delayed enhancement cardiovascular magnetic resonance correlates with clinical measures of myocardial infarction. *Journal of American College of Cardiology* **43**(12):2253–2259.

Janowitz WR, Agatston AS, Kaplan G *et al.* (1993) Differences in prevalence and extent of coronary artery calcium detected by ultrafast computed tomography in asymptomatic men and women. *American Journal of Cardiology* **72**(3):247–254.

Jongbloed MR, Dirksen MS, Bax JJ (2005a) Atrial fibrillation: multi-detector row CT of pulmonary vein anatomy prior to radiofrequency catheter ablation – initial experience. *Radiology* **234**(3):702–709.

Jongbloed MR, Lamb HJ, Bax JJ (2005b) Noninvasive visualization of the cardiac venous system using multislice computed tomography. *Journal of American College of Cardiology* **45**(5):749–753.

Kim TH, Ryu YH, Hur J (2005) Evaluation of right ventricular volume and mass using retrospective ECG-gated cardiac multidetector computed tomography: comparison with first-pass radionuclide angiography. *European Radiology* **15**(9):1987–1993.

Kondos GT, Hoff JA, Sevrukov A (2003) Electron-beam tomography coronary artery calcium and cardiac events: a 37-month follow-up of 5635 initially asymptomatic low- to intermediate-risk adults. *Circulation* **107**(20):2571–2576.

Kopp AF, Schroeder S, Baumbach A (2001) Non-invasive characterisation of coronary lesion morphology and composition by multislice CT: first results in comparison with intracoronary ultrasound. *European Radiology* **11**(9):1607–1611.

Kopp AF, Schroeder S, Kuettner A (2002) Non-invasive coronary angiography with high resolution multidetector-row computed tomography. Results in 102 patients. *European Heart Journal* **23**(21):1714–1725.

Kragel AH, Reddy SG, Wittes JT *et al.* (1989) Morphometric analysis of the composition of atherosclerotic plaques in the four major epicardial coronary arteries in acute myocardial infarction and in sudden coronary death. *Circulation* **80**(6):1747–1756.

Kuettner A (2005) Diagnostic accuracy of noninvasive coronary imaging using 16-detector slice spiral computed tomography with 188 ms temporal resolution. *Journal of American College of Cardiology* **45**(1):123–127.

Kuettner A, Trabold T, Schroeder S (2004) Noninvasive detection of coronary lesions using 16-detector multislice spiral computed tomography technology: initial clinical results. *Journal of American College of Cardiology* **44**(6):1230–1237.

Lardo AC, Cordeiro MA, Fernandes V *et al.* (2004) Contrast-enhanced multidetector computed tomography imaging of acute myocardial infarction: spatial and temporal characterization of myocyte death and microvascular obstruction. *Circulation* **110**(Supplement): III-522.

Lardo AC, Cordeiro MA, Silva C *et al.* (2006) Contrast-enhanced multidetector computed tomography viability imaging after myocardial infarction: characterization of myocyte death, microvascular obstruction, and chronic scar. *Circulation* **113**(3):394–404.

Leber AW, Knez A, Becker A (2004) Accuracy of multidetector spiral computed tomography in identifying and differentiating the composition of coronary atherosclerotic plaques: a comparative study with intracoronary ultrasound. *Journal of American College of Cardiology* **43**(7):1241–1247.

Leber AW, Knez A, von Ziegler F (2005) Quantification of obstructive and nonobstructive coronary lesions by 64-slice computed tomography: a comparative study with quantitative coronary angiography and intravascular ultrasound. *Journal of American College of Cardiology* **46**(1):147–154.

Leschka S, Alkadhi H, Plass A (2005) Accuracy of MSCT coronary angiography with 64-slice technology: first experience. *European Heart Journal* **26**(15):1482–1487.

Ludman PF, Coats AJ, Burger P (1993) Validation of measurement of regional myocardial perfusion in humans by ultrafast x-ray computed tomography. *American Journal of Cardiac Imaging* **7**(4):267–279.

MacMahon H (2005) Guidelines for management of small pulmonary nodules detected on CT scans: a statement from the Fleischner Society. *Radiology* **237**:395–400.

Mahnken AH (2005) Assessment of myocardial viability in reperfused acute myocardial infarction using 16-slice computed tomography in comparison to magnetic resonance imaging. *Journal of American College of Cardiology* **45**(12):2042–2047.

Mollet NR, Cademartiri F, Nieman K (2004) Multislice spiral computed tomography coronary angiography in patients with stable angina pectoris. *Journal of American College of Cardiology* **43**(12):2265–2270.

Newhouse JH (1977) Fluid compartment distribution of intravenous iothalamate in the dog. *Investigative Radiology* **12**(4):364–367.

Newhouse JH, Murphy RX, Jr (1981) Tissue distribution of soluble contrast: effect of dose variation and changes with time. *American Journal of Roentgenology* **136**(3):463–467.

Nieman K, Pattynama PM, Rensing BJ *et al.* (2001) Coronary angiography with multi-slice computed tomography. *Lancet* **357**(9256):599–603.

Nieman K, Cademartiri F, Lemos PA *et al.* (2002a) Reliable noninvasive coronary angiography with fast submillimeter multislice spiral computed tomography. *Circulation* **106**(16):2051–2054.

Nieman K, Rensing BJ, van Geuns RJ (2002b) Non-invasive coronary angiography with multislice spiral computed tomography: impact of heart rate. *Heart* **88**(5):470–474.

Nieman K, Oudkerk M, Rensing BJ (2003) Evaluation of patients after coronary artery bypass surgery: CT angiographic assessment of grafts and coronary arteries. *Radiology* **229**(3):749–756.

Nikolaou K, Knez A, Sagmeister S (2004) Assessment of myocardial infarctions using multidetector-row computed tomography. *Journal of Computer Assisted Tomography* **28**(2):286–292.

Nikolaou K, Sanz J, Poon M (2005) Assessment of myocardial perfusion and viability from routine contrast-enhanced 16-detector-row computed tomography of the heart: preliminary results. *European Radiology* **15**(5):864–871.

O'Rourke RA, Brundage BH, Froelicher VF (2000) American College of Cardiology/American Heart Association Expert Consensus Document on electron-beam computed tomography for the diagnosis and prognosis of coronary artery disease. *Journal of American College of Cardiology* **36**(1):326–340.

Olson MC, Posniak HV, McDonald V *et al.* (1989) Computed tomography and magnetic resonance imaging of the pericardium. *Radiographics* **9**(4):633–649.

Patel S (2005) Non-coronary findings on 16-row multidetector CT coronary angiography. *American Journal of Roentgenology* **184**:S3.

Pugliese F, Mollet NR, Runza G (2006) Diagnostic accuracy of non-invasive 64-slice CT coronary angiography in patients with stable angina pectoris. *European Radiology* 16(3):575–582.

Raff GL, Gallagher MJ, O'Neill WW (2005) Diagnostic accuracy of noninvasive coronary angiography using 64-slice spiral computed tomography. *Journal of American College of Cardiology* 46(3):552–557.

Raggi P, Callister TQ, Cooil B (2000) Identification of patients at increased risk of first unheralded acute myocardial infarction by electron-beam computed tomography. *Circulation* 101(8):850–855.

Ropers D, Baum U, Pohle K (2003) Detection of coronary artery stenoses with thin-slice multi-detector row spiral computed tomography and multiplanar reconstruction. *Circulation* 107(5):664–666.

Rumberger JA, Bell MR, Feiring AJ (1991) Quantitation of myocardial perfusion using fast computed tomography. In: *Cardiac Imaging.*
ML Marcus, DL Skorton, H Shelbert *et al.* (eds.) W.B Saunders, Philadelphia, pp. 688–702.

Rumberger JA, Feiring AJ, Hiratzka LF (1987a) Quantification of coronary artery bypass flow reserve in dogs using cine-computed tomography. *Circulation Research* 61(5):117–123.

Rumberger JA, Feiring AJ, Lipton MG (1987b) Use of ultrafast computed tomography to quantitate regional myocardial perfusion: a preliminary report. *Journal of American College of Cardiology* 9(1):59–69.

Rumberger JA, Schwartz RS, Simons DB, *et al.* (1994) Relation of coronary calcium determined by electron beam computed tomography and lumen narrowing determined by autopsy. *American Journal of Cardiology* 73(16):1169–1173.

Rumberger JA, Simons DB, Fitzpatrick LA *et al.* (1995) Coronary artery calcium area by electron-beam computed tomography and coronary atherosclerotic plaque area. A histopathologic correlative study. *Circulation* 92(8):2157–2162.

Salm LP, Bax JJ, Jukema JW (2005) Comprehensive assessment of patients after coronary artery bypass grafting by 16-detector-row computed tomography. *American Heart Journal* 150(4):775–781.

Schlosser T, Konorza T, Hunold P *et al.* (2004) Noninvasive visualization of coronary artery bypass grafts using 16-detector row computed tomography. *Journal of American College of Cardiology* 44(6):1224–1229.

Schroeder S, Kopp AF, Baumbach A (2001) Noninvasive detection and evaluation of atherosclerotic coronary plaques with multislice computed tomography. *Journal of American College of Cardiology* 37(5):1430–1435.

Schroeder S, Kopp AF, Kuettner A (2002) Influence of heart rate on vessel visibility in noninvasive coronary angiography using new multislice computed tomography: experience in 94 patients. *Clinical Imaging* 26(2):106–111.

Schroeder S, Kuettner A, Leitritz M (2004) Reliability of differentiating human coronary plaque morphology using contrast-enhanced multislice spiral computed tomography: a comparison with histology. *Journal of Computer Assisted Tomography* 28(4):449–454.

Steinberg F (2005) Extracardiac findings at 64-multidetector coronary CTA. Amelia Island, FL: North American Society of Cardiovascular Imaging, 2005.

Tanenbaum SR, Kondos GT, Veselik KE *et al.* (1989) Detection of calcific deposits in coronary arteries by ultrafast computed tomography and correlation with angiography. *American Journal of Cardiology* 63(12):870–872.

Taylor AJ (1992) Sudden cardiac death associated with

isolated congenital coronary artery anomalies. *Journal of American College of Cardiology* 20(3):640–647.

Thomson LE, Kim RJ, Judd RM (2004) Magnetic resonance imaging for the assessment of myocardial viability. *Journal of Magnetic Resonance Imaging* 19(6):771–788.

Trabold T, Buchgeister M, Kuttner A (2003) Estimation of radiation exposure in 16-detector row computed tomography of the heart with retrospective ECG-gating. *RöFo : Fortschritte auf dem Gebiete der Röntgenstrahlen und der Nuklearmedizin* 175(8):1051–1055.

Wayhs R, Zelinger A, Raggi P (2002) High coronary artery calcium scores pose an extremely elevated risk for hard events. *Journal of American College of Cardiology* 39(2):225–230.

Wexler L, Brundage B, Crouse J (1996) Coronary artery calcification: pathophysiology, epidemiology, imaging methods, and clinical implications. A statement for health professionals from the American Heart Association. Writing Group. *Circulation* 94(5):1175–1192.

Willmann JK, Kobza R, Roos JE (2002) ECG-gated multi-detector row CT for assessment of mitral valve disease: initial experience. *European Radiology* 12(11):2662–2669.

Wolfkiel CJ, Ferguson JL, Chomka EV (1987) Measurement of myocardial blood flow by ultrafast computed tomography. *Circulation* 76(6):1262–1273.

Wong ND, Hsu JC, Detrano RC *et al.* (2000) Coronary artery calcium evaluation by electron beam computed tomography and its relation to new cardiovascular events. *American Journal of Cardiology* 86(5):495–498.

Wychulis AR, Connolly DC, McGoon DC (1971) Pericardial cysts, tumors, and fat necrosis. *Journal of Thoracic and Cardiovascular Surgery* 62(2):294–300.

Yamanaka O, Hobbs RE (1990) Coronary artery anomalies in 126,595 patients undergoing coronary arteriography. *Catheterization and Cardiovascular Diagnosis* 21(1):28–40.

CHAPTER 3

Abbott BG, Afshar M, Berger AK *et al.* (2003) Prognostic significance of ischemic electrocardiographic changes during adenosine infusion in patients with normal myocardial perfusion imaging. *Journal of Nuclear Cardiology* 10:9–16.

Abidov A, Bax JJ, Hayes SW *et al.* (2003) Transient ischemic dilation ratio of the left ventricle is a significant predictor of future cardiac events in patients with otherwise normal myocardial perfusion SPECT. *Journal of American College of Cardiology* 42:1818–1825.

Abidov A, Bax JJ, Hayes SW *et al.* (2004) Integration of automatically measured transient ischemic dilation ratio into interpretation of adenosine stress myocardial perfusion SPECT for detection of severe and extensive CAD. *Journal of Nuclear Medicine* 45:1999–2007.

Abidov A, Rozanski A, Hachamovitch R *et al.* (2005) Prognostic significance of dyspnea in patients referred for cardiac stress testing. *New England Journal of Medicine* 353:1889–1898.

Acampa W, Cuocolo A, Sullo P *et al.* (1998) Direct comparison of technetium 99m-sestamibi and technetium 99m-tetrofosmin cardiac single photon emission computed tomography in patients with coronary artery disease. *Journal of Nuclear Cardiology* 5:265–274.

Adachi I, Akagi H, Umeda T *et al.* (2003) Gated blood pool SPECT improves reproducibility of right and left ventricular Fourier phase analysis in radionuclide angiography. *Annals of Nuclear Medicine* 17:711–716.

Akinboboye OO, Idris O, Onwuanyi A *et al.* (2001) Incidence of major cardiovascular events in black patients with normal myocardial stress perfusion study results. *Journal of Nuclear Cardiology* 8:541–547.

Akinboboye O, Nichols K, Yang Y *et al.* (2005) Accuracy of radionuclide ventriculography assessed by magnetic resonance imaging in patients with abnormal left ventricles. *Journal of Nuclear Cardiology* 12:418–427.

Alazraki NP, Krawczynska EG, DePuey EG *et al.* (1994) Reproducibility of thallium-201 exercise SPECT studies. *Journal of Nuclear Medicine* 35:1237–1244.

Alkeylani A, Miller DD, Shaw LJ *et al.* (1998) Influence of race on the prediction of cardiac events with stress technetium-99m sestamibi tomographic imaging in patients with stable angina pectoris. *American Journal of Cardiology* 81:293–297.

Altehoefer C, vom Dahl J, Buell U *et al.* (1994) Comparison of thallium-201 single-photon emission tomography after rest injection and fluorodeoxyglucose positron emission tomography for assessment of myocardial viability in patients with chronic coronary artery disease. *European Journal of Nuclear Medicine* 21:37–45.

Amanullah AM, Berman DS, Hachamovitch R (1997) Identification of severe or extensive coronary artery disease in women by adenosine technetium-99m sestamibi SPECT. *American Journal of Cardiology* 80:132–137.

Araujo LI, Jimenez-Hoyuela JM, McClellan JR *et al.* (2000) Improved uniformity in tomographic myocardial perfusion imaging with attenuation correction and enhanced acquisition and processing. *Journal of Nuclear Medicine* 41:1139–1144.

Ashburn WL, Schelbert HR, Verba JW. (1978) Left ventricular ejection fraction – a review of several radionuclide angiographic approaches using the scintillation camera. *Progress in Cardiovascular Diseases* 20:267–284.

Bacher-Stier C, Sharir T, Kavanagh PB *et al.* (2000) Postexercise lung uptake of 99mTc-sestamibi determined by a new automatic technique: validation and application in detection of severe and extensive coronary artery disease and reduced left ventricular function. *Journal of Nuclear Medicine* 41:1190–1197.

Baer FM, Voth E, Deutsch HJ *et al.* (1996) Predictive value of low dose dobutamine transesophageal echocardiography and fluorine-18 fluorodeoxyglucose positron emission tomography for recovery of regional left ventricular function after successful revascularization. *Journal of American College of Cardiology* 28:60–69.

Banzo I, Pena F J, Allende RH *et al.* (2003) Prospective clinical comparison of non-corrected and attenuation- and scatter-corrected myocardial perfusion SPECT in patients with suspicion of coronary artery disease. *Nuclear Medicine Communications* 24:995–1002.

Bateman TM, Heller GV, McGhie AI *et al.* (2006) Diagnostic accuracy of rest/stress ECG-gated Rb-82 myocardial perfusion PET: comparison with ECG-gated Tc-99m sestamibi SPECT. *Journal of Nuclear Cardiology* 13:24–33.

Batista JF, Pereztol O, Valdes JA *et al.* (1999) Improved detection of myocardial perfusion reversibility by rest-nitroglycerin Tc-99m-MIBI: comparison with TI-201 reinjection. *Journal of Nuclear Cardiology* 6:480–486.

Bax J, Cornel J, Visser F *et al.* (1997a) Prediction of improvement of contractile function in patients with ischemic ventricular dysfunction after revascularization by fluorine-18 fluorodeoxyglucose single-photon emission computed tomography. *Journal of American College of Cardiology* 30:377–383.

Bax JJ, Cornel JH, Visser FC *et al.* (1997b) F18-fluorodeoxyglucose single-photon emission computed tomography predicts functional outcome of dyssynergic myocardium after surgical revascularization. *Journal of Nuclear Cardiology* 4:302–308.

Bax JJ, Wijns W, Cornel JH *et al.* (1997c) Accuracy of currently available techniques for prediction of functional recovery after revascularization in patients with left ventricular dysfunction due to chronic coronary artery disease: comparison of pooled data. *Journal of American College of Cardiology* 30:1451–1460.

Bax JJ, Cornel JH, Visser FC *et al.* (1998) Comparison of fluorine-18-FDG with rest-redistribution thallium-201 SPECT to delineate viable myocardium and predict functional recovery after revascularization. *Journal of Nuclear Medicine* 39:1481–1486.

Benoit T, Vivegnis D, Lahiri A *et al.* (1996) Tomographic myocardial imaging with technetium-99m tetrofosmin. Comparison with tetrofosmin and thallium planar imaging and with angiography. *European Heart Journal* 17:635–642.

Berman DS, Kiat H, Friedman JD (1993) Separate acquisition of rest thallium- 201/stress technetium-99m-sestamibi dual-isotope myocardial single photon emission computed tomography: a clinical validation study. *Journal of American College of Cardiology* 22:1455–1464.

Bodenheimer MM, Banka VS, Fooshee CM *et al.* (1978) Quantitative radionuclide angiography in the right anterior oblique view: comparison with contrast ventriculography. *American Journal of Cardiology* 41:718–725.

Bonow RO, Dilsizian V, Cuocolo A *et al.* (1991) Identification of viable myocardium in patients with chronic coronary artery disease and left ventricular dysfunction. Comparison of thallium scintigraphy with reinjection and PET imaging with 18F-fluorodeoxyglucose. *Circulation* 83:26–37.

Boonyaprapa S, Ekmahachai M, Thanachaikun N *et al.* (1995) Measurement of left ventricular ejection fraction from gated technetium-99m sestamibi myocardial images. *European Journal of Nuclear Medicine* 22:528–531.

Brigger P, Bacharach SL, Srinivasan G *et al.* (1999) Segmentation of gated Tl-SPECT images and computation of ejection fraction: a different approach. *Journal of Nuclear Cardiology* 6:286–297.

Burns RJ, Galligan L, Wright LM *et al.* (1991) Improved specificity of myocardial thallium-201 single-photon emission computed tomography in patients with left bundle branch block by dipyridamole. *American Journal of Cardiology* 68:504–508.

Burt RW, Perkins OW, Oppenheim BE *et al.* (1995) Direct comparison of fluorine-18-FDG SPECT, fluorine-18-FDG PET, and rest thallium-201 SPECT for detection of myocardial viability. *Journal of Nuclear Medicine* 36:176–179.

Calnon DA, Kastner RJ, Smith WH *et al.* (1997) Validation of a new counts-based gated single photon emission computed tomography method for quantifying left ventricular systolic function: comparison with equilibrium radionuclide angiography. *Journal of Nuclear Cardiology* 4:464–471.

Carrel T, Jenni R, Haubold-Reuter S *et al.* (1992) Improvement of severely reduced left ventricular function after surgical revascularization in patients with preoperative myocardial infarction. *European Journal of Cardiothoracic Surgery* 6:479–484.

Casset-Senon D, Philippe L, Babuty D *et al.* (1998) Diagnosis of arrhythmogenic right ventricular cardiomyopathy by fourier analysis of gated blood pool single-photon emission tomography. *American Journal of Cardiology* **82**:1399–1404.

Cerqueira D, Weissman J, Dilsizian V *et al.* (2002) Standardized myocardial segmentation and nomenclature for tomographic imaging of the heart: a statement for healthcare professionals from the Cardiac Imaging Committee of the Council on Clinical Cardiology of the American Heart Association. *Circulation* **105**:539–542.

Chen E, MacIntyre W J, Go RT *et al.* (1997) Myocardial viability studies using fluorine-18-FDG SPECT: a comparison with fluorine-18-FDG PET. *Journal of Nuclear Medicine* **38**:582–586.

Chevalier P, Bontemps L, Fatemi M *et al.* (1999) Gated blood-pool SPECT evaluation of changes after radiofrequency catheter ablation of accessory pathways: evidence for persistent ventricular preexcitation despite successful therapy. *Journal of American College of Cardiology* **34**:1839–1846.

Chow BJW, Wong JW, Yoshinaga K *et al.* (2005) Prognostic significance of dipyridamole-induced ST depression in patients with normal 82Rb PET myocardial perfusion imaging. *Journal of Nuclear Medicine* **46**:1095–1101.

Chua T, Kiat H, Germano G *et al.* (1994) Gated technetium-99m sestamibi for simultaneous assessment of stress myocardial perfusion, postexercise regional ventricular function and myocardial viability. Correlation with echocardiography and rest thallium-201 scintigraphy. *Journal of American College of Cardiology* **23**:1107–1114.

Cooper JA, Neumann PH, McCandless BK (1992) Effect of patient motion on tomographic myocardial perfusion imaging. *Journal of Nuclear Medicine* **33**:1566–1571.

Cramer MJ, Verzijlbergen JF, van der Wall EE *et al.* (1996) Comparison of adenosine and high-dose dipyridamole both combined with low-level exercise stress for 99Tcm-MIBI SPET myocardial perfusion imaging. *Nuclear Medicine Communications* **17**:97–104.

Cramer MJ, van der Wall EE, Verzijlbergen JF *et al.* (1997) SPECT versus planar 99mTc-sestamibi myocardial scintigraphy: comparison of accuracy and impact on patient management in chronic ischemic heart disease. *Quarterly Journal of Nuclear Medicine* **41**:1–9.

Danias PG, Papaioannou GI, Ahlberg AW *et al.* (2004) Usefulness of electrocardiographic-gated stress technetium-99m sestamibi single-photon emission computed tomography to differentiate ischemic from nonischemic cardiomyopathy. *American Journal of Cardiology* **94**:14–19.

Daou D, Delahaye N, Vilain D *et al.* (2002) Identification of extensive coronary artery disease: incremental value of exercise Tl-201 SPECT to clinical and stress test variables. *Journal of Nuclear Cardiology* **9**:161–168.

Daou D, Van Kriekinge SD, Coaguila C *et al.* (2004) Automatic quantification of right ventricular function with gated blood pool SPECT. *Journal of Nuclear Cardiology* **11**:293–304.

De Lorenzo A, Lima RS, Siqueira-Filho AG *et al.* (2002) Prevalence and prognostic value of perfusion defects detected by stress technetium-99m sestamibi myocardial perfusion single-photon emission computed tomography in asymptomatic patients with diabetes mellitus and no known coronary artery disease. *American Journal of Cardiology* **90**:827–832.

DePasquale EE, Nody AC, DePuey EG *et al.* (1988) Quantitative rotational thallium-201 tomography for identifying and localizing coronary artery disease. *Circulation* **77**:316–327.

DePuey EG, Nichols K, Dobrinsky C (1993) Left ventricular ejection fraction assessed from gated technetium-99m-sestamibi SPECT. *Journal of Nuclear Medicine* **34**:1871–1876.

DePuey EG, Rozanski A (1995) Using gated technetium-99m-sestamibi SPECT to characterize fixed myocardial defects as infarct or artifact. *Journal of Nuclear Medicine* **36**:952–955.

DePuey EG, Parmett S, Ghesani M *et al.* (1999) Comparison of Tc-99m sestamibi and Tl-201 gated perfusion SPECT. *Journal of Nuclear Cardiology* **6**:278–285.

DePuey EG, Garcia EV (2001) Updated imaging guidelines for nuclear cardiology procedures. Part 1. *Journal of Nuclear Cardiology* **8**:G5–G58.

Di Carli MF, Davidson M, Little R *et al.* (1994) Value of metabolic imaging with positron emission tomography for evaluating prognosis in patients with coronary artery disease and left ventricular dysfunction. *American Journal of Cardiology* **73**:527–533.

Di Carli MF, Asgarzadie F, Schelbert HR *et al.* (1995) Quantitative relation between myocardial viability and improvement in heart failure symptoms after revascularization in patients with ischemic cardiomyopathy. *Circulation* **92**:3436–3444.

Dilsizian V, Perrone-Filardi P, Arrighi A *et al.* (1993) Concordance and discordance between stress-redistribution-reinjction and rest-redistribution thallium imaging for assessing viable myocardium. Comparison with metabolic activity by positron emission tomography. *Circulation* **88**:941–952.

Dussol B, Bonnet JL, Sampol J *et al.* (2004) Prognostic value of inducible myocardial ischemia in predicting cardiovascular events after renal transplantation. *Kidney International* **66**:1633–1639.

Eitzman D, al-Aouar Z, Kanter HL *et al.* (1992) Clinical outcome of patients with advanced coronary artery disease after viability studies with positron emission tomography. *Journal of American College of Cardiology* **20**:559–565.

Elhendy A, Sozzi FB, Valkema R *et al.* (2000) Dobutamine technetium-99m tetrofosmin SPECT imaging for the diagnosis of coronary artery disease in patients with limited exercise capacity. *Journal of Nuclear Cardiology* **7**:649–654.

Elhendy A, Schinkel AF, van Domburg RT *et al.* (2004) Prognostic value of stress Tc-99m tetrofosmin SPECT in patients with previous myocardial infarction: impact of scintigraphic extent of coronary artery disease. *Journal of Nuclear Cardiology* **11**:704–709.

Everaert H, Franken PR, Flamen P *et al.* (1996) Left ventricular ejection fraction from gated SPET myocardial perfusion studies: a method based on the radial distribution of count rate density across the myocardial wall. *European Journal of Nuclear Medicine* **23**:1628–1633.

Fauchier L, Marie O, Casset-Senon D *et al.* (2003) Ventricular dyssynchrony and risk markers of ventricular arrhythmias in nonischemic dilated cardiomyopathy: a study with phase analysis of angioscintigraphy. *Pacing and Clinical Electrophysiology* **26**:352–356.

Feola M, Biggi A, Ribichini F *et al.* (2002) Predicting cardiac events with Tl201 dipyridamole myocardial scintigraphy in renal transplant recipients. *Journal of Nephrology* **15**:48–53.

Fintel DJ, Links JM, Brinker JA *et al.* (1989) Improved diagnostic performance of exercise thallium-201 single photon emission computed tomography over planar imaging in the diagnosis of coronary artery disease: a receiver operating characteristic analysis. *Journal of American College of Cardiology* **13**:600–612.

Folland ED, Hamilton GW, Larson SM *et al.* (1977) The radionuclide ejection fraction: a comparison of three radionuclide techniques with contrast angiography. *Journal of Nuclear Medicine* **18**:1159–1166.

Fricke E, Fricke H, Weise R *et al.* (2005) Attenuation correction of myocardial SPECT perfusion images with low-dose CT: evaluation of the method by comparison with perfusion PET. *Journal of Nuclear Medicine* **46**:736–744.

Friedman T, Greene A, Iskandrain AS (1982) Exercise thallium-201 myocardial perfusion scintigraphy in women: correlation with coronary arteriography. *American Journal of Cardiology* **49**:1632–1637.

Fuchs RM, Achuff SC, Grunwald L *et al.* (1982) Electrocardiographic localization of coronary artery narrowings: studies during myocardial ischemia and infarction in patients with one-vessel disease. *Circulation* **66**:1168–1176.

Galasko GI, Senior R, Lahiri A (2005) Ethnic differences in the prevalence and aetiology of left ventricular systolic dysfunction in the community: the Harrow heart failure watch. *Heart* **91**:595–600.

Garcia EV, Cooke CD, Van Train KF *et al.* (1990) Technical aspects of myocardial SPECT imaging with technetium-99m sestamibi. *American Journal of Cardiology* **66**:23E–31E.

Geleijnse ML, Elhendy A, van Domburg RT *et al.* (1996) Prognostic significance of normal dobutamine-atropine stress sestamibi scintigraphy in women with chest pain. *American Journal of Cardiology* **77**:1057–1061.

Gerber BL, Vanoverschelde JL, Bol A *et al.* (1996) Myocardial blood flow, glucose uptake, and recruitment of inotropic reserve in chronic left ventricular ischemic dysfunction. Implications for the pathophysiology of chronic myocardial hibernation. *Circulation* **94**:651–659.

Germano G, Kiat H, Kavanagh PB *et al.* (1995) Automatic quantification of ejection fraction from gated myocardial perfusion SPECT. *Journal of Nuclear Medicine* **36**:2138–2147.

Germano G, Kavanagh PB, Waechter P *et al.* (2000) A new algorithm for the quantitation of myocardial perfusion SPECT. I: technical principles and reproducibility. *Journal of Nuclear Medicine* **41**:712–719.

Go RT, Marwick TH, MacIntyre WJ *et al.* (1990) A prospective comparison of rubidium-82 PET and thallium-201 SPECT myocardial perfusion imaging utilizing a single dipyridamole stress in the diagnosis of coronary artery disease. *Journal of Nuclear Medicine* **31**:1899–1905.

Goodgold HM, Rehder JG, Samuels LD, Chaitman BR (1987) Improved interpretation of exercise Tl-201 myocardial perfusion scintigraphy in women: characterization of breast attenuation artifacts. *Radiology* **165**:361–366.

Greco C, Tanzilli G, Ciavolella M *et al.* (1996) Nitroglycerin-induced changes in myocardial sestamibi uptake to detect tissue viability: radionuclide comparison before and after revascularization. *Coronary Artery Disease* **7**:877–884.

Greco C, Ciavolella M, Tanzilli G *et al.* (1998) Preoperative identification of viable myocardium: effectiveness of nitroglycerine-induced changes in myocardial Sestamibi uptake. *Cardiovascular Surgery* **6**:149–155.

Gropler RJ, Geltman EM, Sampathkumaran K *et al.* (1993) Comparison of carbon-11-acetate with fluorine-18-fluorodeoxyglucose for delineating viable myocardium by positron emission tomography. *Journal of American College of Cardiology* **22**:1587–1597.

Grossman GB, Garcia EV, Bateman TM *et al.* (2004) Quantitative Tc-99m sestamibi attenuation-corrected SPECT: development and multicenter trial validation of myocardial perfusion stress gender-independent normal database in an obese population. *Journal of Nuclear Cardiology* **11**:263–272.

Hachamovitch R, Berman DS, Kiat H (1996) Effective risk stratification using exercise myocardial perfusion SPECT in women: gender-related differences in prognostic nuclear testing. *Journal of American College of Cardiology* **28**:34–44.

Hachamovitch R, Berman DS, Shaw LJ *et al.* (1998) Incremental prognostic value of myocardial perfusion single photon emission computed tomography for the prediction of cardiac death: differential stratification for risk of cardiac death and myocardial infarction. *Circulation* **97**:535–543.

Hachamovitch R, Hayes S, Friedman JD *et al.* (2003) Determinants of risk and its temporal variation in patients with normal stress myocardial perfusion scans: what is the warranty period of a normal scan? *Journal of American College of Cardiology* **41**:1329–1340.

Hachamovitch R, Hayes SW, Friedman JD *et al.* (2005) A prognostic score for prediction of cardiac mortality risk after adenosine stress myocardial perfusion scintigraphy. *Journal of American College of Cardiology* **45**:722–729.

Hammermeister KE, DeRouen TA, Dodge HT (1979) Variables predictive of survival in patients with coronary disease. Selection by univariate and multivariate analyses from the clinical, electrocardiographic, exercise, arteriographic, and quantitative angiographic evaluations. *Circulation* **59**:421–430.

Hansen CL, Crabbe D, Rubin S (1996) Lower diagnostic accuracy of thallium-201 SPECT myocardial perfusion imaging in women: an effect of smaller chamber. *Journal of American College of Cardiology* **67**:69–77.

Hase H, Joki N, Ishikawa H *et al.* (2004) Prognostic value of stress myocardial perfusion imaging using adenosine triphosphate at the beginning of haemodialysis treatment in patients with end-stage renal disease. *Nephrology, Dialysis, Transplantation* **19**:1161–1167.

Hays JT, Mahmarian JJ, Cochran AJ, Verani MS (1993) Dobutamine thallium-201 tomography for evaluating patients with suspected coronary artery disease unable to undergo exercise or vasodilator pharmacologic stress testing. *Journal of American College of Cardiology* **21**:1583–1590.

He ZX, Cwajg E, Preslar JS *et al.* (1999) Accuracy of left ventricular ejection fraction determined by gated myocardial perfusion SPECT with Tl-201 and Tc-99m sestamibi: comparison with first-pass radionuclide angiography. *Journal of Nuclear Cardiology* **6**:412–417.

Hecht HS, Mirell SG, Rolett EL, Blahd WH (1978) Left-ventricular ejection fraction and segmental wall motion by peripheral first-pass radionuclide angiography. *Journal of Nuclear Medicine* **19**:17–23.

Heller GV, Bateman TM, Johnson LL *et al.* (2004) Clinical value of attenuation correction in stress-only Tc-99m sestamibi SPECT imaging. *Journal of Nuclear Cardiology* **11**:273–281.

Hendel RC, Berman DS, Cullom SJ *et al.* (1999) Multicenter clinical trial to evaluate the efficacy of correction for photon attenuation and scatter in SPECT myocardial perfusion imaging. *Circulation* **99**:2742–2749.

Hendel RC, Bateman TM, Cerqueira MD *et al.* (2005) Initial clinical experience with regadenoson, a novel selective A2A agonist for pharmacologic stress single-photon emission computed tomography myocardial perfusion imaging. *Journal of American College of Cardiology* **46**:2069–2075.

Herman SD, LaBresh KA, Santos-Ocampo CD *et al.* (1994) Comparison of dobutamine and exercise using technetium-99m sestamibi imaging for the evaluation of coronary artery disease. *American Journal of Cardiology* **73**:164–169.

Higuchi T, Taki J, Nakajima K *et al.* (2004) Left ventricular ejection and filling rate measurement based on the automatic edge detection method of ECG-gated blood pool single-photon emission tomography. *Annals of Nuclear Medicine* **18**:507–511.

Iskander S, Iskandrian AE (1998) Risk assessment using single-photon emission computed tomographic technetium-99m sestamibi imaging. *Journal of American College of Cardiology* **32**:57–62.

Itti E, Rosso J, Hammami H *et al.* (2001) Myocardial tracking, a new method to calculate ejection fraction with gated SPECT: Validation with 201Tl versus planar angiography. *Journal of Nuclear Medicine* **42**:845–852.

Johnson LL, Lawson MA, Blackwell GG *et al.* (1995) Optimizing the method to calculate right ventricular ejection fraction from first-pass data acquired with a multicrystal camera. *Journal of Nuclear Cardiology* **2**:372–379.

Johnson LL, Verdesca SA, Aude WY *et al.* (1997) Postischemic stunning can affect left ventricular ejection fraction and regional wall motion on post-stress gated sestamibi tomograms. *Journal of American College of Cardiology* **30**:1641–1648.

Kapur A, Latus KA, Davies G *et al.* (2002) A comparison of three radionuclide myocardial perfusion tracers in clinical practice: the ROBUST study. *European Journal of Nuclear Medicine and Molecular Imaging* **29**:1608–1616.

Kiat H, Maddahi J, Roy LT *et al.* (1989) Comparison of technetium 99m methoxy isobutyl isonitrile and thallium 201 for evaluation of coronary artery disease by planar and tomographic methods. *American Heart Journal* **117**:1–11.

Kim SJ, Kim IJ, Kim YS, Kim YK (2005) Gated blood pool SPECT for measurement of left ventricular volumes and left ventricular ejection fraction: comparison of 8 and 16 frame gated blood pool SPECT. *International Journal of Cardiovascular Imaging* **21**:261–266.

Kirac S, Wackers FJ, Liu YH (2000) Validation of the Yale circumferential quantification method using 201Tl and 99mTc: a phantom study. *Journal of Nuclear Medicine* **41**:1436–1441.

Kjaer A, Cortsen A, Rahbek B *et al.* (2002) Attenuation and scatter correction in myocardial SPET: improved diagnostic accuracy in patients with suspected coronary artery disease. *European Journal of Nuclear Medicine and Molecular Imaging* **29**:1438–1442.

Klodas E, Miller TD, Christian TF *et al.* (2003) Prognostic significance of ischemic electrocardiographic changes during vasodilator stress testing in patients with normal SPECT images. *Journal of Nuclear Cardiology* **10**:4–8.

Knuuti MJ, Saraste M, Nuutila P *et al.* (1994) Myocardial viability: fluorine-18-deoxyglucose positron emission tomography in prediction of wall motion recovery after revascularization. *American Heart Journal* **127**:785–796.

Kober L, Torp-Pedersen C, Pedersen OD *et al.* (1996) Importance of congestive heart failure and interaction of congestive heart failure and left ventricular systolic function on prognosis in patients with acute myocardial infarction. *American Journal of Cardiology* **78**:1124–1128.

Kostkiewicz M, Olszowska M, Przewlocki T *et al.* (2003) Prognostic value of nitrate enhanced Tc99m MIBI SPECT study in detecting viable myocardium in patients with coronary artery disease. *International Journal of Cardiovascular Imaging* **19**:129–135.

Leslie WD, Tully SA, Yogendran MS *et al.* (2005) Prognostic value of automated quantification of 99mTc-sestamibi myocardial perfusion imaging. *Journal of Nuclear Medicine* **46**:204–211.

Lima RSL, Watson DD, Goode AR *et al.* (2003) Incremental value of combined perfusion and function over perfusion alone by gated SPECT myocardial perfusion imaging for detection of severe three-vessel coronary artery disease. *Journal of the American College of Cardiology* **42**:64–70.

Links JM, DePuey EG, Taillefer R, Becker LC (2002) Attenuation correction and gating synergistically improve the diagnostic accuracy of myocardial perfusion SPECT. *Journal of Nuclear Cardiology* **9**:183–187.

Liu YH, Sinusas AJ, DeMan P *et al.* (1999) Quantification of SPECT myocardial perfusion images: methodology and validation of the Yale-CQ method. *Journal of Nuclear Cardiology* **6**:190–204.

Liu YH, Sinusas AJ, Khaimov D *et al.* (2005) New hybrid count- and geometry-based method for quantification of left ventricular volumes and ejection fraction from ECG-gated SPECT: methodology and validation. *Journal of Nuclear Cardiology* **12**:55–65.

Lucignani G, Paolini G, Landoni C *et al.* (1992) Presurgical identification of hibernating myocardium by combined use of technetium-99m hexakis 2-methoxyisobutylisonitrile single photon emission tomography and fluorine-18 fluoro-2-deoxy-D-glucose positron emission tomography in patients with coronary artery disease. *European Journal of Nuclear Medicine* **19**:874–881.

Machecourt J, Longere P, Fagret D *et al.* (1994) Prognostic value of thallium-201 single-photon emission computed tomographic myocardial perfusion imaging according to extent of myocardial defect. Study in 1,926 patients with follow-up at 33 months. *Journal of American College of Cardiology* **23**:1096–1106.

Maes AF, Borgers M, Flameng W *et al.* (1997) Assessment of myocardial viability in chronic coronary artery disease using technetium-99m sestamibi SPECT. Correlation with histologic and positron emission tomographic studies and functional follow-up. *Journal of American College of Cardiology* **29**:62–68.

Mahmarian JJ, Boyce TM, Goldberg RK *et al.* (1990) Quantitative exercise thallium-201 single photon emission computed tomography for the enhanced diagnosis of ischemic heart disease. *Journal of American College of Cardiology* **15**:318–329.

Mahmarian JJ, Moye LA, Verani MS *et al.* (1995) High reproducibility of myocardial perfusion defects in patients undergoing serial exercise thallium-201 tomography. *American Journal of Cardiology* **75**:1116–1119.

Mahmood S, Gupta NK, Gunning M *et al.* (1994) 201Tl myocardial perfusion SPET: adenosine alone or combined with dynamic exercise. *Nuclear Medicine Communications* **15**:586–592.

Manrique A, Faraggi M, Vera P *et al.* (1999) 201Tl and 99mTc-MIBI gated SPECT in patients with large perfusion defects and left ventricular dysfunction: comparison with equilibrium radionuclide angiography. *Journal of Nuclear Medicine* **40**:805–809.

Marie PY, Danchin N, Durand JF *et al.* (1995) Long-term prediction of major ischemic events by exercise thallium-

201 single-photon emission computed tomography. Incremental prognostic value compared with clinical, exercise testing, catheterization and radionuclide angiographic data. *Journal of American College of Cardiology* **26**:879–886.

Martin WH, Delbeke D, Patton JA *et al.* (1995) FDG-SPECT: correlation with FDG-PET. *Journal of Nuclear Medicine* **36**:988–995.

Marwick T, Willemart B, D'Hondt AM *et al.* (1993) Selection of the optimal nonexercise stress for the evaluation of ischemic regional myocardial dysfunction and malperfusion. Comparison of dobutamine and adenosine using echocardiography and 99mTc-MIBI single photon emission computed tomography. *Circulation* **87**:345–354.

Marwick TH, MacIntyre WJ, Lafont A *et al.* (1992) Metabolic responses of hibernating and infarcted myocardium to revascularization. A follow-up study of regional perfusion, function, and metabolism. *Circulation* **85**:1347–1353.

Marwick TH, D'Hondt AM, Mairesse GH *et al.* (1994) Comparative ability of dobutamine and exercise stress in inducing myocardial ischaemia in active patients. *British Heart Journal* **72**:31–38.

Marwick TH, Shan K, Patel S *et al.* (1997) Incremental value of rubidium-82 positron emission tomography for prognostic assessment of known or suspected coronary artery disease. *American Journal of Cardiology* **80**:865–870.

Masood Y, Liu YH, Depuey G *et al.* (2005) Clinical validation of SPECT attenuation correction using x-ray computed tomography-derived attenuation maps: multicenter clinical trial with angiographic correlation. *Journal of Nuclear Cardiology* **12**:676–686.

Mieres JH, Shaw LJ, Hendel RC (2003) Consensus statement from the American Society of Nuclear Cardiology Task Force on Women and Heart Disease. The role of myocardial perfusion imaging in the clinical evaluation of coronary artery disease in women. *Journal of Nuclear Cardiology* **10**:95–101.

Milcinski M, Henze E, Lietzenmayer R *et al.* (1991) Reproducibility of quantitative hexakis-2-methoxyisobutylisonitrile single photon emission tomography in stable coronary artery disease. *European Journal of Nuclear Medicine* **18**:17–22.

Mowatt G, Brazzelli M, Gemmell H *et al.* (2005) Systematic review of the prognostic effectiveness of SPECT myocardial perfusion scintigraphy in patients with suspected or known coronary artery disease and following myocardial infarction. *Nuclear Medicine Communications* **26**:217–229.

Multicenter Postinfarction Research Group (1983) Risk stratification and survival after myocardial infarction. *New England Journal of Medicine* **309**:331–367.

Najm YC, Timmis AD, Maisey MN *et al.* (1989) The evaluation of ventricular function using gated myocardial imaging with Tc-99m MIBI. *European Heart Journal* **10**:142–148.

Narayanan MV, King MA, Pretorius PH *et al.* (2003) Human-observer receiver-operating-characteristic evaluation of attenuation, scatter, and resolution compensation strategies for (99m)Tc myocardial perfusion imaging. *Journal of Nuclear Medicine* **44**:1725–1734.

Navare SM, Wackers FJ, Liu YH (2003) Comparison of 16-frame and 8-frame gated SPET imaging for determination of left ventricular volumes and ejection fraction. *European Journal of Nuclear Medicine and Molecular Imaging* **30**:1330–1337.

Nichols K, Humayun N, De Bondt P *et al.* (2004) Model

dependence of gated blood pool SPECT ventricular function measurements. *Journal of Nuclear Cardiology* **11**:282–292.

O'Connor CM, Hathaway WR, Bates ER *et al.* (1997) Clinical characteristics and long-term outcome of patients in whom congestive heart failure develops after thrombolytic therapy for acute myocardial infarction: development of a predictive model. *American Heart Journal* **133**:663–673.

Patel AD, Abo-Auda WS, Davis JM *et al.* (2003) Prognostic value of myocardial perfusion imaging in predicting outcome after renal transplantation. *American Journal of Cardiology* **92**:146–151.

Patel GM, Hauser TH, Parker JA *et al.* (2004) Quantitative relationship of stress Tc-99m sestamibi lung uptake with resting Tl-201 lung uptake and with indices of left ventricular dysfunction and coronary artery disease. *Journal of Nuclear Cardiology* **11**:408–413.

Pitman AG, Kalff V, Van Every B *et al.* (2005) Contributions of subdiaphragmatic activity, attenuation, and diaphragmatic motion to inferior wall artifact in attenuation-corrected Tc-99m myocardial perfusion SPECT. *Journal of Nuclear Cardiology* **12**:401–409.

Pohost GM, Zir LM, Moore RH *et al.* (1977) Differentiation of transiently ischemic from infarcted myocardium by serial imaging after a single dose of thallium-201. *Circulation* **55**:294–302.

Romanens M, Gradel C, Saner H, Pfisterer M (2001) Comparison of 99mTc-sestamibi lung/heart ratio, transient ischaemic dilation and perfusion defect size for the identification of severe and extensive coronary artery disease. *European Journal of Nuclear Medicine* **28**:907–910.

Sakamoto K, Nakamura T, Zen K *et al.* (2004) Identification of exercise-induced left ventricular systolic and diastolic dysfunction using gated SPECT in patients with coronary artery disease. *Journal of Nuclear Cardiology* **11**:152–158.

Samady H, Wackers FJ, Joska TM *et al.* (2002) Pharmacologic stress perfusion imaging with adenosine: role of simultaneous low-level treadmill exercise. *Journal of Nuclear Cardiology* **9**:188–196.

Sandler MP, Patton JA (1996) Fluorine 18-labeled fluorodeoxyglucose myocardial single-photon emission computed tomography: an alternative for determining myocardial viability. *Journal of Nuclear Cardiology* **3**:342–349.

Sandler MP, Bax JJ, Patton JA *et al.* (1998) Fluorine-18-fluorodeoxyglucose cardiac imaging using a modified scintillation camera. *Journal of Nuclear Medicine* **39**:2035–2043.

Santana-Boado C, Candell-Riera J, Castell C (1998) Diagnostic accuracy of technetium-99m-MIBI myocardial SPECT in women and men. *Journal of Nuclear Medicine* **39**:751–755.

Schinkel AF, Elhendy A, Biagini E *et al.* (2005) Prognostic stratification using dobutamine stress 99mTc-tetrofosmin myocardial perfusion SPECT in elderly patients unable to perform exercise testing. *Journal of Nuclear Medicine* **46**:12–18.

Senior R, Kaul S, Raval U, Lahiri A (2002) Impact of revascularization and myocardial viability determined by nitrate-enhanced Tc-99m sestamibi and Tl-201 imaging on mortality and functional outcome in ischemic cardiomyopathy. *Journal of Nuclear Cardiology* **9**:454–462.

Shaw LJ, Hendel R, Borges-Neto S *et al.* (2003) Prognostic value of normal exercise and adenosine (99m)Tc-tetrofosmin SPECT imaging: results from the multicenter registry of 4,728 patients. *Journal of Nuclear Medicine* 44:134–139.

Shaw LJ, Hendel RC, Cerquiera M *et al.* (2005) Ethnic differences in the prognostic value of stress technetium-99m tetrofosmin gated single-photon emission computed tomography myocardial perfusion imaging. *Journal of American College of Cardiology* 45:1494–1504.

Singal PK, Iliskovic N (1998) Doxorubicin-induced cardiomyopathy. *New England Journal of Medicine* 339:900–905.

Slomka PJ, Nishina H, Berman DS *et al.* (2005) Automated quantification of myocardial perfusion SPECT using simplified normal limits. *Journal of Nuclear Cardiology* 12:66–77.

Smanio PE, Watson DD, Segalla DL *et al.* (1997) Value of gating of technetium-99m sestamibi single-photon emission computed tomographic imaging. *Journal of American College of Cardiology* 30:1687–1692.

Smith WH, Kastner RJ, Calnon DA *et al.* (1997) Quantitative gated single photon emission computed tomography imaging: a counts-based method for display and measurement of regional and global ventricular systolic function. *Journal of Nuclear Cardiology* 4:451–463.

Srinivasan G, Kitsiou A, Bacharach S *et al.* (1998) [^{18}F]Fluorodeoxyglucose single photon emission computed tomography. Can it replace PET and thallium SPECT for the assessment of myocardial viability? *Circulation* 97:843–850.

Tamaki N, Yonekura Y, Mukai T *et al.* (1984) Stress thallium-201 transaxial emission computed tomography: quantitative versus qualitative analysis for evaluation of coronary artery disease. *Journal of American College of Cardiology* 4:1213–1221.

Tamaki N, Yonekura Y, Yamashita K *et al.* (1989) Positron emission tomography using fluorine-18 deoxyglucose in evaluation of coronary artery bypass grafting. *American Journal of Cardiology* 64:860–865.

Tamaki N, Kawamoto M, Tadamura E *et al.* (1995) Prediction of reversible ischemia after revascularization. Perfusion and metabolic studies with positron emission tomography. *Circulation* 91:1697–1705.

Tillisch J, Brunken R, Marshall R *et al.* (1986) Reversibility of cardiac wall-motion abnormalities predicted by positron tomography. *New England Journal of Medicine* 314:884–888.

Tzonevska A, Tzvetkov K, Dimitrova M, Piperkova E (2005) Assessment of myocardial viability with (99m)Tc-sestamibi - gated SPET images in patients undergoing percutaneous transluminar coronary angioplasty. *Hellenic Journal of Nuclear Medicine* 8:48–53.

Udelson JE, Heller GV, Wackers FJ *et al.* (2004) Randomized, controlled dose-ranging study of the selective adenosine A2A receptor agonist binodenoson for pharmacological stress as an adjunct to myocardial perfusion imaging. *Circulation* 109:457–464.

Utsunomiya D, Tomiguchi S, Shiraishi S *et al.* (2005) Initial experience with X-ray CT based attenuation correction in myocardial perfusion SPECT imaging using a combined SPECT/CT system. *Annals of Nuclear Medicine* 19:485–489.

Vaduganathan P, He ZX, Raghavan C *et al.* (1996) Detection of left anterior descending coronary artery stenosis in patients with left bundle branch block: exercise, adenosine or dobutamine imaging? *Journal of American College of Cardiology* 28:543–550.

Vaduganathan P, He ZX, Vick GW, 3rd *et al.* (1999) Evaluation of left ventricular wall motion, volumes, and ejection fraction by gated myocardial tomography with technetium 99m-labeled tetrofosmin: a comparison with cine magnetic resonance imaging. *Journal of Nuclear Cardiology* 6:3–10.

Vallejo E, Dione DP, Bruni WL *et al.* (2000a) Reproducibility and accuracy of gated SPECT for determination of left ventricular volumes and ejection fraction: experimental validation using MRI. *Journal of Nuclear Medicine* 41:874–882; discussion 883–876.

Vallejo E, Dione DP, Sinusas AJ, Wackers FJ (2000b) Assessment of left ventricular ejection fraction with quantitative gated SPECT: accuracy and correlation with first-pass radionuclide angiography. *Journal of Nuclear Cardiology* 7:461–470.

Van Kriekinge SD, Berman DS, Germano G (1999) Automatic quantification of left ventricular ejection fraction from gated blood pool SPECT. *Journal of Nuclear Cardiology* 6:498–506.

Van Tosh A, Garza D, Roberti R *et al.* (1995) Serial myocardial perfusion imaging with dipyridamole and rubidium-82 to assess restenosis after angioplasty. *Journal of Nuclear Medicine* 36:1553–1560.

Vanhove C, Franken PR, Defrise M, Bossuyt A (2003) Comparison of 180 degrees and 360 degrees data acquisition for determination of left ventricular function from gated myocardial perfusion tomography and gated blood pool tomography. *European Journal of Nuclear Medicine and Molecular Imaging* 30:1498–1504.

Voth E, Baer FM, Theissen P *et al.* (1994) Dobutamine 99mTc-MIBI single-photon emission tomography: non-exercise-dependent detection of haemodynamically significant coronary artery stenoses. *European Journal of Nuclear Medicine* 21:537–544.

Wackers F (2005) Coronary artery disease: exercise stress. In: *Clinical Nuclear Cardiology*. B Zaret, GA Beller (eds.). Elsevier Mosby, Philadelphia, pp. 215–232.

Wackers FJ, Berger HJ, Johnstone DE *et al.* (1979) Multiple gated cardiac blood pool imaging for left ventricular ejection fraction: validation of the technique and assessment of variability. *American Journal of Cardiology* 43:1159–1166.

Wackers FJ, Young LH, Inzucchi SE *et al.* (2004) Detection of silent myocardial ischemia in asymptomatic diabetic subjects: the DIAD study. *Diabetes Care* 27:1954–1961.

Weiss AT, Berman DS, Lew AS *et al.* (1987) Transient ischemic dilation of the left ventricle on stress thallium-201 scintigraphy: a marker of severe and extensive coronary artery disease. *Journal of American College of Cardiology* 9:752–759.

Williams KA, Taillon LA (1996) Left ventricular function in patients with coronary artery disease assessed by gated tomographic myocardial perfusion images. Comparison with assessment by contrast ventriculography and first-pass radionuclide angiography. *Journal of American College of Cardiology* 27:173–181.

Williams KA, Schneider CM (1999) Increased stress right ventricular activity on dual isotope perfusion SPECT: a sign of multivessel and/or left main coronary artery disease. *Journal of American College of Cardiology* 34:420–427.

Williams KA, Hill KA, Sheridan CM (2003) Noncardiac findings on dual-isotope myocardial perfusion SPECT. *Journal of Nuclear Cardiology* 10:395–402.

Worsley DF, Fung AY, Coupland DB *et al.* (1992) Comparison of stress-only *vs.* stress/rest with technetium-99m methoxyisobutylisonitrile myocardial perfusion imaging. *European Journal of Nuclear Medicine* 19:441–444.

Yang KT, Chen HD (1994) A semi-automated method for edge detection in the evaluation of left ventricular function using ECG-gated single-photon emission tomography. *European Journal of Nuclear Medicine* **21**:1206–1211.

Yao SS, Qureshi E, Nichols K *et al.* (2004) Prospective validation of a quantitative method for differentiating ischemic versus nonischemic cardiomyopathy by technetium-99m sestamibi myocardial perfusion single-photon emission computed tomography. *Clinical Cardiology* **27**:615–620.

Zaret BL, Strauss HW, Hurley PJ *et al.* (1971) A noninvasive scintiphotographic method for detecting regional ventricular dysfunction in man. *New England Journal of Medicine* **284**:1165–1170.

Zaret BL, Wackers FJ, Terrin ML *et al.* (1995) Value of radionuclide rest and exercise left ventricular ejection fraction to access survival of patients following thrombolytic therapy for acute myocardial infarction: results of the Thrombolysis in Myocardial Infarction (TIMI) phase II study. *Journal of American College of Cardiology* **26**:73–79.

Zarich SW, Cohen MC, Lane SE *et al.* (1996) Routine perioperative dipyridamole 201Tl imaging in diabetic patients undergoing vascular surgery. *Diabetes Care* **19**:355–360.

Zellweger MJ, Hachamovitch R, Kang X *et al.* (2004) Prognostic relevance of symptoms versus objective evidence of coronary artery disease in diabetic patients. *European Heart Journal* **25**:543–550.

CHAPTER 4

Cheitlin MD, Armstrong WF, Aurigemma GP *et al.* (2003) ACC/AHA/ASE 2003 Guideline update for the clinical application of echocardiography: summary article: a report of the American College of Cardiology/American Heart Association Task Force on practice guidelines (ACC/AHA/ASE committee to update the 1997 guidelines for the clinical application of echocardiography. *Journal of the American College of Cardiology* **42**:954–970.

Lang RM, Bierig M, Devereaux RB *et al.* (2005) Recommendation for chamber quantification: A report from the American Society of Echocardiography's Guidelines and Standards Committee and the Chamber Quantification Writing Group, developed in conjunction with the European Association of Echocardiography, a branch of the European Society of Echocardiography. *Journal of the American Society of Echocardiography* **18**:1440–1463.

Lucas FL, Wennberg DE, Malenka DJ (1999) Variation in the use of echocardiography. *Effective Clinical Practice* **2**:71–75.

Schiller NB, Shah PM, Crawford M *et al.* (1989) Recommendations for quantitation of the left ventricle by two-dimensional echocardiography. American Society of Echocardiography Committee on Standards, Subcommittee on Quantitation of Two-Dimensional Echocardiograms. *Journal of the American Society of Echocardiography* **2**:358–367.

Zoghbi WA, Enriquez-Sarano M, Foster E, Grayburn PA (2005) American Society of Echocardiography. Recommendations for evaluation of the severity of native valvular regurgitation with two-dimensional and Doppler echocardiography. *Journal of the American Society of Echocardiography* **16**:777–802.

CHAPTER 5

Auffermann W, Olofsson P, Stoney R, Higgins CB (1987) MR imaging of complications of aortic surgery. *Journal of Computed Assisted Tomography* **11**:982–989.

Aurigemma G, Reichek N, Schiebler M, Axel L (1990) Evaluation of mitral regurgitation by cine magnetic resonance imaging. *American Journal of Cardiology* **66**:621–625.

Axel L and Dougherty L (1989) MR imaging of motion with spatial modulation of magnetization. *Radiology* **171**:841–845.

Bakker CJ, Hoogeveen RM, Hurtak WF *et al.* (1997) MR-guided endovascular interventions: susceptibility-based catheter and near-real-time imaging technique. *Radiology* **202**:273–276.

Banki JH, Meiners LC, Barentsz JO and Witkamp TD (1992) Detection of aortic dissection by magnetic resonance imaging in adults with Marfan's syndrome. *International Journal of Cardiac Imaging* **8**:249–254.

Beerbaum P, Korperich H, Esdorn H *et al.* (2003) Atrial septal defects in pediatric patients: noninvasive sizing with cardiovascular MR imaging. *Radiology* **228**:361–369.

Bisset GS, III, Strife JL, Kirks DR, Bailey WW (1987) Vascular rings: MR imaging. *American Journal of Roentgenology* **149**:251–256.

Bouchard A, Higgins CB, Byrd BF III *et al.* (1985) Magnetic resonance imaging in pulmonary arterial hypertension. *American Journal of Cardiology* **56**:938–942.

Boxt LM (1996) MR imaging of pulmonary hypertension and right ventricular dysfunction. *Magnetic Resonance Imaging Clinics of North America* **4**:307–325.

Boxt LM (2004) Magnetic resonance and computed tomographic evaluation of congenital heart disease. *Journal of Magnetic Resonance Imaging* **19**:827–847.

Boxt LM, Katz J, Kolb T *et al.* (1992) Direct quantitation of right and left ventricular volumes with nuclear magnetic resonance imaging in patients with primary pulmonary hypertension. *Journal of American College of Cardiology* **19**:1508–1515.

Buser PT, Auffermann W, Holt WW *et al.* (1989) Noninvasive evaluation of global left ventricular function with use of cine nuclear magnetic resonance. *Journal of American College of Cardiology* **13**:1294–1300.

Carr JC, Simonetti O, Bundy J *et al.* (2001) Cine MR angiography of the heart with segmented true fast imaging with steady-state precession. *Radiology* **219**:828–834.

Caruthers SD, Lin SJ, Brown P *et al.* (2003) Practical value of cardiac magnetic resonance imaging for clinical quantification of aortic valve stenosis: comparison with echocardiography. *Circulation* **108**:2236–2243.

Casolo GC, Zampa V, Rega L *et al.* (1992) Evaluation of mitral stenosis by cine magnetic resonance imaging. *American Heart Journal* **123**:1252–1260.

Cerqueira MD, Weissman NJ, Dilsizian V *et al.* (2002) Standardized myocardial segmentation and nomenclature for tomographic imaging of the heart: a statement for healthcare professionals from the Cardiac Imaging Committee of the Council on Clinical Cardiology of the American Heart Association. *Circulation* **105**:539–542.

Chiles C, Woodard PK, Gutierrez FR, Link KM (2001) Metastatic involvement of the heart and pericardium: CT and MR imaging. *Radiographics* **21**:439–449.

Choi YH, Park JH, Choe YH, Yoo SJ (1994) MR imaging of Ebstein's anomaly of the tricuspid valve. *American Journal of Roentgenology* **163**:539–543.

Choudhury RP, Fuster V, Badimon JJ *et al.* (2002) MRI and characterization of atherosclerotic plaque: emerging applications and molecular imaging. *Arteriosclerosis, Thrombosis, and Vascular Biology* **22**:1065–1074.

Chowdhury UK, Pradeep KK, Patel CD *et al.* (2006)

Noninvasive assessment of repaired tetralogy of Fallot by magnetic resonance imaging and dynamic radionuclide studies. *Annals of Thoracic Surgery* **81**:1436–1442.

Corrado D, Fontaine G, Marcus FI *et al.* (2000) Arrhythmogenic right ventricular dysplasia/cardiomyopathy: need for an international registry. Study Group on Arrhythmogenic Right Ventricular Dysplasia/Cardiomyopathy of the Working Groups on Myocardial and Pericardial Disease and Arrhythmias of the European Society of Cardiology and of the Scientific Council on Cardiomyopathies of the World Heart Federation. *Circulation* **101**:E101–E106.

Correia LC, Atalar E, Kelemen MD *et al.* (1997) Intravascular magnetic resonance imaging of aortic atherosclerotic plaque composition. *Arteriosclerosis, Thrombosis, and Vascular Biology* **17**:3626–3632.

Corti R, Fuster V, Fayad ZA *et al.* (2005) Effects of aggressive versus conventional lipid-lowering therapy by simvastatin on human atherosclerotic lesions: a prospective, randomized, double-blind trial with high-resolution magnetic resonance imaging. *Journal of American College of Cardiology* **46**:106–112.

Cowley CG, Orsmond GS, Feola P *et al.* (2005) Long-term, randomized comparison of balloon angioplasty and surgery for native coarctation of the aorta in childhood. *Circulation* **111**:3453–3456.

Cullen JH, Horsfield MA, Reek CR *et al.* (1999) A myocardial perfusion reserve index in humans using first-pass contrast-enhanced magnetic resonance imaging. *Journal of American College of Cardiology* **33**:1386–1394.

De Cobelli F, Pieroni M, Esposito A *et al.* (2006) Delayed gadolinium-enhanced cardiac magnetic resonance in patients with chronic myocarditis presenting with heart failure or recurrent arrhythmias. *Journal of American College of Cardiology* **47**:1649–1654.

Desai MY, Bluemke DA (2005) Atherosclerosis imaging using MR imaging: current and emerging applications. *Magnetic Resonance Imaging Clinics of North America* **13**:171–180, vii.

Desai MY, Rodriguez A, Wasserman BA *et al.* (2005) Association of cholesterol subfractions and carotid lipid core measured by MRI. *Arteriosclerosis, Thrombosis, and Vascular Biology* **25**:e110–e111.

Diethelm L, Dery R, Lipton MJ, Higgins CB (1987) Atrial-level shunts: sensitivity and specificity of MR in diagnosis. *Radiology* **162**:181–186.

Dinsmore RE, Wismer GL, Levine RA *et al.* (1984) Magnetic resonance imaging of the heart: positioning and gradient angle selection for optimal imaging planes. *American Journal of Roentgenology* **143**:1135–1142.

Doherty NE III, Seelos KC, Suzuki J *et al.* (1992) Application of cine nuclear magnetic resonance imaging for sequential evaluation of response to angiotensin-converting enzyme inhibitor therapy in dilated cardiomyopathy. *Journal of American College of Cardiology* **19**:1294–1302.

Duro AC, Villa JA, Rienzu MA *et al.* (2000) [Criss-cross heart with discordant atrioventricular connection and arterial ventricle]. *Revista Española de Cardiología* **53**:1121.

Durongpisitkul K, Tang NL, Soongswang J *et al.* (2004) Predictors of successful transcatheter closure of atrial septal defect by cardiac magnetic resonance imaging. *Pediatric Cardiology* **25**:124–130.

Edwards MB, Taylor KM, Shellock FG (2000) Prosthetic heart valves: evaluation of magnetic field interactions, heating, and artifacts at 1.5 T. *Journal of Magnetic Resonance Imaging* **12**:363–369.

Fayad ZA, Nahar T, Fallon JT *et al.* (2000) *In vivo* magnetic resonance evaluation of atherosclerotic plaques in the human thoracic aorta: a comparison with transesophageal echocardiography. *Circulation* **101**:2503–2509.

Fenchel M, Helber U, Kramer U *et al.* (2005) Detection of regional myocardial perfusion deficit using rest and stress perfusion MRI: a feasibility study. *American Journal of Roentgenology* **185**:627–635.

Fernandes VR, Polak JF, Edvardsen T *et al.* (2006) Subclinical atherosclerosis and incipient regional myocardial dysfunction in asymptomatic individuals: the Multi-Ethnic Study of Atherosclerosis (MESA). *Journal of American College of Cardiology* **47**:2420–2428.

Flamm SD, VanDyke CW, White RD (1996) MR imaging of the thoracic aorta. *Magnetic Resonance Imaging Clinics of North America* **4**:217–235.

Fogel MA (2005) Is routine cardiac catheterization necessary in the management of patients with single ventricles across staged Fontan reconstruction? No! *Pediatric Cardiology* **26**:154–158.

Fogel MA, Donofrio MT, Ramaciotti C *et al.* (1994) Magnetic resonance and echocardiographic imaging of pulmonary artery size throughout stages of Fontan reconstruction. *Circulation* **90**:2927–2936.

Fogel MA, Weinberg PM, Hoydu A *et al.* (1997) The nature of flow in the systemic venous pathway measured by magnetic resonance blood tagging in patients having the Fontan operation. *Journal of Thoracic and Cardiovascular Surgery* **114**:1032–1041.

Fogel MA, Weinberg PM, Rychik J *et al.* (1999) Caval contribution to flow in the branch pulmonary arteries of Fontan patients with a novel application of magnetic resonance presaturation pulse. *Circulation* **99**:1215–1221.

Friedrich MG, Strohm O, Schulz-Menger J *et al.* (1998) Contrast media-enhanced magnetic resonance imaging visualizes myocardial changes in the course of viral myocarditis. *Circulation* **97**:1802–1809.

Fujita N, Duerinekx AJ, Higgins CD (1993) Variation in left ventricular regional wall stress with cine magnetic resonance imaging: normal subjects versus dilated cardiomyopathy. *American Heart Journal* **125**:1337–1345.

Fujita N, Chazouilleres AF, Hartiala JJ *et al.* (1994) Quantification of mitral regurgitation by velocity-encoded cine nuclear magnetic resonance imaging. *Journal of American College of Cardiology* **23**:951–958.

Gerber BL, Garot J, Bluemke DA *et al.* (2002) Accuracy of contrast-enhanced magnetic resonance imaging in predicting improvement of regional myocardial function in patients after acute myocardial infarction. *Circulation* **106**:1083–1089.

Geskin G, Kramer CM, Rogers WJ *et al.* (1998) Quantitative assessment of myocardial viability after infarction by dobutamine magnetic resonance tagging. *Circulation* **98**:217–223.

Geva T, Sandweiss BM, Gauvreau K *et al.* (2004) Factors associated with impaired clinical status in long-term survivors of tetralogy of Fallot repair evaluated by magnetic resonance imaging. *Journal of American College of Cardiology* **43**:1068–1074.

Globits S, Higgins CB (1995) Assessment of valvular heart disease by magnetic resonance imaging. *American Heart Journal* **129**:369–381.

Glogar D, Globits S, Neuhold A, Mayr H (1989) Assessment of mitral regurgitation by magnetic resonance imaging. *Magnetic Resonance Imaging* **7**:611–617.

Greenberg SB, Crisci KL, Koenig P *et al.* (1997) Magnetic resonance imaging compared with echocardiography in the evaluation of pulmonary artery abnormalities in children with tetralogy of Fallot following palliative and corrective surgery. *Pediatric Radiology* **27**:932–935.

Gutberlet M, Oellinger H, Ewert P *et al.* (2000) [Pre- and postoperative evaluation of ventricular function, muscle mass and valve morphology by magnetic resonance tomography in Ebstein's anomaly]. *RöFo: Fortschritte auf dem Gebiete der Röntgenstrahlen und der Nuklearmedizin* **172**:436–442.

Hasenkam JM, Ringgaard S, Houlind K *et al.* (1999) Prosthetic heart valve evaluation by magnetic resonance imaging. *European Journal of Cardiothoracic Surgery* **16**:300–305.

Heidenreich PA, Steffens J, Fujita N *et al.* (1995) Evaluation of mitral stenosis with velocity-encoded cine-magnetic resonance imaging. *American Journal of Cardiology* **75**:365–369.

Ho VB, Kinney JB, Sahn DJ (1995) Ruptured sinus of Valsalva aneurysm: cine phase-contrast MR characterization. *Journal of Computed Assisted Tomography* **19**:652–656.

Hundley WG, Li HF, Willard JE *et al.* (1995) Magnetic resonance imaging assessment of the severity of mitral regurgitation. Comparison with invasive techniques. *Circulation* **92**:1151–1158.

Hundley WG, Hamilton CA, Thomas MS *et al.* (1999) Utility of fast cine magnetic resonance imaging and display for the detection of myocardial ischemia in patients not well suited for second harmonic stress echocardiography. *Circulation* **100**:1697–1702.

Ishida N, Sakuma H, Motoyasu M *et al.* (2003) Noninfarcted myocardium: correlation between dynamic first-pass contrast-enhanced myocardial MR imaging and quantitative coronary angiography. *Radiology* **229**:209–216.

Judd RM, Lugo-Olivieri CH, Arai M *et al.* (1995) Physiological basis of myocardial contrast enhancement in fast magnetic resonance images of 2-day-old reperfused canine infarcts. *Circulation* **92**:1902–1910.

Kalil FR, de Albuquerque CP (1995) Magnetic resonance imaging in Chagas' heart disease. *Sao Paulo Medical Journal* **113**:880–883.

Kato S, Kawata T, Kuwata H *et al.* (2004) [Cardiac liposarcoma at the right ventricular outflow tract (RVOT) following lipomatous hypertrophy of the interatrial septum (LHIS); report of a case]. *Kyobu Geka* **57**:143–146.

Kersting-Sommerhoff BA, Diethelm L, Teitel DF *et al.* (1989) Magnetic resonance imaging of congenital heart disease: sensitivity and specificity using receiver operating characteristic curve analysis. *American Heart Journal* **118**:155–161.

Kim D, Gilson WD, Kramer CM, Epstein FH (2004) Myocardial tissue tracking with two-dimensional cine displacement-encoded MR imaging: development and initial evaluation. *Radiology* **230**:862–871.

Kim RJ, Wu E, Rafael A *et al.* (2000) The use of contrast-enhanced magnetic resonance imaging to identify reversible myocardial dysfunction. *New England Journal of Medicine* **343**:1445–1453.

Kramer CM, Lima JA, Reichek N *et al.* (1993) Regional differences in function within noninfarcted myocardium during left ventricular remodeling. *Circulation* **88**:1279–1288.

Kramer CM, Reichek N, Ferrari VA *et al.* (1994) Regional heterogeneity of function in hypertrophic cardiomyopathy. *Circulation* **90**:186–194.

Kramer CM, Rogers WJ, Theobald TM *et al.* (1996) Remote noninfarcted region dysfunction soon after first anterior myocardial infarction. A magnetic resonance tagging study. *Circulation* **94**:660–666.

Kramer CM, Malkowski MJ, Mankad S *et al.* (2002) Magnetic resonance tagging and echocardiographic response to dobutamine and functional improvement after reperfused myocardial infarction. *American Heart Journal* **143**:1046–1051.

Krinsky GA, Rofsky NM, DeCorato DR *et al.* (1997) Thoracic aorta: comparison of gadolinium-enhanced three-dimensional MR angiography with conventional MR imaging. *Radiology* **202**:183–193.

La Noce A, Stoelben S, Scheffler K *et al.* (2002) B22956/1, a new intravascular contrast agent for MRI: first administration to humans – preliminary results. *Academic Radiology* **9**(Suppl2):S404–S406.

Lardo AC, McVeigh ER, Jumrussirikul P *et al.* (2000) Visualization and temporal/spatial characterization of cardiac radiofrequency ablation lesions using magnetic resonance imaging. *Circulation* **102**:698–705.

Lauerma K, Virtanen KS, Sipila LM *et al.* (1997) Multislice MRI in assessment of myocardial perfusion in patients with single-vessel proximal left anterior descending coronary artery disease before and after revascularization. *Circulation* **96**:2859–2867.

Leung DA, Debatin JF, Wildermuth S *et al.* (1995) Intravascular MR tracking catheter: preliminary experimental evaluation. *American Journal of Roentgenology* **164**:1265–1270.

Lim HE, Yong HS, Shin SH *et al.* (2004) Early assessment of myocardial contractility by contrast-enhanced magnetic resonance (ceMRI) imaging after revascularization in acute myocardial infarction (AMI). *Korean Journal of Internal Medicine* **19**:213–219.

Lima JA, Judd RM, Bazille A *et al.* (1995) Regional heterogeneity of human myocardial infarcts demonstrated by contrast-enhanced MRI. Potential mechanisms. *Circulation* **92**:1117–1125.

Lin SJ, Brown PA, Watkins MP *et al.* (2004) Quantification of stenotic mitral valve area with magnetic resonance imaging and comparison with Doppler ultrasound. *Journal of American College of Cardiology* **44**:133–137.

Link KM, Loehr SP, Baker DM, Lesko NM (1993) Magnetic resonance imaging of the thoracic aorta. Semin. *Seminars in Ultrasound, CT, and MR* **14**:91–105.

Lorenz CH (2000) The range of normal values of cardiovascular structures in infants, children, and adolescents measured by magnetic resonance imaging. *Pediatric Cardiology* **21**:37–46.

Lorenz CH, Walker ES, Morgan VL *et al.* (1999) Normal human right and left ventricular mass, systolic function, and gender differences by cine magnetic resonance imaging. *Journal of Cardiovascular Magnetic Resonance* **1**:7–21.

Luna A, Ribes R, Caro P *et al.* (2005) Evaluation of cardiac tumors with magnetic resonance imaging. *European Radiology* **15**:1446–1455.

Lund TE (2001) fcMRI – mapping functional connectivity or correlating cardiac-induced noise? *Magnetic Resonance Medicine* **46**:628–629.

MacGowan GA, Shapiro EP, Azhari H *et al.* (1997) Noninvasive measurement of shortening in the fiber and cross-fiber directions in the normal human left ventricle and in idiopathic dilated cardiomyopathy. *Circulation* **96**:535–541.

Mader MT, Poulton TB, White RD (1997) Malignant tumors of the heart and great vessels: MR imaging appearance. *Radiographics* **17**:145–153.

Mahrholdt H, Goedecke C, Wagner A *et al.* (2004) Cardiovascular magnetic resonance assessment of human myocarditis: a comparison to histology and molecular pathology. *Circulation* 109:1250–1258.

Mankad S, Khalil R, Kramer CM (2003) MRI for the diagnosis of myocardial ischemia and viability. *Current Opinions in Cardiology* 18:351–356.

Maron BJ, Gottdiener JS, Epstein SE (1981) Patterns and significance of distribution of left ventricular hypertrophy in hypertrophic cardiomyopathy. A wide angle, two dimensional echocardiographic study of 125 patients. *American Journal of Cardiology* 48:418–428.

Masui T, Finck S, Higgins CB (1992) Constrictive pericarditis and restrictive cardiomyopathy: evaluation with MR imaging. *Radiology* 182:369–373.

McCrohon JA, Moon JC, Prasad SK *et al.* (2003) Differentiation of heart failure related to dilated cardiomyopathy and coronary artery disease using gadolinium-enhanced cardiovascular magnetic resonance. *Circulation* 108:54–59.

McNamara MT, Higgins CB (1986) Magnetic resonance imaging of chronic myocardial infarcts in man. *American Journal of Roentgenology* 146:315–320.

Meleca MJ, Hoit BD (1995) Previously unrecognized intrapericardial hematoma leading to refractory abdominal ascites. *Chest* 108:1747–1748.

Mitchell L, Jenkins JP, Watson Y *et al.* (1989) Diagnosis and assessment of mitral and aortic valve disease by cine-flow magnetic resonance imaging. *Magnetic Resonance Medicine* 12:181–197.

Mitsumori LM, Hatsukami TS, Ferguson MS *et al.* (2003) *In vivo* accuracy of multisequence MR imaging for identifying unstable fibrous caps in advanced human carotid plaques. *Journal of Magnetic Resonance Imaging* 17:410–420.

Moore CC, Lugo-Olivieri CH, McVeigh ER *et al.* (2000) Three-dimensional systolic strain patterns in the normal human left ventricle: characterization with tagged MR imaging. *Radiology* 214:453–466.

Murray JG, Manisali M, Flamm SD *et al.* (1997) Intramural hematoma of the thoracic aorta: MR image findings and their prognostic implications. *Radiology* 204:349–355.

Nazarian S, Bluemke DA, Lardo AC *et al.* (2005) Magnetic resonance assessment of the substrate for inducible ventricular tachycardia in nonischemic cardiomyopathy. *Circulation* 112:2821–2825.

Nielsen JC, Powell AJ, Gauvreau K *et al.* (2005) Magnetic resonance imaging predictors of coarctation severity. *Circulation* 111:622–628.

Nienaber CA, von Kodolitsch Y, Nicolas V *et al.* (1993) The diagnosis of thoracic aortic dissection by noninvasive imaging procedures. *New England Journal of Medicine* 328:1–9.

Niwa K, Tashima K, Terai M *et al.* (1989) Contrast-enhanced magnetic resonance imaging of cardiac tumors in children. *American Heart Journal* 118:424–425.

Norton KI, Tong C, Glass RB *et al.* (2006) Cardiac MR imaging assessment following tetralogy of fallot repair. *Radiographics* 26:197–211.

Ohnishi S, Fukui S, Kusuoka H *et al.* (1992) Assessment of valvular regurgitation using cine magnetic resonance imaging coupled with phase compensation technique: comparison with Doppler color flow mapping. *Angiology* 43:913–924.

Osman NF, Prince JL (2000) Visualizing myocardial function using HARP MRI. *Physics in Medicine and Biology* 45:1665–1682.

Pan L, Lima JA, Osman NF (2003) Fast tracking of cardiac motion using 3D-HARP. *Information Processing in Medical Imaging* 18:611–622.

Panting JR, Gatehouse PD, Yang GZ *et al.* (2001) Echo-planar magnetic resonance myocardial perfusion imaging: parametric map analysis and comparison with thallium SPECT. *Journal of Magnetic Resonance Imaging* 13:192–200.

Parga JR, Avila LF, Bacal F *et al.* (2001) Partial left ventriculectomy in severe idiopathic dilated cardiomyopathy: assessment of short-term results and their impact on late survival by magnetic resonance imaging. *Journal of Magnetic Resonance Imaging* 13:781–786.

Parsons JM, Baker EJ, Anderson RH *et al.* (1990) Morphological evaluation of atrioventricular septal defects by magnetic resonance imaging. *British Heart Journal* 64:138–145.

Pflugfelder PW, Landzberg JS, Cassidy MM *et al.* (1989) Comparison of cine MR imaging with Doppler echocardiography for the evaluation of aortic regurgitation. *American Journal of Roentgenology* 152:729–735.

Poon M, Fuster V, Fayad Z (2002) Cardiac magnetic resonance imaging: a 'one-stop-shop' evaluation of myocardial dysfunction. *Current Opinions in Cardiology* 17:663–670.

Prince MR, Narasimham DL, Jacoby WT *et al.* (1996) Three-dimensional gadolinium-enhanced MR angiography of the thoracic aorta. *American Journal of Roentgenology* 166:1387–1397.

Rebergen S, Ottenkamp J, Doornbos J *et al.* (1993) Postoperative pulmonary flow dynamics after Fontan surgery: assessment with nuclear magnetic resonance velocity mapping. *Journal of American College of Cardiology* 21:123–131.

Rebergen SA, Helbing WA, van der Wall EE *et al.* (1995) MR velocity mapping of tricuspid flow in healthy children and in patients who have undergone Mustard or Senning repair. *Radiology* 194:505–512.

Richardson P, McKenna W, Bristow M *et al.* (1996) Report of the 1995 World Health Organization/International Society and Federation of Cardiology Task Force on the Definition and Classification of cardiomyopathies. *Circulation* 93:841–842.

Rickers C, Seethamraju RT, Jerosch-Herold M *et al.* (2003) Magnetic resonance imaging guided cardiovascular interventions in congenital heart diseases. *Journal of Interventional Cardiology* 16:143–147.

Rochitte CE, Lima JA, Bluemke DA *et al.* (1998) Magnitude and time course of microvascular obstruction and tissue injury after acute myocardial infarction. *Circulation* 98:1006–1014.

Rochitte CE, Oliveira PF, Andrade JM *et al.* (2005) Myocardial delayed enhancement by magnetic resonance imaging in patients with Chagas' disease: a marker of disease severity. *Journal of American College of Cardiology* 46:1553–1558.

Roman MJ, Rosen SE, Kramer-Fox R *et al.* (1993) Prognostic significance of the pattern of aortic root dilation in the Marfan syndrome. *Journal of American College of Cardiology* 22:1470–1476.

Rosen BD, Gerber BL, Edvardsen T *et al.* (2004) Late systolic onset of regional LV relaxation demonstrated in three-dimensional space by MRI tissue tagging. *American Journal of Physiology. Heart and Circulatory Physiology* 287:H1740–H1746.

Russo V, Buttazzi K, Renzulli M, Fattori R (2006) Acquired diseases of the thoracic aorta: role of MRI and MRA. *European Journal of radiology* 16:852–865.

Sakuma H, Fujita N, Foo TK *et al.* (1993) Evaluation of left ventricular volume and mass with breath-hold cine MR imaging. *Radiology* **188**:377–380.

Sampson C, Kilner PJ, Hirsch R *et al.* (1994) Venoatrial pathways after the Mustard operation for transposition of the great arteries: anatomic and functional MR imaging. *Radiology* **193**:211–217.

Sayad DE, Willett DL, Hundley WG *et al.* (1998) Dobutamine magnetic resonance imaging with myocardial tagging quantitatively predicts improvement in regional function after revascularization. *American Journal of Cardiology* **82**:1149–1151, A10.

Schaefer S, van Tyen R, Saloner D (1992) Evaluation of myocardial perfusion abnormalities with gadolinium-enhanced snapshot MR imaging in humans. Work in progress. *Radiology* **185**:795–801.

Schalla S, Saeed M, Higgins CB *et al.* (2005) Balloon sizing and transcatheter closure of acute atrial septal defects guided by magnetic resonance fluoroscopy: assessment and validation in a large animal model. *Journal of Magnetic Resonance Imaging* **21**:204–211.

Schulz-Menger J, Strohm O, Waigand J *et al.* (2000) The value of magnetic resonance imaging of the left ventricular outflow tract in patients with hypertrophic obstructive cardiomyopathy after septal artery embolization. *Circulation* **101**:1764–1766.

Sechtem U, Tscholakoff D, Higgins CB (1986a) MRI of the abnormal pericardium. *American Journal of Roentgenology* **147**:245–252.

Sechtem U, Tscholakoff D, Higgins CB (1986b) MRI of the normal pericardium. *American Journal of Roentgenology* **147**:239–244.

Seelos KC, Funari M, Chang JM *et al.* (1992) Magnetic resonance imaging in acute and subacute mediastinal bleeding. *American Heart Journal* **123**:1269–1272.

Shellock FG, Kanal E (1994) Guidelines and recommendations for MR imaging safety and patient management. III. Questionnaire for screening patients before MR procedures. The SMRI Safety Committee. *Journal of Magnetic Resonance Imaging* **4**:749–751.

Shunk KA, Lima JA, Heldman AW *et al.* (1999) Transesophageal magnetic resonance imaging. *Magnetic Resonance Medicine* **41**:722–726.

Shunk KA, Garot J, Atalar E *et al.* (2001) Transesophageal magnetic resonance imaging of the aortic arch and descending thoracic aorta in patients with aortic atherosclerosis. *Journal of American College of Cardiology* **37**:2031–2035.

Smedema JP, Snoep G, van Kroonenburgh MP *et al.* (2005) Evaluation of the accuracy of gadolinium-enhanced cardiovascular magnetic resonance in the diagnosis of cardiac sarcoidosis. *Journal of American College of Cardiology* **45**:1683–1690.

Sondergaard L, Hildebrandt P, Lindvig K *et al.* (1993a) Valve area and cardiac output in aortic stenosis: quantification by magnetic resonance velocity mapping. *American Heart Journal* **126**:1156–1164.

Sondergaard L, Lindvig K, Hildebrandt P *et al.* (1993b) Quantification of aortic regurgitation by magnetic resonance velocity mapping. *American Heart Journal* **125**:1081–1090.

Sparrow PJ, Kurian JB, Jones TR, Sivanathan MU (2005) MR Imaging of cardiac tumors. *Radiographics* **25**(s):1255–1276.

Srichai MB, Axel L (2005) Magnetic resonance imaging in the management of pericardial disease. *Current Treatment Options in Cardiovascular Medicine* **7**:449–457.

Strach K, Meyer C, Schild H, Sommer T (2006) Cardiac

stress MR imaging with dobutamine. *European Radiology* **16**:2728–2738.

Sueyoshi E, Sakamoto I, Okimoto T *et al.* (2006) Cardiac amyloidosis: typical imaging findings and diffuse myocardial damage demonstrated by delayed contrast-enhanced MRI. *Cardiovascular Interventional Radiology* **29**:710–712.

Tadamura E, Yamamuro M, Kubo S *et al.* (2005) Effectiveness of delayed enhanced MRI for identification of cardiac sarcoidosis: comparison with radionuclide imaging. *American Journal of Roentgenology* **185**:110–115.

Tandri H, Calkins H, Nasir K *et al.* (2003) Magnetic resonance imaging findings in patients meeting task force criteria for arrhythmogenic right ventricular dysplasia. *Journal of Cardiovascular Electrophysiology* **14**:476–482.

Tandri H, Saranathan M, Rodriguez ER *et al* (2005) Noninvasive detection of myocardial fibrosis in arrhythmogenic right ventricular cardiomyopathy using delayed-enhancement magnetic resonance imaging. *Journal of the American College of Cardiology* **45**:98–103.

Ungkanont K, Friedman EM, Sulek M (1998) A retrospective analysis of airway endoscopy in patients less than 1-month old. *Laryngoscope* **108**:1724–1728.

Van Der TA, Barenbrug P, Snoep G *et al.* (2002) Transmural gradients of cardiac myofiber shortening in aortic valve stenosis patients using MRI tagging. *American Journal of Physiology. Heart and Circulatory Physiology* **283**:H1609–H1615.

van Rossum AC, Visser FC, Sprenger M *et al.* (1988a) Evaluation of magnetic resonance imaging for determination of left ventricular ejection fraction and comparison with angiography. *American Journal of Cardiology* **62**:628–633.

van Rossum AC, Visser FC, van Eenige MJ *et al.* (1988b) Magnetic resonance imaging of the heart for determination of ejection fraction. *International Journal of Cardiology* **18**:53–63.

vanden Driesen RI, Slaughter RE, Strugnell WE (2006) MR findings in cardiac amyloidosis. *American Journal of Roentgenology* **186**:1682–1685.

Vilacosta I, Gomez J, Dominguez J *et al.* (1995) Massive pericardiac hematoma with severe constrictive pathophysiologic complications after insertion of an epicardial pacemaker. *American Heart Journal* **130**:1298–1300.

Vriend JW, Mulder BJ (2005) Late complications in patients after repair of aortic coarctation: implications for management. *International Journal of Cardiology* **101**:399–406.

Wagner S, Auffermann W, Buser P *et al.* (1989) Diagnostic accuracy and estimation of the severity of valvular regurgitation from the signal void on cine magnetic resonance images. *American Heart Journal* **118**:760–767.

Ward CJ, Mullins CE, Nihill NR *et al.* (1995) Use of intravascular stents in systemic venous and systemic venous baffle obstructions. Short-term follow-up results. *Circulation* **91**:2948–2954.

Weissleder R, Moore A, Mahmood U *et al.* (2000) *In vivo* magnetic resonance imaging of transgene expression. *Nature Medicine* **6**:351–355.

Welch TJ, Stanson AW, Sheedy PF *et al.* (1990) Radiologic evaluation of penetrating aortic atherosclerotic ulcer. *Radiographics* **10**:675–685.

Wendt M, Busch M, Wetzler R *et al.* (1998) Shifted rotated keyhole imaging and active tip-tracking for interventional procedure guidance. *Journal of Magnetic Resonance Imaging* **8**:258–261.

Westenberg JJ, Danilouchkine MG, Doornbos J et al. (2004) Accurate and reproducible mitral valvular blood flow measurement with three-directional velocity-encoded magnetic resonance imaging. *Journal of Cardiovascular Magnetic Resonance* 6:767–776.

Westenberg JJ, Doornbos J, Versteegh MI et al. (2005) Accurate quantitation of regurgitant volume with MRI in patients selected for mitral valve repair. *European Journal of Cardiothoracic Surgery* 27:462–466.

White CS (1995) MR evaluation of the pericardium. *Topics in Magnetic Resonance Imaging* 7:258–266.

White RD, Higgins CB (1989) Magnetic resonance imaging of thoracic vascular disease. *Journal of Thoracic Imaging* 4:34–50.

White RD, Obuchowski NA, Gunawardena S et al. (1996) Left ventricular outflow tract obstruction in hypertrophic cardiomyopathy: presurgical and postsurgical evaluation by computed tomography magnetic resonance imaging. *American Journal of Cardiac Imaging* 10:1–13.

Wildermuth S, Dumoulin CL, Pfammatter T et al. (1998) MR-guided percutaneous angioplasty: assessment of tracking safety, catheter handling and functionality. *Cardiovascular Interventional Radiology* 21:404–410.

Wilke NM, Jerosch-Herold M, Zenovich A et al. (1999) Magnetic resonance first-pass myocardial perfusion imaging: clinical validation and future applications. *Journal of Magnetic Resonance Imaging* 10:676–685.

Wu KC (2003) Myocardial perfusion imaging by magnetic resonance imaging. *Current Cardiology Reports* 5:63–68.

Wu KC, Zerhouni EA, Judd RM et al. (1998) Prognostic significance of microvascular obstruction by magnetic resonance imaging in patients with acute myocardial infarction. *Circulation* 97:765–772.

Wu KC, Heldman AW, Brinker JA et al. (2001) Microvascular obstruction after nonsurgical septal reduction for the treatment of hypertrophic cardiomyopathy. *Circulation* 104:1868.

Yang X, Atalar E, Li D et al. (2001) Magnetic resonance imaging permits *in vivo* monitoring of catheter-based vascular gene delivery. *Circulation* 104:1588–1590.

Yoo SJ, Lim TH, Park IS et al. (1991) Defects of the interventricular septum of the heart: en face MR imaging in the oblique coronal plane. *American Journal of Roentgenology* 157:943–946.

Yuan C, Zhang SX, Polissar NL et al. (2002) Identification of fibrous cap rupture with magnetic resonance imaging is highly associated with recent transient ischemic attack or stroke. *Circulation* 105:181–185.

Zerhouni EA, Parish DM, Rogers WJ et al. (1988) Human heart: tagging with MR imaging – a method for noninvasive assessment of myocardial motion. *Radiology* 169:59–63.

CHAPTER 6

Barbash IM, Chouraqui P, Baron J et al. (2003) Systemic delivery of bone marrow-derived mesenchymal stem cells to the infarcted myocardium: feasibility, cell migration, and body distribution. *Circulation* 108(7):863–868.

Battegay EJ (1995) Angiogenesis: mechanistic insights, neovascular diseases, and therapeutic prospects. *Journal of Molecular Medicine* 73(7):333–346.

Behm C, Lindner J (2006) Cellular and molecular imaging with targeted contrast ultrasound. *Ultrasound Quarterly* 22(1):67–72.

Blankenberg FG, Katsikis PD, Tait JF et al. (1998) *In vivo* detection and imaging of phosphatidylserine expression during programmed cell death. *Proceedings of the National Academy of Sciences of the United States of America* 95(11):6349–6354.

Brooks P, Clark R, Cheresh D (1994a) Requirement of vascular integrin alpha v beta 3 for angiogenesis. *Science* 264(5158):569–571.

Brooks P, Montgomery A, Rosenfeld M et al. (1994b) Integrin alpha v beta 3 antagonists promote tumor regression by inducing apoptosis of angiogenic blood vessels. *Cell* 79(7):1157–1164.

Brumley CL, Kuhn JA (1995) Radiolabeled monoclonal antibodies. *AORN Journal* 62(3):343–350, 353–355; quiz 356–358, 361–362.

Cerqueira M, Udelson J (2003) Lake Tahoe Invitation Meeting 2002. *Journal of Nuclear Cardiology* 10(2):223–256.

Chang GY, Xie X, Wu JC (2006) Overview of stem cells and imaging modalities for cardiovascular diseases. *Journal of Nuclear Cardiology* 13(4):554.

Chen IY, Wu JC, Min JJ et al. (2004) Micro-positron emission tomography imaging of cardiac gene expression in rats using bicistronic adenoviral vector-mediated gene delivery. *Circulation* 109(11):1415–1420.

Choy G, Choyke P, Libutti SK (2003) Current advances in molecular imaging: noninvasive *in vivo* bioluminescent and fluorescent optical imaging in cancer research. *Molecular Imaging* 2(4):303.

Dobrucki WL, Sinusas AJ (2005) *Journal of Nuclear Medicine and Molecular Imaging* 49:106–115.

Dumont EA, Reutelingsperger CP, Smits JF et al. (2001) Real-time imaging of apoptotic cell-membrane changes at the single-cell level in the beating murine heart. *Nature Medicine* 7(12):1352–1325.

Ferrara N, Gerber H, LeCouter J (2003) The biology of VEGF and its receptors. *Nature Medicine* 9(6):669–676.

Fraser AG, Buser P, Bax JJ et al.(2006) The future of cardiovascular imaging and noninvasive diagnosis. *European Journal of Echocardiography* 7:268–273.

Haas TL, Madri JA (1999) Extracellular matrix-driven matrix metalloproteinase production in endothelial cells: implications for angiogenesis. *Trends in Cardiovascular Medicine* 9(3–4):70–77.

Harris T, Kalogeropoulos S, Nguyen T et al. (2003) Design, synthesis, and evaluation of radiolabeled integrin v 3 receptor antagonists for tumor imaging and radiotherapy. *Cancer Biotherapy and Radiopharmaceuticals* 18(4):631–645.

Haubner R, Wester H, Reuning U et al. (1999) Radiolabeled alpha(v)beta3 integrin antagonists: a new class of tracers for tumor targeting. *Journal of Molecular Medicine* 40(6):1061–1071.

Haubner R, Wester H, Burkhart F et al. (2001a) Glycosylated RGD-containing peptides: tracer for tumor targeting and angiogenesis imaging with improved biokinetics. *Journal of Molecular Medicine* 42(2):326–336.

Haubner R, Wester H, Weber W et al. (2001b) Noninvasive imaging of alpha(v)beta3 integrin expression using 18F-labeled RGD-containing glycopeptide and positron emission tomography. *Cancer Research* 61(5):1781–1785.

Hua J, Dobrucki LW, Sadeghi MM et al. (2005) Noninvasive imaging of angiogenesis with a 99mTc-labeled peptide targeted at alphavbeta3 integrin after murine hindlimb ischemia. *Circulation* 111(24):3255–3260.

Kolodgie F, Petrov A, Virmani R et al. (2003) Targeting of apoptotic macrophages and experimental atheroma with radiolabeled annexin V: a technique with potential for noninvasive imaging of vulnerable plaque. *Circulation* 108:3134–3139.

Lanza GM, Winter PM, Caruthers S D *et al.* (2004) Magnetic resonance molecular imaging with nanoparticles. *Journal of Nuclear Cardiology* **11**(6):733.

Lee KH, Jung KH, Song S H *et al.* (2005) Radiolabeled RGD uptake and alphav integrin expression is enhanced in ischemic murine hindlimbs. *Journal of Molecular Medicine* **46**(3):472–478.

Leong-Poi H, Christiansen J, Klibanov AL *et al.* (2003) Noninvasive assessment of angiogenesis by ultrasound and microbubbles targeted to [alpha]v-integrins. *Circulation* **107**(3):455–460.

Lindsey ML, Escobar GP, Dobrucki LW *et al.* (2006) Matrix metalloproteinase-9 gene deletion facilitates angiogenesis after myocardial infarction. *American Journal of Physiology. Heart and Circulatory Physiology* **290**(1):H232–239.

Link JM, Stratton JR, Levy W *et al.* (2003) PET measures of pre- and post-synaptic cardiac beta adrenergic function. *Nuclear Medicine and Biology* **30**(8):795–803.

Lu E, Wagner WR, Schellenberger U *et al.* (2003) Targeted *in vivo* labeling of receptors for vascular endothelial growth factor: approach to identification of ischemic tissue. *Circulation* **108**(1):97–103.

McAteer J, Song J, Dobrucki L *et al.* (2005) Targeted radiotracer imaging of myocardial matrix metalloproteinase activity post-myocardial infarction. *Circulation* **11**:761.

Meoli DF, Sadeghi MM, Krassilnikova S *et al.* (2004) Noninvasive imaging of myocardial angiogenesis following experimental myocardial infarction. *Journal of Clinical Investigation* **113**(12):1684–1691.

Morawski AM, Lanza GA, Wickline SA (2005) Targeted contrast agents for magnetic resonance imaging and ultrasound. *Current Opinion in Biotechnology* **16**(1):89.

Narula J, Petrov A, Ditlow C *et al.* (1997) Maximizing radiotracer delivery to experimental atherosclerotic lesions with high-dose, negative charge-modified Z2D3 antibody for immunoscintigraphic targeting. *Journal of Nuclear Cardiology* **4**:226–233.

Narula J, Acio ER, Narula N *et al.* (2001) Annexin-V imaging for noninvasive detection of cardiac allograft rejection. *Nature Medicine* **7**(12):1347–1352.

Piao D, Sadeghi MM, Zhang J *et al.* (2005) Hybrid positron detection and optical coherence tomography system: design, calibration, and experimental validation with rabbit atherosclerotic models. *Journal of Biomedical Optics* **10**(4):44010.

Sadeghi MM, Krassilnikova S, Zhang J *et al.* (2004) Detection of injury-induced vascular remodeling by targeting activated [alpha]v[beta]3 integrin *in vivo*. *Circulation* **110**(1):84–90.

Sadeghi MM, Bender JR (2007) Activated [alpha]v[beta]3 integrin targeting in injury-induced vascular remodeling. *Trends in Cardiovascular Medicine* **17**(1):5.

Sahul Z, Song J, McAteer J *et al.* (2006) Non-invasive evaluation of regional myocardial strain and activation of matrix metalloproteinases. *Journal of American College of Cardiology* **47**:114a–115a.

Schafers M, Riemann B, Kopka K *et al.* (2004) Scintigraphic imaging of matrix metalloproteinase activity in the arterial wall *in vivo*. *Circulation* **109**(21):2554–2559.

Schwartz M, Schaller M, Ginsberg M *et al.* (1995) Integrins: emerging paradigms of signal transduction. I. *Annual Review of Cell and Developmental Biology* **11**:549–599.

Sinusas A (2004) Imaging of angiogenesis. *Journal of Nuclear Cardiology* **11**(5):617–633.

Sipkins D, Cheresh D, Kazemi M *et al.* (1998) Detection of tumor angiogenesis *in vivo* by alphaVbeta3-targeted magnetic resonance imaging. *Nature Medicine* **4**(5):623–626.

Strauss HW, Narula J, Blankenberg FG (2000) Radioimaging to identify myocardial cell death and probable injury. *Lancet* **356**(9225):180–181.

Strauss HW, Mari C, Patt BE *et al.* (2006) Intravascular radiation detectors for the detection of vulnerable atheroma. *Journal of the American College of Cardiology* **47**(8Suppl1):C97.

Su H, Hu X, Bourke B *et al.* (2003) Detection of myocardial angiogenesis in chronic infarction with a novel technetium-99m labeled peptide targeted at avß3 integrin. *Circulation* **108**:SIV278–279.

Su H, Spinale FG, Dobrucki LW *et al.* (2005) Noninvasive targeted imaging of matrix metalloproteinase activation in a murine model of postinfarction remodeling. *Circulation* **112**(20):3157–3167.

Tseng H, Link J, Stratton J *et al.* (2001) Cardiac receptor physiology and its application to clinical imaging: present and future. *Journal of Nuclear Cardiology* **8**:390–409.

Wickline SA, Neubauer AM, Winter P *et al.* (2006) Applications of nanotechnology to atherosclerosis, thrombosis, and vascular biology. *Arteriosclerosis, Thrombosis, and Vascular Biology* **26**(3):435–441.

Winter PM, Morawski AM, Caruthers SD *et al.* (2003) Molecular imaging of angiogenesis in early-stage atherosclerosis with [alpha]v[beta]3-integrin-targeted nanoparticles. *Circulation* **108**(18):2270–2274.

Zhu Q, Piao D, Sadeghi MM *et al.* (2003) Simultaneous optical coherence tomography imaging and beta particle detection. *Optics Letters* **28**(18):1704–1706.

INDEX